# Integrative Psychotherapy

## The Art and Science of Relationship

**JANET P. MOURSUND**
*University of Oregon*
*Associate Professor Emerita*

**RICHARD G. ERSKINE**
*Institute for Integrative Psychotherapy,*
*New York City*

THOMSON
™
BROOKS/COLE

AUSTRALIA • CANADA • MEXICO • SINGAPORE • SPAIN
UNITED KINGDOM • UNITED STATES

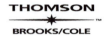

Executive Editor: *Lisa Gebo*
Editorial Assistant: *Sheila Walsh*
Marketing Manager: *Caroline Concilla*
Marketing Assistant: *Mary Ho*
Project Manager, Editorial Production:
 *Stephanie Zunich*
Print/Media Buyer: *Doreen Suruki*
Permissions Editor: *Sue Ewing*
Production Service: *Shepherd, Inc.*

Text Designer: *Jeanne Calabrese*
Copy Editor: *Jeanne Patterson*
Cover Designer: *Cheryl Carrington*
Cover Photo: *Andy Roberts/Stone/Getty Images*
Cover Printer: *Transcontinental Printing*
Compositor: *Shepherd, Inc.*
Printer: *Transcontinental Printing*

Printed in Canada

1  2  3  4  5  6  7  06  05  04  03  02

For more information about our products,
contact us at:
**Thomson Learning Academic Resource Center**
**1-800-423-0563**
For permission to use material from this text,
contact us by: **Phone:** 1-800-730-2214
**Fax:** 1-800-730-2215
**Web:** http://www.thomsonrights.com

**Library of Congress Control Number:**
2002111296

ISBN 0-534-51355-7

**Brooks/Cole–Thomson Learning**
**511 Forest Lodge Road**
**Pacific Grove, CA 93950**
**USA**

**Asia**
Thomson Learning
5 Shenton Way #01-01
UIC Building
Singapore 068808

**Australia/New Zealand**
Thomson Learning
102 Dodds Street
Southbank, Victoria
Australia 3006

**Canada**
Nelson
1120 Birchmount Road
Toronto, Ontario M1K 5G4
Canada

**Europe/Middle East/Africa**
Thomson Learning
High Holborn House
50/51 Bedford Row
London WC1R 4LR
United Kingdom

**Latin America**
Thomson Learning
Seneca, 53
Colonia Polanco
11560 Mexico D.F.
Mexico

**Spain**
Paraninfo
Calle/Magallanes, 25
28015 Madrid, Spain

# Contents

# Preface

A book—any new book—is an invitation to a cooperative venture. The book's author offers ideas, facts, and conclusions; the reader reaches out to grasp and take in all of that information. As in all cooperative ventures, it is useful for each participant to have an idea of what the other is trying to accomplish. In our venture together, we authors assume that you, the reader, are interested in learning how to be a better counselor or psychotherapist, as well as (possibly) doing well in a course that uses this book as a text. To be successful, you need to know something of what we are trying to do and how we intend to do it. That is what the first part of this preface is about.

First, we must confess that the title of the book—*Integrative Psychotherapy*—is something of a misnomer. As you will discover, there are many varieties of integrative psychotherapy, and this book concerns itself with only one of them. As the subtitle suggests, ours is a relationship-focused integrative psychotherapy. We decided, though, that *Relationship-Focused Integrative Psychotherapy* would have been a bit cumbersome and opted for a shorter, if less accurate, title.

The book is divided into three parts: Theoretical Foundations, Therapeutic Interventions, and The Transcript (a verbatim, annotated transcript of a full therapy session). While it might be tempting to skip the theoretical section and leap right into the chapters about actual psychotherapy, we recommend against it. What we have to say about therapy will be much more meaningful in the context of a theoretical background—how we believe people function, how they get that way, and how they can be helped to change. Chapter 1 provides an introduction to the notion of relationship-focused integrative psychotherapy and its connections to the whole developing array of psychotherapeutic approaches. Chapter 2 presents a sort of anatomy of human functioning, discussing the sorts of problems and challenges that people deal with and often bring to psychotherapy. It is a here-and-now sort of chapter, asserting that all human behavior is grounded in relationships and addressing the ways in which relationships affect who and how we are as people. In contrast, chapter 3 concerns itself with human development, the paths we all follow as we go through our lives. It talks about how things can go right for us, and how they can go wrong, and how those rights and wrongs can influence our ways of being in the world months and years later.

In the second major section of the book, we turn to the process of relationship-focused integrative psychotherapy: given what we believe about how people function and how they get to be the way they are, what a therapist can do to help them live fuller, happier, more contactful lives. Do please notice that word "contactful;" the basic premise of our work is that *contact,* with self and with others, is what healthy functioning is all about. The work of therapy is designed to help clients restore full contact with all of the parts of themselves, with the other people in their lives, and with the world around them. Chapter 4 provides an overview of this approach, along with some of the other basic assumptions of a relationship-focused psychotherapy.

Chapter 5 and chapter 6 take us more deeply into the nature of the therapeutic relationship, the relationship within which the client experiences a new sort of interpersonal contact. Chapter 5 discusses how to establish and maintain a therapeutic relationship, and chapter 6 explores the three major facets of such a relationship that we believe to be central to the healing process: inquiry, attunement, and therapeutic involvement. In chapter 7, we discuss some of the issues to be dealt with as therapy begins; chapter 8 takes us further into the process of deepening the client's awareness of and contact with self and others. Chapter 9 is perhaps the most pragmatic part of the book, as it deals with specific interventions that tend to further the client's growth. Chapter 10 brings us back again to the most important "intervention"—the relationship between client and therapist and how that relationship itself can be used in the therapeutic process. Finally, chapter 11 discusses the end of therapy and how it can best be managed so that clients continue to grow and heal even after they terminate their work with the therapist.

Throughout the book, we have struggled with the issue of clinical examples. Most significant therapeutic events generally build over a series of transactions and lose much of their meaningfulness when plucked, a few sentences at a time, from the therapeutic fabric. How, then, can we present examples that truly represent the concepts we are trying to describe? How can we convey the ongoing, evolving quality of a relationship-focused integrative psychotherapy?

Our solution has been to provide the reader not with individual, out-of-context examples (although a few such examples have been retained) but with a verbatim transcript of an entire therapy session. The final section of the book—chapter 12—contains this transcript. The session was not chosen specifically to illustrate the concepts introduced in the earlier part of the book; nor were the earlier chapters written to fit the transcript we selected. Rather, the transcript was chosen almost at random from audio recordings available to us; it has been a confirmation and a delight to rediscover how closely our actual work fits the theory we have been developing and professing over the years.

The transcript is annotated with comments about both therapist interventions and client responses, and the annotations, in turn, are keyed to pages in previous chapters where relevant theoretical and clinical material is presented in greater detail. We had originally planned to insert references to the transcript chapter as footnotes throughout the entire book. The footnotes began to feel intrusive, however, interrupting the flow of the narrative, and we removed them. The reader who would like to move back and forth, from text to transcript example, can still do so: the "Transcript Linkage Index" correlates important concepts, together with the page numbers on which they are discussed, with transcript segments. Using this linkage index, the reader can find embedded examples of most of the ideas presented in the first 11 chapters of the book.

In the last several decades, we have all been sensitized to the gender-pronoun issue: the English language does not have a gender-neutral pronoun, and the use of "he" and "him" to refer to people in general is no longer acceptable. We have found that using "he or she" and "her or him" as a solution to this problem is awkward, and have instead chosen to refer consistently to the therapist as "she" and the client as "he." This usage not only helps the reader keep track of who is being referred to, but also tends to counteract the bias that assumes men to have senior or higher-status positions than women—a bias that still exists, though largely at an unconscious level, among many people in our culture.

Another linguistic challenge for us was the "counseling" or "psychotherapy" distinction. This book is intended for both counselors and psychotherapists, as well as for psychiatrists, clinical social workers, psychiatric nurse practitioners, and pastoral counselors. But, again, the continual use of "psychotherapy and counseling," and "counselor or psychotherapist" becomes cumbersome and intrusive. We decided to use "psychotherapy" (and, occasionally, simply "therapy") as a shorthand way of referring to all counseling and therapeutic activities. We hope that you, as a part of our cooperative venture, will frequently remind yourself that this usage is indeed a kind of shorthand and that our ideas are intended to apply to all of the many varieties and settings of counseling and psychotherapy.

Finally, you may notice that we have not included a chapter on multicultural issues. There are no guidelines in these pages for working with individuals from various cultural backgrounds, no generalizations about this group or that. We believe that such generalizations can be dangerous to therapists, in that they tend to create a sort of false confidence: a belief that the therapist does know and understand her client without having to fully explore his world, her response to him, and the in-between that client and therapist create through their work together. Similarities and differences among individuals are more profound and significant than similarities and differences between groups—whatever the basis for the grouping.

As we learn to attune ourselves to the cognitive, affective, behavioral, rhythmic, and developmental aspects of each client, putting aside our own preconceptions and simply listening to and resonating with him, issues of race, age, and gender become—not unimportant—but an integral part of the unique fabric of the therapeutic relationship. The key word here is *unique*: cultural generalizations can too easily slide into cultural stereotypes, stereotypes that undermine our growing appreciation of each client's uniqueness. Rather than espouse a politically correct (and all too often superficial) concern with multiculturalism, we invite the reader to learn from every client the beliefs and values they have acquired through contact with caregivers and comrades, through dealing with opportunities and with oppression.

Culture is a two-way street. While it is true that understanding a client's cultural background can help us to understand how he deals with his world and the people in it, it is equally true that we can only truly understand his culture *as he experiences it* by learning about him: his needs, wants, fears, and expectations, how he makes and rejects contact, how he relates to self and others. The most sincere respect for cultural differences emerges from a respect for each individual and from an honest acknowledgment that we know that individual only insofar as he chooses to share of himself with us—and that only through the lens of what we ourselves have been and are now. Rather than trying to learn about any group in the abstract, we believe therapists are better served by allowing our clients to teach us what we need to know and by never assuming that we know before we have been taught.

A number of people should be recognized and thanked for their help in making this book possible. First on the list is Rebecca Trautmann, who has played a major part in the development of our ideas over the years. Next are the members of the Professional Development Seminar (Institute for Integrative Psychotherapy, New York, New York, and Kent, Connecticut), to whom the book is dedicated: their questions, comments, criticisms, and insights have been invaluable in shaping our thinking, and their love and support have helped us through many snags and stuck spots. The staff of the Sacred Heart Medical Center in Eugene, Oregon, have shown extraordinary patience in allowing the use of their facilities for writing and editing. Our reviewers Chris Faiver, John Carroll University; Susan W. Gray, Barry University; Cindy Juntunen, University of North Dakota; Ellyn Kaschak, San Jose State University; Pamela M. Kiser, Elon University; Jennifer Kukis, Lorain County Community College; Christopher McCarthy, University of Texas at Austin; and H. Edward Stone, Lee University have been both helpful and encouraging. Our own editor, Lisa Gebo, and production editors Stephanie Zunich at Brooks/Cole and Peggy Francomb at Shepherd, Inc., have performed yeoman services as the book has worked its way through the steps and stages of the publication process. To all, a most heartfelt thanks!

# Development of Integrative Psychotherapy

# CHAPTER 1

As a relative beginner in the field of psychotherapy, you are almost surely looking for some specific, practical guidelines about how to work with your clients. People are coming to you for help. They are dealing with an often bewildering array of problems, and you want to be useful. You need to know what to do and when to do it. And you may well be tired of discussions of theory, of endless talk about how problems arise or about the different ways that different scholars look at such problems.

While we, the authors, would like to plunge right into a discussion of how to do good therapy (we, too, are most fascinated by this topic), some other issues need to be dealt with before we do so. Psychotherapy does not happen in a vacuum. It is practiced in a current cultural setting, a current view of the nature of therapy, and within the context of other therapies currently being practiced. Any approach to psychotherapy inevitably overlaps to some extent with other approaches that are being used and have been used in the past. This is partly because all therapists are looking at the same kinds of data (confused people, angry people, people in pain) and drawing their conclusions from those data, and partly because therapists talk to each other, read about each other's ideas, and take from those ideas whatever seems useful to them.

To fully understand a given therapeutic approach, then, it is necessary to understand where that approach comes from, what ideas it has built upon, and how it is similar to and different from the approaches suggested by other theories. In this first chapter, we review the way in which modern psychotherapy has evolved since Sigmund Freud (1938) wrote his landmark *The Interpretation of Dreams* more than 100 years ago. We look briefly at some of the major ways in which psychotherapy is practiced now, in the 21st century. We discuss the impact of managed care—arguably the most significant external factor in current psychotherapy practice—on the therapeutic process. With all this as background, we are then ready to lay out for you our own view of psychotherapy: how it comes to be needed, how it can be helpful to people, what we actually do with our clients, and how we decide to do it.

## THE ROOTS AND BEYOND

It all started with Freud. Of course, Freud did study with others, and activities much like psychotherapy have been going on for much longer than 100 years. Some of the procedures carried out in the ancient Greek temples sound quite psychotherapeutic; shamans around the world have been practicing their art for untold centuries; and, in many cultures, elders are expected to counsel the young. But in terms of a recognized profession with its own identity, and with enormous implications for Western thought as well as medical practice, psychotherapy did start with Freud. He not only developed a new way of looking at psychological problems and a new way of working with people who suffered from such problems, but also was able to gather around himself a group of creative, competent therapists who carried the notion of a "talking cure" back to their own colleagues and students—and the psychoanalytic movement was born.

Although modern therapists may take issue with many of the details of Freud's theories, there is no doubt that his ideas about the importance of talking and of being listened to continue to influence the way all therapists work. Freud took seriously the notion of the *unconscious*—the notion that a person can perceive, think, hope, or fear without being consciously aware of those perceptions and thoughts and hopes and fears. He developed a methodology to bring to awareness that which had previously been out of awareness: *free association* and the basic rule that nothing must be censored, nothing thought too trivial or irrelevant to tell the therapist about. He prescribed for the therapist a state of "evenly hovering attention" (Freud, 1959/1912) as a way of taking in all of the multiple communications provided by a client. This idea that "The Doctor" might do well to listen more and talk less was quite revolutionary in the authority-oriented Austrian culture of his time. Freud suggested—and his daughter Anna (1937) developed the concept further—that people erect psychological defenses to protect themselves from the pain of knowing their own internal process. He gave therapists a model of child psychological development, a model based on the then radical notion that children, as much as adults, experience sexual needs and drives and that child sexuality involves a much broader range of objects and activities than we allow ourselves as adults.

Finally, he introduced the concept of *transference:* the feelings we had as children toward important people (and especially toward our caregivers) are transferred onto the person of the therapist, and a great deal of what we experience in the psychotherapy relationship—and other relationships, too—may have as much to do with how we were in those old relationships as it does with here-and-now reality. All of these ideas pervade most modern approaches to psychotherapy, even though they may be in the background rather than the primary focus of treatment. Whether therapists are working with adults, children, couples, families, groups—whatever the client population, it is safe to say that therapy and counseling, as they are now known, could not have come to be without the ideas that Freud developed.

## Next Steps

Almost as important as Freud's work were the contributions of his colleagues, the psychoanalysts and psychotherapists who helped spread the word about this new way of treating emotional pain. Each of them took Freud's ideas and shaped them to fit their own views of the world. Some changed the original ideas very little, passing them on to their own students much as Freud had originally presented them. Others made very significant changes, changes that eventually led to their leaving Freud's original group and going their own way. Notable among these latter pioneers were Carl Jung, with his ideas about the collective unconscious, and Alfred Adler, who insisted that people can be understood better in terms of what they strive toward in the future than in terms of what has happened to them in the past. But even as these and other dissidents moved away from psychoanalytic orthodoxy, forming their own schools of therapy and training their own cadres of students, they were still part of the great overall pattern: the growing acceptance of a link between one's emotional state and one's physical well-being, a connection between feelings and behavior, and a conviction that emotional health could be restored (or at least improved) simply by *talking* with a trained therapist.

Up until around the middle of the 20th century, psychoanalysis in its various forms *was* psychotherapy. Virtually nothing else existed. If you wanted help for an emotional problem, you found yourself an analyst—a Freudian or a Jungian or an Adlerian, perhaps, but nevertheless an analyst. To be sure, a few others were trying to develop alternative ways of dealing with psychic pain, but none of them came close to being as influential in the development of psychotherapy as the psychoanalysts and those who studied with them.

## Branching Out

The defining event of the mid-1900s was World War II. It interrupted many developing lines of theory and research by sending the theorists and the researchers off to fight, to flee for their lives, or to support those who *were* fighting. The war was a highly effective distractor from the concerns of psychotherapy in general and of psychoanalysis in particular. When one is engaged in a struggle to determine the fate of the world, the early memories of a well-to-do client are likely to seem relatively unimportant! But with the end of the war came a resurgence of interest in psychology and psychotherapy, a resurgence fueled by the thousands of shell-shocked veterans (who would now be said to have post-traumatic stress syndrome) who needed psychiatric assistance.

During these psychologically fertile years of the 1940s and 1950s, new schools of thought were taking hold in the U.S. psychotherapeutic community. Two of these, as radically different from each other as they were from the ideas of the psychoanalysts, were to leave their own indelible marks on the psychotherapeutic landscape. Each has become a part of the thinking—the psychological worldview—of virtually every therapist in practice today. These two schools of thought were behaviorism and learning theory on the one hand, and the client-centered therapy of Carl Rogers on the other.

Learning theory, of course, was not exactly new. Psychologists, and philosophers before them, have always been interested in just how it is that people learn. Behaviorism, though, put a new twist on the study of learning: instead of probing the phenomenology of the learning organism, trying to understand the learning process by looking at it from the inside out, they chose to look at what that learning organism actually *did*. By limiting themselves to observables, to behaviors that could be described and counted and verified by other observers, they hoped to build a truly scientific body of theory, one based on measurable, quantifiable events rather than on one's subjective experience. Once this theory was in place and it was clearly known what sorts of stimuli led to what sorts of behaviors, it would be a relatively simple matter to apply these rules to the treatment of behavioral disorders. Notice the wording here—*behavioral* disorders. For these theorists, emotional pain was the result—not the cause—of dysfunctional behavior. Freud and the psychoanalysts tried to improve behavior by interpreting their patients' thoughts and feelings. The behaviorists asserted that thoughts and feelings would be improved by changing one's behavior. It is hard to imagine two points of view more fundamentally different than these; yet each has survived (in modified form), and many if not most therapists today borrow liberally from both.

Then there was Carl Rogers, the young professor at the University of Chicago who wrote the book with such a strange title: *Client-Centered Therapy* (1951). Rogers was not interested in manipulating feelings in order to change behaviors, and he was not interested in manipulating behaviors in order to change feelings. He was not interested in manipulating anything at all. He believed that people have the capacity and the right to determine for themselves how they want to grow and change. Given the proper psychological climate, said Rogers, people discover on their own how to heal their pain and how to become the best they can possibly be. He asserted that three ingredients make up such a psychological climate: openness and honesty (he called this *congruence*), unconditional acceptance, and empathic understanding. When therapists learn how to provide those, their patients—Rogers called them *clients* in order to get away from the doctor-as-authority quality of the medical model—will naturally and instinctively begin to grow and heal.

## The "Human Potential" Decades

By the beginning of the 1960s, the center of psychological and psychotherapeutic thought had shifted from Europe to the United States. Poised at the brink of one of the most turbulent, creative, exciting, frustrating, rebellious decades that the United States had ever known, psychotherapy was still largely limited to the three approaches we have been discussing: the "old guard" psychoanalysts, the new-to-the-scene behaviorists, and Rogerians. But those Big Three were about to explode into tens, scores, maybe even hundreds of new approaches. The 1960s and the 1970s were the decades of the human potential movement, of the quest for self-actualization, of a belief that everyone had a right to "do his own thing." They were also, of course, the decades that saw young men being sent to fight and die in a war they did not understand; decades that were riddled with mistrust of and cynicism about nearly everything; and decades in which the United States finally began, in pain and tragedy, to face squarely the evils of racial inequality. In short, they were decades of tremendous paradox and social upheaval. Small wonder that the paradoxes and the upheavals were reflected in the world of psychotherapy and that new approaches to emotional healing sometimes seemed to be springing up on every street corner.

# MODERN PSYCHOTHERAPIES

The world of psychotherapy as it exists today has grown out of those turbulent times. Some of the "new" therapies have survived, and some have not. All—the new and the old—have changed, as research and experience have shed even more light on how people become disturbed and what sorts of things help them to heal. Even the kinds of disturbances that bring people to psychotherapy have changed: new times bring new "diseases of choice," new culturally supported ways of expressing emotional pain. And the tremendous burgeoning of drug therapy has meant that many people now treat their depression or anxiety with pills and that therapists work much more closely with physicians, developing a treatment regimen that combines psychopharmacology with psychotherapy.

## Managed Care

A major event in determining the kinds of therapy that are generally available today is the advent of managed care. Therapists now must fight their way through an alphabet soup of PPOs, HMOs, and PCPs and must often obtain permission from insurance providers for every session they schedule with a client. Not only is the number of sessions regulated, but increasingly even the kind of treatment that must be provided for a given diagnostic category is being standardized and prescribed for practitioners (Erskine, 1998). In a discussion of the psychotherapeutic implications of managed care, Weiss and Weiss (1998) comment, "The rise of the managed care approach to controlling health care costs has made it next to impossible to work in any kind of real depth with the majority of people whose insurance will only cover the psychological equivalent of first aid" (pp. 45–46). Some therapists, concerned over the likelihood of having to curtail services to people in need of help and also over the ethical implications of reporting confidential information about their clients to insurance companies, choose not to deal with the managed care system at all and work only with clients who can afford to pay out of pocket for their therapy. Others remain within the system, even though this usually means that their clients will have fewer sessions, spaced farther apart, than either client or therapist would wish, and that writing reports and filling out forms will require time that could better be spent in more therapeutic activities.

Managed care is still evolving, and no one can predict what its ultimate effect on the provision of psychotherapy will be. What is certain, though, is that every therapist, whether providing short- or long-term care, must develop a way of working with clients that fits the client's needs, the therapist's own personal style, and the demands and limitations of the client's financial resources.

## The New "Big Three"

What theoretical approaches are available from which to choose, as therapists try to craft their own personal approaches to psychotherapy? First, psychoanalytic ideas still shape much of the therapy done today. Those ideas have evolved and changed, of course; analysts now may embrace *neo-Freudianism* or *object-relations theory* or *self-psychology,* but they are still working from a basically psychodynamic perspective. Moreover, Freud's ideas about unconscious processes, the importance of human development, and the centrality of the therapeutic relationship are a part of the thinking of many practitioners who do not identify themselves formally with one of the analytic schools. In these opening years of the 21st century, there seems to be a resurgence of interest in depth therapies, therapies that attempt to deal with long-standing emotional patterns as opposed to more obvious behavioral concerns. And all of these depth therapies, to a greater or lesser extent, are based on ideas that have grown out of psychoanalysis.

The behavioral approach to therapy has grown and prospered. Linked now with advances in cognitive psychology, *cognitive behaviorism* has become the darling of managed care because it lends itself to short-term work and because its therapeutic goals can be specified in objective and observable language. Managed care organizations like to know in very specific terms what results they are paying for and how long it will take clients to achieve those results. Cognitive behaviorism and its numerous offspring—the rational emotive therapy of Albert Ellis (1997), Beck's cognitive therapy (1991), and the BASIC ID model proposed by Lazarus (1989), to mention only a few—promise this kind of specificity; and, while they cannot always deliver what they promise, they probably do so as well as most and better than many other approaches.

Carl Rogers' client-centered therapy (1951), perhaps bowing to a concern for political correctness, is now known as *person-centered,* and it is difficult to find a therapist whose work has not been shaped by it. Every modern psychotherapy training program expects its students to master the skills of active listening, and these skills are based largely on the "accurate empathy" that Rogers and his students believed to be critical to psychotherapeutic success. Most therapists use Rogers' ideas about empathy, congruence, and positive regard—in essence, ideas about the fundamental importance of the therapeutic relationship—as a foundation for whatever additional therapeutic ideas and techniques they may use.

## Newer Therapies

Perhaps the best known of the next generation of psychotherapy frameworks (putting aside, for the moment, the various branches of cognitive behaviorism) are the Gestalt therapy of Fritz and Laura Perls (Perls, Hefferline, & Goodman, 1951) and Eric Berne's transactional analysis (1961). Both of these approaches developed theoretical concepts that have migrated into the general body of psychotherapeutic thought. Berne's descriptions of ego states, for instance, and the concepts of strokes and of "life script" have been adopted by many non-TA therapists; the Perlses' ideas about contact and the "safe emergency," and their empty chair techniques are widely used within a variety of theoretical approaches.

Many other approaches have been developed as well. Bioenergetics links physical and emotional phenomena and advocates working with the body in order to bring about psychological change (Lowen, 1976). Primal therapy is best known for its focus on the psychological effects of the earliest of all human experiences: birth itself (Janov, 1970). In psychodrama, first developed in a group context, clients act out the roles of important people in their lives and in the lives of other people in the group (Moreno, 1964). Neuro–Linguistic programming (NLP) is/was an odd conglomerate of techniques (Bandler & Grinder, 1975); it grew and flourished for a decade or so and then began to wither away. Again and again, approaches to therapy have sprung up, gained a significant following, and died back a few years later, each leaving its own contribution to our evolving understanding of psychological change.

Some approaches take their identity not so much from their theoretical base as from the clients they serve. Couples therapy and family therapy are notable examples here; a whole body of theory, with associated strategies and interventions, has developed out of therapists' efforts to help these "conglomerate clients" to deal with both their individual difficulties and the difficulties involved in their relationships with each other. The National Training Laboratories developed theory and associated strategies for helping people from the workplace enhance their personal and occupational effectiveness. And generically labeled group therapists have concerned themselves (logically enough) with providing therapy to clients in small group settings.

When therapists are confronted with such a multiplicity of therapeutic possibilities, a temptation always exists to go beyond simply using an approach that fits for oneself, and to become a therapeutic disciple of that approach. Discipleship involves a kind of theoretical tunnel vision, an unwillingness to consider anything but the One Way of the approach one has decided to espouse. "Isolated language systems and rival definitions encourage clinicians to wrap themselves in semantic cocoons from which they cannot escape and which others cannot penetrate" (Norcross, 1990, p. 218). Fortunately, recent years have seen a decline in this sort of theoretical rigidity; therapists appear to be increasingly willing to learn not only from colleagues who share their views (and prejudices) but also from others who see things quite differently.

## ECLECTICISM AND INTEGRATION

Aware of the limitations of each of the major schools of psychology and also aware of the danger of being co-opted into uncritical discipleship, many practitioners are now choosing to build their own, unique ways of doing therapy, taking what seems to them the best and most effective techniques from a variety of approaches. Therapeutic eclecticism has become more common than adherence to any one school and is, indeed, almost a school in itself; much has been written about how to choose from one's therapeutic tool kit the strategy that will be most effective with a given client at a particular moment in therapy. Norcross and Newman (1992) point out that "Eclecticism focuses on predicting for whom interventions will work; the foundation is actuarial rather than theoretical" (p. 11). Norcross (1995) urges therapists to adapt such an eclectic stance to ". . . widen our therapeutic repertoire and embrace multiple techniques and theories . . . specifically [to] know when and where to use these multiple techniques and theories" (p. 503).

The problem with this sort of eclecticism is that it is not always based on a sound and consistent theoretical framework. "If it works, use it" seems to be the motto of eclecticism; eclectics see no particular need for an encompassing and coherent theory from which their practice flows. While we, the authors of this book, applaud the pragmatic concern of the eclectics, we believe that theory, too, is important. A well-developed theory of therapy helps the practitioner to plan interventions so that they form a logical progression, to examine her own behavior in the context of its theoretical implications, and to ensure that all of the client's needs are taken into account as the therapy progresses. Selecting the best from among therapies that have been shown to be effective is a fine idea; but these "bests" should be integrated into a theoretically consistent understanding of the nature of psychotherapeutic change and of how such change can be facilitated. An integrative—as contrasted with eclectic—therapy "provides internally compatible understandings of personality functioning, change, and technique" (Frank, 1991, p. 540). Such a theory allows the practitioner to select interventions and strategies from a variety of approaches, weaving them into a logically coherent network that supports and informs the work at any given moment. Say Norcross and Newman (1992), discussing the difference between eclecticism and theoretical integration, "Theoretical integration involves a commitment to a conceptual or theoretical creation beyond a technical blend of methods. The goal is to create a conceptual framework that synthesizes the best elements of two or more approaches to therapy. Integration, however, aspires to more than a simple combination; it seeks an emergent theory that is more than the sum of its parts, and that leads to new directions for practice and research" (pp. 11–12).

Integrative psychotherapy may well be the wave of the future. Already, professional journals and professional societies have arisen that are devoted to developing and advancing integrative theories. Integrative therapists may behave quite differently from each other in their actual work with clients, but all have in common a commitment to "attend seriously to what has been observed by proponents of *all* the major schools and to incorporate those observations and the methods they have spawned into a framework that is comprehensive, coherent, and continually evolving" (Wachtel, 1990, p. 235). Integrative psychotherapists share a belief in the interdependence of theory and practice, a conviction that the best therapy is supported by theory, and that the best theory leads to effective practice. The intent of this book is to present such an integrative theory, together with the means of implementing it in our work with clients. The integrative theory that we have developed has at its center the therapeutic relationship, and the therapy that emerges uses the therapeutic relationship as the primary vehicle for change and growth.

## PRINCIPLES OF RELATIONSHIP-FOCUSED INTEGRATIVE PSYCHOTHERAPY

Relationship-focused integrative psychotherapy, as we conceptualize and practice it, is integrative in two ways. The first of these is the theoretical integration we have been discussing: a coherent and consistent merging of ideas from a variety of sources. Secondly, the therapy is intended to facilitate psychological integration within the client, bringing together previously fragmented and isolated aspects of the self into a unified whole. We base our approach on two fundamental principles. One of these principles is that all aspects of human functioning—affect, behavior, cognition, physiology—are interdependent and mutually causative. The second is that relationship is the very stuff of being human, and that human activity can only be understood in the context of relationship. Let us consider each of these assertions in turn.

### The Interdependence of Aspects of Human Functioning

Historically, different theories have stressed the importance and/or the primacy of different aspects of human experience. Freud and his followers tended to focus on something they called *drives*—a metaphorical concept, one that finds only questionable support in today's scientific climate. For Freud, people were *driven* by some internal forces, and thwarting those drives led to anxiety and other uncomfortable internal states. Behavior was *caused* by drives or by one's efforts to resist them. What goes on internally, in other words, was thought to cause what people do externally.

Behaviorism, in contrast, focuses on external behavior. For the radical behaviorist, no aspect of a person is relevant unless it can be measured and verified by independent observers. Reading a book, for instance, or making love or laughing or weeping, can be observed, and independent observers would most likely agree as to what they are observing. The length of time an observable behavior persists, how often it occurs in a given time span, and the events that precede or follow it can be described and measured with relative accuracy. Behaviorists assert that these externally observable events are the only legitimate targets for scientific exploration or therapeutic effort. Internal experiences, feelings like anxiety and depression, or thinking patterns like confusion or obsession, may occur, but they cannot be reliably measured: perhaps what you experience when you are "anxious" is totally different from someone else's experience of "anxiety" and, indeed, is closer to what your neighbor or roommate would call "confusion." There is no way for anyone to actually know another person's internal experience, because internal experiences are necessarily subjective. Internal events occur, to be sure; but, because they *are* internal and not objectively observable, they should not be made the focus of research or of therapy. Focus your therapy on that which can be seen, say the behaviorists. Help people change their problematic behaviors; then you and they will both be able to gauge how well you have succeeded. Moreover, when problematic behaviors are changed, reports of internal discomfort tend to decrease. Radical behaviorism asserts that internal events do not cause external behaviors; quite the reverse, external and observable behaviors are the cause of internal states.

Cognitive behaviorism provides yet another view: feelings do not cause behavior, nor does behavior cause feelings. Instead, *thinking*—cognition—lies at the root of both our behaviors and our emotional experience. Whatever the situation in which we find ourselves, it is our thoughts about that situation that determine both what we do and how we feel about it. This being so, it follows that therapy should address itself to cognitive processes. Changing how a client thinks will change both his behaviors and his emotional experience.

## Pulling It All Together

So, do thoughts cause both feelings and behaviors? Do behaviors cause both feelings and thoughts? Do feelings cause both thoughts and behaviors? For a relationship-focused integrative psychotherapist, yes, yes, and yes; and no, no, and no. No simple, one-way, cause-and-effect relationships exist in human functioning; rather, all aspects interact, affecting and being affected by all the others. Our external behaviors do affect the way we think and feel; but how we think and feel affects how we behave and even how our bodies function. Changing how we think about something can certainly change how we feel about it and what we do about it; but it is equally true that a shift in our emotional response will lead to different cognitions and behaviors. And our physiology has a profound effect on our thoughts, our feelings, and our actions; and thoughts and feelings and actions in turn affect our physiology.

The very language we use to describe ourselves bears witness to this fundamental interdependence. When we look closely at the words for different arenas of human function, their meanings begin to blur. Take *behavior,* for instance; ordinarily, and in the preceding discussion, we take it to mean some kind of action. Likewise, inaction; *not* doing something is a *behavior,* is it not? What about internal behaviors? If *behaving* is what I do, isn't *worrying* or *fantasizing* or *thinking about a problem* a behavior? *Behavior* is not the only word that tends to shift and flow when we look closely at it; *emotions* and *feelings* are elusive, too. It is hard to imagine an emotion that does not have a cognitive component. What I feel about something is determined by the meaning I give it, and meanings are cognitive. Moreover, what I feel about something (and even the meaning I give it) is also a physiological thing; feelings are dealt with in specific parts of the brain and are closely linked to chemical events in the body. Basch (1976), noting this confusion around the nature of feelings, has suggested that we use the word *affect* to refer to the simple physiological experience of a particular chemical configuration and reserve *emotion* for a cognitively monitored event. Emotion, he says, involves recollection of past events and of our physiological reponses to those events. It represents the coming together of a here-and-now physiological experience and our associations to previous similar experiences. Nathanson (1996) summarizes this distinction neatly: "Affect is biology, while emotion is biography" (p. 13).

Not only is our experience of emotion strongly affected by our cognitions and our physiology, but also our cognition is influenced by our affective experience. Says Nathanson (1996), "It is only when affect makes us pay attention to a stimulus that we may be said to be conscious of it; in the language of affect theory, consciousness itself occurs only when some mental content has been assembled with an affect to gain access to our highest cognitive functions" (p. 3). If there is no emotional response, in other words, there is no consciousness; and without consciousness, there is no cognition.

As is shown in later chapters, one of the happy consequences of this interrelatedness of all human functioning is that changing one aspect of ourselves generally results in changes elsewhere. Therapists are not required to work only with behaviors (as the radical behaviorists would have them do) or primarily with cognitions (as many cognitive behaviorists recommend) or to regard emotions as the ultimate battleground of the human condition. We are free to move in wherever we are invited, to help the client explore the avenues that are least defended, with the certain knowledge that everything is related to everything else. However, lest we become too complacent, we must remind ourselves that interrelatedness also means that dysfunction and pain in one aspect of human process are likely to spread and affect every other aspect. Therapists need to make sure that, in choosing the avenue of least resistance to begin the work with a client, they are not overlooking potholes and broken pavement elsewhere. Eventually, those potholes will need to be repaired; dealing with other parts of the client's experience will make the repairing easier but will not substitute for it.

## RELATIONSHIP

All of the facets of human experience that we have discussed occur in the context of relationship. To be human is to be in constant relationship with other humans, in actuality or in fantasy. Relationship-focused integrative psychotherapy asserts that literally no human activity can be relationship-free. Even the most reclusive hermit is solitary only in contrast to and with knowlege of relationship: a fish, swimming in water, does not know that it is wet because *wetness* has meaning only as it is contrasted with *not wet;* and just so, *no relationship* can be meaningful only when it is contrasted with *relationship.*

In an even more basic sense, to be a thinking, feeling human being absolutely requires relationship with others. Without relationship, there can be no cognition. Midgely (1998) speaks almost poetically of the connection between thinking and relationship: "Thought involves communication. Cartesian beings, isolated in their separate shells of alien matter, could never even have discovered each other's existence. What thinks has to be the whole person, living in a public world" (p. 164). Similarly, it is impossible to imagine emotion without relationship, for emotion (in contrast to affect, a private physiological phenomenon) is itself a form of communication (Erskine & Trautmann, 1997/1996). Nathanson's characterization (1996) of emotion as biography certainly implies this, for biography is in essence a history of relationships. Our relationships, good and bad, long and short, actual and fantasized, are the single most influential factor in our development as human creatures.

Considering the pervasiveness of relationships in human experience, one may well wonder whether developing relationsnhips with others may be, in fact, the fundamental task of each individual. Perhaps relationship is not just a psychological need but a biological one as well, as Mitchell (1993) asserts: "Attachment is not . . . derived from more basic biological needs; attachment is itself a basic biological need, wired into the species as fundamentally as is nest-building behavior in a bird" (p. 22). It is no accident that people think, feel, and act in relationship to others; our relationship hunger has evolved with us down through the eons. I am not just an *I*—I am part of many *we*s, and my I-ness depends upon the quality of each *we* in which I participate.

For far too long, psychotherapists have underemphasized or even ignored relationship as a fundamental aspect of human nature. Psychotherapy has been all too often a celebration of the *I,* an oxymoronic search for individual health and growth. The so-called Gestalt Prayer is sometimes seen as an example of this misguided emphasis on individuality: "I do my thing and you do your thing. I am not in this world to live up to your expectations, and you are not in this world to live up to mine. You are you, and I am I. And if by chance we find each other, it's beautiful. If not, it can't be helped" (Perls, 1969a). In contrast to this view, relationship-focused integrative psychotherapy recognizes relationship as a necessary complement to individuality. Individuality and relationship are two sides of the same coin. An individual is him- or herself because of his or her relationships; a relationship is itself because of the individuals who comprise it. Neither can exist without the other.

## A Relational Psychotherapy

The interrelatedness of all aspects of human functioning, cradled within and depending upon relationships between individuals: this is the complex and exciting system that a relationship-focused integrative psychotherapist must enter and within which the seeds of change are sown. Gold (1996) sums up the common characteristics of integrative psychotherapeutic approaches:

> Theoretical integration involves the synthesis of novel models of personality functioning, psychopathology, and psychological change from the concepts of two or more traditional systems. Integrative theories . . . generally attempt to explain psychological phenomena in interactional terms, by looking for the ways in which environmental, motivational, cognitive and affective factors influence and are influenced by each other. Causation is usually assumed to be multidirectional and to include conscious and covert factors, and most theoretical integrations include a focus on the ways that individuals re-create past patterns and experiences in the present." (p. 13)

To this description, we add a focus on relationships, both as they have brought the client to his present situation and as a means for bringing about changes in that situation. Such a focus is increasingly supported by research. In 1999 a special task force of the American Psychological Association's Division of Psychotherapy was commissioned to "identify, operationalize, and disseminate information on empirically supported [therapy] relationships" (Norcross, 2001, pp. 347–348), and the findings of this task force have been published in a special edition of *Psychotherapy*. Briefly, they found that "among those factors most closely associated with therapist activity . . . client-therapist relationship factors are most significant in contributing to positive therapy outcome" (Lambert & Barley, 2001, p. 358). Our primary challenge as therapists is to create, maintain, and utilize a therapeutic relationship for the benefit of our clients.

Where do we begin, though, when all causation is multidirectional and there seems to be no single, clear starting point? How do we use the client's relationships—with us, and with others—in the healing process? How do we create a therapeutic environment in which it is safe for our clients to bring past relational patterns and experiences into awareness and to allow that awareness to change the nature of their interactions with self and others?

The key to all of these concerns is that phrase, "create a therapeutic environment." In relationship-focused integrative psychotherapy, the therapist enters consciously and purposefully into relationship with the client and, in so doing, creates a psychological environment in which the relationship itself supports and encourages change. Relationship-focused integrative psychotherapists do not sit back, safely uninvolved, interpreting the client's words and behaviors or assigning tasks or parceling out rewards for "progress." Instead, they enter fully into the therapeutic arena, sharing their own responses and emotions, allowing themselves to be genuinely affected by what is happening between themselves and this client. In so doing, they offer the client a new kind of relationship, a relationship that invites awareness and disarms defensiveness. Not only do they stress "the contribution and mutual interplay of expanded aware-ness and the corrective [emotional] experience in and out of therapy, within the setting of a positively toned, safe, and accepting therapeutic relationship" (Gold, 1996, p. 59), but they make themselves responsible for the creation, nurturance, and utilization of that relationship as a healing instrument.

## The Therapeutic Relationship

The relationship between client and therapist is unique, unlike any other rela-tionship that humans enter into. To be sure, other relationships may be "ther-apeutic" in that they foster growth and change; being in relationship with someone who cares about you, respects you, shares your pain, and celebrates your successes does support growth and healing. But there is a *demand* qual-ity in most naturally occurring relationships, a kind of conditionality: the rela-tionship will continue only if each partner is generally satisfied with the behavior of the other, only if each gains something for him- or herself out of being together. Why do I stay in relationship with you? Because that relation-ship is satisfying to me, because you give me something that I need and/or enjoy. Friendships, collegial associations, and romantic relationships are all built upon variations of this kind of mutual gain.

A therapeutic relationship, in contrast, is focused on and has its very exis-tence in a commitment to the well-being of *one* person, the client. It is not *mutual,* for the therapist (although often gaining satisfaction from the inter-action) is not there to please herself. The goal of a therapeutic relationship is for the *client* to get what is needed for his growth. Any growth or pleasure for the therapist is a side effect, a bonus, not a part of the therapeutic contract. Moreover, the therapeutic relationship is different from other relationships in which there is a "one-way" sort of expectation, such as that between a teacher and student or a lawyer and client, for in these contractual arrangements the teacher or lawyer is not expected to be fully emotionally engaged, using his or her own openness and vulnerability to foster the client's growth.

This business of establishing and maintaining a therapeutic relationship requires a delicate balance—involved but not demanding, vulnerable but not weak, willing to share self-awareness but not thrusting that self-awareness upon the client. Poised between overconcern (which invites the client to behave so as to please the therapist) and underconcern (which attenuates the relationship and leaves the client feeling unsupported), the relationship-focused integrative psychotherapist occupies a paradoxical space in which she cares genuinely about the client's well-being but supports with equal genuine-ness the client's right to grow—or not grow—at his own pace.

Note that this concern with relationship is not unique to integrative psy-chotherapies. Therapists who espouse other approaches, too, rely upon the relationship between client and therapist to support the specific techniques and interventions that they utilize. Indeed, it is our assertion that *all* therapy and counseling can and should be based upon a sound therapeutic relationship and that the principles of establishing and maintaining such a relationship are relevant to any practitioner, working in any setting.

One's own joy or pain can be fully experienced only in the context of an intimate bond, past or present, with another person. It may well be that the absence of such intimate bonding is the critical factor in creating the kinds of trauma and distress that bring people to psychotherapy (we have much more to say about this in later chapters); it seems certain that the kind of intimate bonding that occurs within the therapeutic relationship can be instrumental in healing trauma and distress. The therapist's willingness to share the client's experience as he discovers it, to be fully present and involved and human in the relationship, is what relationship-focused integrative psychotherapy is all about. That willingness, combined with the skill and knowledge needed to assist the client to venture ever further into the hidden or walled-off parts of self, is the essence of the psychotherapeutic task.

## SUMMARY

From a somewhat arbitrary beginning point marked by the work of Sigmund Freud, psychotherapy has developed literally hundreds of approaches to the cure of psychological distress. A number of Freud's colleagues, notably Alfred Adler and Carl Jung, began the proliferation process; the behavioral therapies and Carl Rogers' client-centered therapy also offered new ways of working with troubled individuals. The demand for psychotherapy continued to spur new developments after World War II, and the human potential movement of the 1960s and 1970s brought even more diversity to the field. Today, a major force for change has been the advent of managed care, with its demand for shorter-term treatment and objective, verifiable results.

As the number of competing approaches has increased, many therapists have adopted eclectic styles, borrowing techniques from a variety of psychotherapeutic schools. Others also borrow from more than one source but insist that their importations be held together by a consistent theoretical base; this is the integrative approach.

Relationship-focused integrative psychotherapy assumes a fundamental interrelatedness among all aspects of human functioning: cognition, affect, behavior, and physiology. It is based on a conviction that, just as relationship shapes the development of all of these aspects, so relationship is the basic therapeutic mechanism by which they can be changed and healed.

# 2 CHAPTER | Script, Repression, and Contact Distortion

To say that relationships are a central factor in promoting change in psychotherapy is all well and good—but it does not take us very far in terms of understanding what, specifically, is happening with our clients and what, specifically, we can do about it. The purpose of this chapter is to bring some sort of order into the complex and ever-changing system of thoughts, feelings, actions, physiology, and relationship that comprise human functioning: to provide a framework within which we can begin to understand how the different facets of self and others are related and how we as therapists can most effectively intervene in those systems.

In writing the preceding paragraph, we (the authors) were again forced to recognize the limitations of language in describing the wonderful interrelated complexity of humans in relationship. Even finding a word to designate what we therapists deal with is so difficult: *human behavior* doesn't do it, because there is much more to being a human than overt behavior. *Human activity* has the same problem; some of one's most significant experiences may come when one's body is at rest. *Human processes* may come closest, though the phrase feels awkward and has a mechanistic flavor. What we need to look at and talk about is all the things that people do, internally and externally: things that can be observed by others and things that can only be reported; things of which one is aware and things of which one is unaware; beliefs and attitudes and hopes and fears and all the myriad ways in which we make contact and draw back from contact with ourselves and with others.

This process of being human is a dauntingly complex arena. To begin to understand what we are dealing with, we need to simplify things, pare away some of the details so that we can get a sense of the underlying structure. If we are to see the forest, we must ignore some of the trees—at least for a while. Every description of how people function is a kind of schematic, a map that emphasizes some things and ignores others. Even though "the map is not the territory" (Watzlawick, Weakland, & Fisch, 1974), maps are still useful when we are trying to find our way through a complicated world. As noted in chapter 1, some psychologists have drawn their maps in a way that emphasizes observable behavior as the most important data of human functioning. Some have been more interested in cognition, and some have placed emotions in the foreground. Some have been primarily concerned with the effect of the past on what one is and does in the present, while others look to the future—to goals and expectations—as the best way to make sense out of what is happening to a person here and now.

The relationship-focused integrative psychotherapy map has derived primarily from four theoretical perspectives: transactional analysis, Gestalt therapy, client-centered therapy, and behaviorism. It also borrows significantly from psychoanalytic self-psychology, from object relations theory, and from neo-Reichian body therapy. Each of these models, we believe, offers important insights into human nature: how people come to be the way they are and do the things they do. We have added to these borrowings our own clinical observations and conclusions. By now, this synthesis of ideas has become a part of us, of our overall way of looking at people, and it is quite impossible to say with certainty where each idea came from. We shall do our best to credit the major sources, and we apologize in advance for the instances in which we may have so thoroughly incorporated a concept that we no longer can remember its origin.

All of the theories that have shaped our thinking—all of the maps of human functioning—acknowledge, in one way or another, what relationship-focused integrative psychotherapists believe to be the central fact and primary influence on each human being: that we are social creatures who have our being within a sea of relationships. A person comes to be an individual, uniquely different from every other individual, through his or her relationships with others. Mitchell (1992) urges us, as therapists, to "get away from a search for presocial or extrasocial roots of the core or true self and focus on what it means at any particular moment to be experiencing and using oneself more or less authentically" (p. 19). As Mitchell asserts, the "true self" does not exist in a vacuum; it is formed out of the social relationships in which one participates. Authenticity is a social phenomenon, rooted in social experience. As we turn our attention to questions of why someone acts/feels/thinks/senses the way he or she does, and how that person came to be that way, we must remember that the person we are looking at is, at every moment, living within a matrix of relationships. Just as the background of a picture gives meaning and substance to the figure in the foreground, so each individual draws meaning and substance from the network of relationships within which he or she is grounded.

More often than not, people are unaware of the extent to which they are shaped by their relationships. They may pay lip service to how much they have learned from a parent or to the influence of a teacher, a neighbor, or a particular friend. But what they (and we ourselves) know consciously—and can remember—is just the tip of the iceberg. Perhaps the most important influences of all, those that give a person his or her fundamental sense of selfhood and continuity, occur before the acquisition of language. Without words to symbolize the quality of a learning experience, the nature of that experience is soon lost to conscious awareness. Yet such out-of-awareness shaping lies at the very heart of our sense of self, of others, and of the world around us. That sense of self-with-others-in-world, in turn, gives meaning to our ongoing experiencing.

Think for a moment of what it would be like to live in a world in which past social experience did not shape your understanding of here-and-now occurrences. You wake to an alarm clock. What is that noise? What does it mean? You hear a voice saying "Come on, it's time to get up." Leaving aside the problem of understanding language—and language-learning is always a social process—you have no idea who this person is, or what he wants; you do not know if he's happy, sad, scared of you, or angry with you, because you have not learned to interpret nonverbal signals. You do not know what is expected of you, whether your day will be good or bad (indeed, the notion of a *good* or *bad* day or even the abstract idea of *the day to come* is foreign to you; all those ideas, along with their affective contexts, are acquired socially), or where you are, or whether you want to be there.

All of this information, the knowings that we simply take for granted in our everyday lives, has been acquired over the years of our existence. The great preponderance of it has been acquired in a social context. Those few things that were not socially learned are colored and made significant by their social surround. A child who touches a hot stove, for instance, learns that a red stove burns fingers—and can learn this with nobody else around. But how people respond to the child's being burned will shape the child's emotional response to the experience. For one child, getting burned fingers is a temporary discomfort to be soothed by a cuddle, a sympathetic voice, and some cool lotion; for another, it is a matter of personal inadequacy and shame, acquired through the experience of a sharp scolding and a disapproving frown.

## SCHEMAS AND SCRIPT

So much socially mediated learning occurs in a person's lifetime that capturing all of it in words would be virtually impossible, even if language could be adequate to describe the emotional nuances of each learning experience. Given the tremendous body of information that each of us acquires, we must also have a way of structuring that information, of grouping it so that whatever is needed to understand a here-and-now situation is available without having to sort through oceans of not-so-relevant material. Indeed, we do create such structures; called *schemas,* they make up an internal system of categories and procedures that allow us to navigate through and make sense of the confusion of data available to us at any given moment. Our schemas are the patterns we use to generalize events into classes (it has four legs, eats grass, and says "moo," so it's a cow; he's 7 feet tall and wears baggy shorts and runs down the floor bouncing a big round thing, so he's a basketball player). Schemas "embody the rules and categories that order raw experience into coherent meaning. All knowledge and experience is packaged in schemas. Schemas are the ghost in the machine, the intelligence that guides information as it flows through the mind" (Goleman, 1985, p. 75).

Some schemas are relatively simple: how to walk or pick up an object or brush your teeth. Others are complex blends of definitions and emotions and memories: the idea of *father* or the meanings and implications of *whispering,* for instance. Schemas are the raw ingredients of our expectations, our dreams, our wishes, our imaginings. They determine our external behavior (the way to get into Suzie's house is to take the sidewalk around to the back door, so I go to the back without even checking to see if the front is open), our perceptions (I don't even notice that the front door is slightly ajar), and our thoughts (in my thinking at that moment, the house has only one door and that door is in the back).

In a very real sense, everything we do in our lives shapes and adds to our collection of schemas. We are constantly gathering new information and comparing it with previous experience. Does it fit? Fine; schema confirmed and strengthened. Does it clash? Maybe I saw/heard/understood wrong, or maybe I'm missing some important piece, or maybe—last resort!—my schema needs readjusting. Poppell (1988) talks about *hypotheses,* using this term essentially as we have used *schema:* "Every act of cognition, every perception, is the confirmation or the refutation of a hypothesis about the world, about the phenomenal appearance or the behavior of others, or about oneself. The hypothesis is an active production of the cognitive person, even if—particularly at the moment of cognition—he is himself unconscious of this" (p. 66). Not only is the person unaware that he has produced a hypothesis, but he is also unaware that the hypothesis is being tested or that he may over time distort perceptions, memories, emotional reactions, and even overt behaviors in order to protect himself from having to revise it. Again, all of this activity takes place within a rich, flowing, ever-present stream of social relationships.

The phrase *hypothesis testing* is a bit misleading in that it suggests an activity that is primarily—if not entirely—cognitive. Schemas have a cognitive component, to be sure, but they are much more. They include emotions, behaviors, and physiological responses as well. A schema involves the whole person; it is a seamless blend of all of the aspects of one's experience. Schemas emerge from the interaction of one's internal and external worlds, and they in turn affect how we think and feel about those internal and external worlds and what we do with them. Our schemas shape our experiencing, and our experiencing creates our schemas.

If a schema were an isolated bit of experiencing, a solitary chunk of self in world, it would be an interesting but not particularly useful psychological concept. What makes schemas all-important to us as therapists is that they can be strung together into larger patterns or *scripts* (Berne, 1972; Perls, 1973). Unlike schemas, which are necessary if we are to function efficiently in a complex world, scripts tend to limit our ability to adapt to new situations creatively and constructively. "Scripts," says Atwood, "are plans that people have about what they are doing and what they are going to do. [People] justify actions that are in agreement with their scripts and challenge those that are not. Scripts are the 'blueprints for behavior' that specify the whos, whats, whens, and whys of behavior" (1999, p. 13). Scripts are the old habits, the familiar ways of relating to people, the unquestioned, knee-jerk reactions that prevent us from growing and changing and forming new kinds of relationships. They are self-perpetuating: because of our patterns of thinking, feeling, and reacting in a certain way, we create the very situations that the script predicts (Erskine & Zalcman, 1997/1979).

More about the development of script is found in chapter 3; for now, let us concern ourselves with how script operates in the here and now of a client's life. First, script is always out of awareness: script-bound behavior feels like a natural and inevitable response to what the world gives us. In actuality, though, our script helps to bring about our experiences and shapes our phenomenological world to fit our expectations. "Scripts," says Nathanson (1993), "are sets of rules for the management of scenes that are inevitable or desired or feared or despised but nonetheless will always assemble in predictable forms." Those forms are predictable precisely because of the rules we use to manage them. It is a circular process, one that interferes with making genuine, spontaneous contact with other people: "managed scenes" are the antithesis of spontaneity and authenticity. One of the primary tasks of psychotherapy is to help people interrupt their old script patterns, the patterns that trap them in pain-producing and isolating behaviors, and find new and more satisfying ways of relating to themselves and to other people.

## THE FUNCTION OF SCRIPT

Script patterns are familiar, easy to drop into. They have the same sort of comfort as an old, well-worn piece of furniture—not very attractive, perhaps, maybe a bit lumpy, but they are what we are used to and we would feel rather lost without them. When we are under stress, when we feel threatened, script patterns give us a well-rehearsed way to respond; they free us from the necessity of figuring out what to do next. Hite (1996) points out that scripts help us to manage the affect that we feel when our experience of the external world collides with our internal feelings, wants, and expectations. An affective reaction can be disconcerting, even frightening—especially if we have been taught that it is bad or dangerous to feel that way—and running through a familiar, automatic script pattern can occupy us until the affect cools down a bit.

Remember, too, that the choice of sliding into a familiar script pattern is not a conscious one. By the time a constellation of beliefs, feelings, and behaviors has formed into a schema and then become part of a script pattern, the whole thing has dropped out of awareness. Behaving in a script-bound way does not feel at all like a *choice;* rather, it appears to be the only possible way to react. As a child, I may have been (marginally) aware that I was suppressing my anger at being treated unfairly and feeling sad instead; as an adult, the response of sadness—and the thoughts and behaviors that go with it—is immediate, automatic, and unquestioned. It is very difficult to even think about changing something that feels both natural and inevitable, and that is the quality that we experience in our script behavior.

## Predictability, Identity, Consistency, Stability

Script, then, is maintained at two levels: by the absence of any other imaginable way of doing/feeling/thinking and by the immediate psychological benefits provided by moving into an old script pattern. These benefits fall into four major categories: *predictability, identity, consistency,* and *stability*—PICS, for short (Erskine, Moursund, & Trautmann, 1999). By telling us what to expect and then helping us to behave so as to make those expectations come true, script makes life *predictable*. In a predictable world, one knows what's coming and can get ready for it or perhaps even avoid it; if the world is unpredictable, one can not prepare oneself ahead of time for the bad things that might happen. Through script, we avoid unpleasant surprises. We may not like those script beliefs and feelings, or the behaviors that they lead us into, or the responses we get as a result; but, at least, we will not be taken by surprise. We can brace ourselves to bear it: after all, we've been there before.

The second benefit of script is that of maintaining *identity*. Identity gives us a focus, a sense of place in the world. It is our "passport" to relationship. Identity is, in a sense, a special kind of predictability—predictability of one's own self, one's own being. Stein and Young (1997) see the need to protect one's sense of identity as the primary factor in a client's maintaining his script. Without a sense of identity, we would experience no continuity of self from one moment to the next, no sense that we are the same person as we move from one situation to another. The experience of continuity, in turn, contributes to identity, allows knowledge of self as an ongoing entity. "I yam what I yam," says Robin Williams in the movie *Popeye:* "I" remains "I," the same "I," regardless of the changes that may occur around me. Hanging on to script-bound ways of thinking, of experiencing emotion, and of interacting with the world around us allows us to keep that sense of "I."

Third, is *consistency*. Humans are organizing animals. As we have already noted, without a set of organizing schemas, our lives would be a jumble of unrelated events occurring in a meaningless kaleidoscope of settings. Scripts organize our schemas into even more meaningful patterns, so that our experiences make sense to us. Maintaining those scripts allows us to keep our behaviors and those of others organized and consistent, to keep some kind of structure in our world. This structuring, in turn, makes predictability and identity possible and helps us to manage the anxiety of dealing with new and unfamiliar circumstances.

A fourth major script benefit is *stability*. Stability really should come first in the list: predictability, identity, and consistency are possible only if one can maintain some sense of control, some sense of being in charge of oneself. Without our scripts, we run the risk of being flooded by a rush of emotions, needs, memories, and perceptions—hopelessly confused, whirled away, drowning in our own ungovernable process. In popular parlance, this is being "crazy." Our script patterns allow us to feel sane and stable, and with that sanity and stability comes the possibility of maintaining a consistent, predictable identity in a consistent and predictable world.

## MAINTAINING THE SCRIPT SYSTEM

Script patterns are begun because they serve useful purposes. As is shown in chapter 3, a script pattern originates as a solution to a problem; it is a way of dealing with some situation that is causing discomfort or is experienced as dangerous. It is only when the pattern is rigidified, automatic, and out of awareness that it becomes dysfunctional, interfering with our ability to grow and change, to act spontaneously and creatively, to be fully ourselves, and to enter into authentic relationships with others. Script-bound individuals live in a constant tension between the pseudosafety provided by their script behaviors and the problems that those very script behaviors create. Our task, as therapists, is to help clients break through the script so that they have full access to both internal and external resources—so that they can develop new ways of being in the world that are effective for them now, in this place and at this time and in their current relationships. However, script patterns are not easily overcome. Because they serve such important psychological functions, people strongly resist giving them up. The resistance, like the script itself, is out of awareness.

Stein and Young (1997), who use the term *schema* to refer to what we have designated as *script*, say that a schema will be resistant to change to the degree that it "develops early and is central to the person's view of him- or herself and others" (p. 162). When it has been acquired early and is an intrinsic part of one's sense of self, script becomes a pole around which new bits of information, the experiences of one's life, are organized. As we take in new data, we filter and distort our perceptions so that they will fit with what we already believe. Just as someone who has just bought a new car tends to notice advertisements for the kind of car he or she bought and to ignore or dispute the claims of other makes and models, so we are selective in our remembering of experiences. The things that fit our script expectations are kept, stored away for future reference; the things that do not fit are distorted or denied— if they are noticed at all. Thus we structure our experiencing to create an ongoing reinforcement of the beliefs that underlie the script.

**Figure 2.1** | A Self-Perpetuating Script System

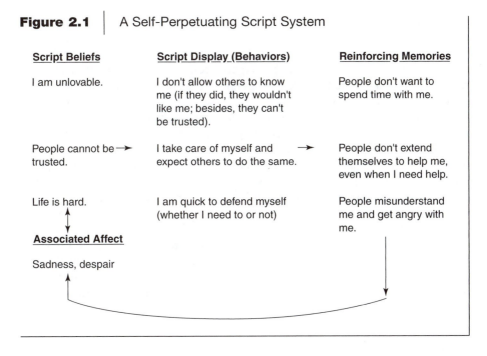

| Script Beliefs | Script Display (Behaviors) | Reinforcing Memories |
|---|---|---|
| I am unlovable. | I don't allow others to know me (if they did, they wouldn't like me; besides, they can't be trusted). | People don't want to spend time with me. |
| People cannot be trusted. | I take care of myself and expect others to do the same. | People don't extend themselves to help me, even when I need help. |
| Life is hard. | I am quick to defend myself (whether I need to or not) | People misunderstand me and get angry with me. |

**Associated Affect**

Sadness, despair

Not only does this selectivity operate in our perception and our memories, but it is also active in our behaviors. The client, says Fosshage (1992), may hope that people will relate to him in a new and different way but nevertheless expects that nothing will change. Because of that expectation, he organizes his behavior and interactions in ways that feel protective but elicit the same old unwanted reactions from others, thus creating a sequence of "repetitious relational experiences" (p. 34). The whole system becomes self-perpetuating, with each element serving to strengthen and reinforce the others.

In previous writings (Erskine & Zalcmann, 1997; Erskine & Moursund, 1988, 1999) we have used the notion of a *script system* to illustrate the self-fulfilling quality of script. Figure 2.1 is an example of this system. The client in this illustration holds a number of script beliefs, acquired over years of early neglect and deprivation: that he is unlovable, that people cannot be trusted, that life is hard. These beliefs are associated with feelings of sadness and despair. When one of the script beliefs is activated, he experiences the associated feelings; when circumstances stimulate similar feelings, he is reminded of the script beliefs. The script beliefs and affects, in turn, lead him to behave in predictable ways; he does not form close relationships, does not reach out to people, and is suspicious and defensive. In response to these behaviors, the other people in his life tend to be distant; they don't enjoy his company, don't seek him out, and are easily annoyed and frustrated with him. The client remembers many instances of these kinds of social responses, and, as shown in the figure, his memories serve to strengthen his script beliefs.

A circular pattern such as this has no real beginning. Each part is preceded by something else; each aspect is both a cause and an effect. Behaviors are reinforced by their consequences, but the consequences are determined by the behaviors. Even when the expected consequences do not occur in reality, they are often fantasized. The client imagines that people will respond to him in the old, painful ways, ways predicted by script. Over time, even those fantasies become a part of the system; that is, the memories act as reinforcers too, as if the fantasy had actually happened. The fantasy, arising out of the other elements of the system, becomes a cause as well as an effect. To make matters worse, the whole pattern is out of awareness, unavailable for updating or revision. The client is unaware of his pattern; for him, this is the world—the only possible world—and his ways of responding to it are the only possible responses. Says Wachtel (1990), ". . . [U]nconscious processes, so important in influencing how we construe and experience events and how we behave in response to them, are in turn understandable as also a response *to* those same events. Close inspection reveals that, far from persisting in spite of any input from everyday reality, and far from being simply unrealistic and infantile, these unconscious processes can be seen as being maintained by the very circumstances they bring about" (p. 236).

## Repression

In 1937, Anna Freud wrote *The Ego and the Mechanisms of Defense.* In this book, she expanded on her father's concept of defense mechanisms as the ways in which people ward off anxiety. The list of specific defense mechanisms is familiar to students of psychoanalytic thought—repression, denial, displacement, isolation, rationalization, reaction formation, and undoing are among the most commonly referred to—and we shall not, in this volume, deal with their many permutations and combinations. One of them, however, is of particular importance in understanding how the script system is maintained and how psychotherapists can help clients overthrow it. This is the process known as *repression.*

Repression is the most basic of the defense mechanisms; all of the others flow from it and can be seen as elaborations of it. Repression is a process of active holding back, active not-knowing. "The essence of repression," say Stolorow and Atwood (1989), "lies simply in the function of rejecting and keeping something out of consciousness" (p. 105). Script is, by definition, out of awareness, and repression is a key to keeping it that way. All of the other defense mechanisms described by Freud and his followers involve repression, in that all defenses require that we curtail or distort our awareness of self and/or others.

Repression is different from suppression; it is not merely a matter of turning our attention away from some thought or behavior, of choosing to do or think about something else. A scene in Margaret Mitchell's novel, *Gone With The Wind,* describes Scarlett, the heroine, faced with the terrible challenge of surviving in a world turned upside down by civil war; she uses suppression to deal with her pain and fear. "I'll think about that tomorrow," she declares. Scarlett chooses to not-know, to actively hold something out of awareness.

Unlike repression, however, suppression is a conscious process. Scarlett knows exactly what she is doing when she decides not to think about her problems. Repression, in contrast, is a holding-back process that has gone underground. The repressed material is not thought of—and cannot be thought of. It is no longer available to conscious awareness. It is not simply forgotten, in the way that we forget thousands of unimportant details of our lives—the phone number you looked up just a few minutes ago, for instance, or the color of the shirt that Robert was wearing in class last week. We forget unimportant things; we repress important ones. Repression happens for a reason, and the reason has to do with the significance of that which is repressed. It is "the failure to recall consciously something that is both significant and for which the inability to recall is apparently *motivated*. That motivation may be conscious or unconscious, and it may be internally or externally driven" (Freyd, 1996, p. 15). But, while the motivation for repression may be conscious, the repression itself is not; the process, like the repressed material, is unknown to its author.

Repression may begin as suppression and turn into repression when the habit of suppression has become so automatic that it is no longer noticed and one no longer has a choice about whether or not to be aware of the suppressed/repressed material; or it may be a more sudden acquisition, as when some experience is so unacceptable, so pain-filled, that it must be kept out of awareness from the outset. In either case, gradual or immediate, it always involves some sort of tightening up, of holding in that which needs to be expressed externally (Perls, Hefferline, & Goodman, 1951).

Repression can appear in a number of guises, depending on what sort of thing is being repressed. *Denial* is repression of thinking or of one's ability to think. Choosing, like Scarlett, not to think about a problem can be the first step in losing the ability to even know that the problem exists. *Disavowal,* in contrast, is the repression of emotion or of the ability to feel emotions. Many people report that they "went numb" in an emotional crisis. Temporary disavowal of emotion may be an important survival response in a crisis situation in which one must act quickly and decisively. A parent caring for a critically ill child may have to put aside his or her own feelings of fear and sadness in order to be there for the child; later, when the crisis has passed, the emotions may come streaming back. If they do not, the choice of not feeling has moved underground, out of awareness; it is no longer a temporary coping mechanism but has become part of the person's permanent defensive pattern. A third sort of repression is *desensitization,* which involves the repression of physical sensation. Those who have had to diet may have learned to desensitize themselves to sensations of hunger; others may be desensitized to sexual feelings or to a variety of other body sensations. Desensitization and disavowal often go hand in hand; people whose scripts demand that they not experience certain emotions frequently maintain their disavowal by tuning out their bodies entirely. Such people live "from the neck up"; theirs is an almost exclusively cognitive world in which relationships tend to be superficial and one-dimensional. Repression is serious business, because it cripples our ability to use our full selves in interactions with the world around us. "Whatever we call it," says

Freyd, "—repression, dissociation, psychological defense, denial, amnesia, unawareness, or betrayal blindness—the failure to know some significant and negative aspect of reality is an aspect of human experience that remains at once elusive and of central importance" (1996, p. 16).

All three forms of repression—denial, disavowal, and desensitization—interfere with relationships in that they prevent one from being fully present, fully responsive, to another. Not only do they affect relationships, but (again, in a circular pattern) they are created by and grow out of relational experiences. Freud and his fellow analysts believed that repressed material always involves either an unacceptable impulse from within the person, or an unbearable trauma or the memory of a trauma coming from outside. Relationship-focused integrative psychotherapists see relationships as central in initiating and maintaining repression. An emotion, thought, or action may be "unacceptable" in the context of some important relationship that would be lost or damaged were the emotion or thought or action to be allowed into awareness; a traumatic experience is repressed because being fully aware of it would in some way threaten a needed relationship. Fairbairn, one of the early object-relations theorists, appears to support this assertion: ". . . [A]t the core of the repressed is not a trauma, a memory, or an impulse, but a relationship . . . which could not be contained in awareness and in continuity with other experiences of the self" (Mitchell, 1988, p. 27).

Perhaps the ultimate repression occurs when a part of the self must be kept out of awareness. Such dissociation can come about in at least two ways. In one, some configuration of thoughts, desires, fears, emotions, and behaviors is experienced as *me* but is unacceptable; to be this sort of *me* would mean losing my relationship with valued others (who would reject me if they knew I was like this) and even with myself (I detest and reject those aspects of myself). So I split myself; I keep the acceptable parts available to awareness and call them *myself*, and I banish the unacceptable parts into the limbo of unawareness. Another sort of division or splitting can occur when a person, usually during childhood, experiences extreme trauma. In order to escape the pain (physical or emotional or both) of the trauma, the person simply leaves psychologically—*dissociates* from the experience—so that it does not have to happen to him or her. The child's body may still be there, being abused, but his or her real sense of self is somewhere else. In the absence of a protective, comforting, and accepting relationship, where the child can talk through the traumatic experience and eventually recover the traumatized and split-off part, the dissociation becomes a relatively permanent feature of the child's personality organization (Erskine, 1997b, 1997d).

Remember, too, that the whole process of splitting and dividing goes on out of awareness; if one were aware of it, it simply would not work. How could I keep myself from knowing and experiencing and owning something of which I am already aware? Gaining awareness of a split, then, and of the quality of the split-off part, is an important part of recovering one's sense of self and one's ability to relate to others as a whole person. Dissociation, Bromberg (1998) asserts, is hurtful because it "limits and often forecloses one's ability to hold and reflect upon different states of mind with a single experience of me-ness" (p. 7). The dissociating person literally does not know who he or she is. Moreover, like all defenses, because dissociation goes on out of awareness, it can be continued long after it ceases to be needed. The trauma may be long past, or the person may have long outgrown the need to keep some aspect of self from being known, but the defense cannot be given up because the person does not even know it is there. Says Sigmund (1998), "It is the unconscious nature of [the] initial splitting that results in the dissociative survival adapta-tion being carried forward in life even when the initial persecutors are no longer harming the person and he or she is no longer in the original persecu-tory environment" (p. 26).

Script patterns and repression go together; each supports the other. The various kinds of repression protect the script, and the script often dictates the ways in which repression will be used. It is a cruel paradox that script and repression, originally developed in order to maintain contact with significant others and to preserve the integrity of the self, eventually cut us off from both self and others. Nor are these patterns the exclusive province of people who are "disturbed" or "mentally ill"; all of us, in the process of growing up, devel-oped solutions that seemed necessary at the time but are no longer useful to us as adults. To the degree that we have incorporated those old solutions into our being and continue to follow their patterns without being aware of doing so, we are using repression and are trapped in script.

## Contact Disruption and Introjection

The authors of Gestalt therapy (Perls, Hefferline, & Goodman, 1951) discuss defenses and script behavior from yet another perspective: they look at defen-sive phenomena in terms of how people distort and disrupt contact. Script pat-terns and repression are ways of interrupting our contact with self and others—that is, awareness of our internal processes and openness to those around us—but contact disruption is also a way of supporting repression and maintaining script. According to Perls and his colleagues, five major ways are used to interrupt contact with others: projection, introjection, retroflection, confluence, and egotism.

It is beyond the scope of this volume to provide a full discussion of Perls' concept of contact disruption. Briefly, though, in *projection,* one projects a part of oneself onto the other person and then interacts with that projected part rather than with the real person behind the projection. *Introjection* is the converse of projection: here, in order to avoid conflict with another, the per-son takes in a part of that other, internalizing the conflict and thus making it more manageable. When one *retroflects,* one refuses to express oneself out-wardly but, rather, focuses on some internal dialogue, some conversation between two parts of oneself, instead of on the dialogue with another person. In *confluence,* one melds with the other, allowing no space and no differences—and, thus, little possibility of contact or conflict, both of which require the coming together of two or more distinct entities. Finally, *egotism* makes the individual so central and so important that others simply do not exist as the same sort of being and contact with them is impossible. For a more detailed description, the reader is referred to Perls, Hefferline, and Goodman's *Gestalt Therapy: Excitement and Growth in the Human Personality (1951)*; and Polster and Polster, *Gestalt Therapy Integrated (1973)*.

All of the contact-disruption processes are important in understanding how people distort awareness, but introjection is of special interest in a therapeutic approach that focuses on relationships. Introjection involves an out-of-awareness taking on of the beliefs, feelings, motivations, behaviors, and defenses of another person. It is an unconscious defensive identification with another that occurs in the absence of need-fulfilling contact (Erskine, 1997/1994). Say Stolorow and Atwood (1989), "The essence of introjection . . . lies in the substitution of some part of the psychic reality of an invalidating other for the child's own experience" (p. 372). The other person's "psychic reality" is his worldview, including his perception of the child. The child takes in that other person's view of him- or herself and others—according to Stolorow and Atwood, a view that is invariably negative and invalidating of the child—and adopts it as his or her own.

While relationship-focused integrative psychotherapists agree that the introjected other is often negative and critical, we define introjection somewhat more broadly: introjection occurs in the absence of need-fulfilling contact. One takes in some part of someone outside the self—emotions, attitudes, reactions, prejudices—without integrating that part into the overall personality, and responds to and with that part as if it were indeed part of oneself. As children, we may introject our caregivers' beliefs, values, emotional responses, and physical habits. Comments like "You laugh just like your mother" or "You're just as stubborn as your dad" attest to the frequency with which such introjection occurs. Adults, too, introject; how many young therapists have introjected the beliefs and values and mannerisms of their supervisors? How often does one family member pick up the emotional pattern of a spouse or a sibling?

Introjection is much more than simple imitation. As we have noted, it is a form of defense. It serves to reduce the possibility of conflict between the introjecting individual and the person upon whom that introjecting individual depends. To avoid conflict with a benevolent other (upon whom we rely but who cannot always meet our needs perfectly) or with a malevolent other (with whom conflict is dangerous), we defensively and unconsciously identify with the other, becoming like the other by taking the other into ourselves. All of this is out of awareness, of course; consciously, we may absolutely reject the notion that we would want to be at all like that other person. Introjection is a matter of survival—survival of the self, and survival of the self in relationship. Taking a part of the other into oneself, making oneself like that other, is a kind of survival insurance. It internalizes the conflict resulting from the lack of need fulfillment or the threat of that lack; when the conflict is internalized, it can—seemingly—be managed more easily or at least with less anxiety and pain (L. Perls, 1978).

The special interest that relationship-focused integrative psychotherapists have in introjection arises because an introject can function as an almost independent part of the personality, a separate entity with whom quasi-relationships can be formed. It sits within the psyche like a foreign lump, often impervious to the kinds of learning and growing in which the rest of the person is engaged. When activated, it responds as that introjected other was perceived to respond years ago. It is a kind of psychic time capsule, rigidly repeating the same old, unchanging patterns over and over again. When an introject is acquired by a child, it is defined by a child's perceptions of the world. It may be acquired at times of high stress, when one is unable to see the complexities and the depth of the other but, rather, introjects a kind of caricature of that other's process. These distorted, caricature-like aspects of the introjected other operate internally as one side of an internal dialog, and externally in transactions with other people. Because the introject is separate, isolated, it is protected from being affected by later relationships, and it is relatively impervious to therapeutic interventions that are aimed at other parts of the self.

## THE CONSEQUENCES OF SCRIPT, REPRESSION, AND CONTACT DISRUPTION

Many of our schemas are a necessary part of our psychic equipment. Operating out of awareness, they help us to move about our world from moment to moment, recognizing classes of events and dealing with those events efficiently. Defensive script patterns, maintained through repression and contact disruption and rigidified to the point where they can no longer be modified or discarded in the face of changing circumstances, are not helpful and are usually harmful. Because they block us from full awareness of internal and external events, these processes limit our ability to function spontaneously and creatively. They keep out feelings and thoughts and memories; they may split off whole aspects of self; and they cripple relationships with others. Ultimately, they result in the problems and symptoms that people bring to psychotherapy.

One of the more common consequences of scripting is the experience of internal dialog. Because repression and contact disruption, as well as the script they support, always involve blocking access to some aspect of self, people operating out of script are divided: one or more parts of themselves are no longer fully integrated within the whole psyche. Such division may result in dialogue between the repressed part(s) and the part that is experienced as *me*. Self-criticism ("that was a really stupid thing to say"), second-guessing ("did I do that right? should I have done something else instead?"), and self-restraining ("better not try that; it won't work anyhow") are common forms of this internal dialogue. The dialogues, and the behaviors and emotions that accompany them, are self-reinforcing; out of awareness, they chug along like an old two-cycle engine, drowning out the sounds of the real world and polluting one's contact with self and with others. Even though the engine distorts an individual's perceptions and dictates his or her responses, he or she does not know what is happening. People are not conscious of "the repetitive (looping) nature of the negativistic internal dialogues, nor are they aware that there are painful consequences to themselves, other persons, the situation, or the environment from the unconscious acting out that occurs as a direct result of these dialogues" (Sigmund, 1998, p. 24).

Hammen and Goodman-Brown (1990) talk about the cost of defensive patterns in terms of self-depletion. As one learns to defend by blocking access to some part of self, the self comes to be sensed as incompetent or deficient or dangerous. This is even more true when the original stimulus was critical or abusive and the defense involved introjection of the criticism and abuse: now there is a part of *me* that knows how bad another part of me is. One's sense of self-worth is eroded by the internal dialogue, by the behaviors that result from the dialogue, and even by the effort needed to maintain the whole pattern. By far the most pervasive consequence of script and the defenses that maintain it is loss of contact. Both basic survival (in a social world) and quality of life depend upon the continual moment-by-moment interplay between external and internal stimuli and upon the ability to be aware of and respond to those stimuli. Awareness of and response to internal and external stimuli means contact—contact with self, in all its aspects, and contact with the world around us and the people in that world. Script, by limiting contact both internally and externally, interferes with the quality of life and, in its most toxic forms, with survival itself.

A self divided, its parts not in contact with each other, is inevitably in conflict. With internal contact, one may have many different wants, needs, dreams, and fears; one sorts these out, prioritizes them, makes adjustments and compromises. Without such contact, the differing wants and needs are at war with each other. There is no communication, no working things out, only a constant tension, a feeling of not trusting oneself, and a growing sense of misery and hopelessness. That which originally was defended against has become a minor figure in this drama of despair; the script itself is now the enemy. But, hiding out of awareness, script and its associated defenses are impervious to change. They continue to operate, spewing out their poisons, even though their original usefulness has long been overshadowed by the damage they do.

External contact, too, is crippled by repression, contact disruption, and script. People learn to not see or not understand the things that might challenge their script beliefs. They remember events in ways that support those beliefs. Things are overlooked, stumbled over, misplaced; people seem to be uncaring, or overprotective, or vicious—whatever the script calls for. True contact with those other people cannot be made (because the whole self is not available to make that contact), so there is no way to correct the misperception. Over time, our functioning shapes our social environment. Script gradually eats away at our relationships until the other people in our life are no longer interested in being in contact with us.

# THE WIDENING SPIRAL

Schemas rigidify into script; script is supported by repression and contact disruption. Script shapes the way in which one processes information, so that new data are used to reinforce and further harden the script, rather than challenge it. Ideas and perceptions and responses that might threaten the script are blocked out of awareness, and the divisions within the self increase. Script creates a widening spiral in which distortions and disruptions reach out to affect more and more of one's problem-solving abilities, one's relationships, one's sense of self.

This widening spiral of script affects every modality of human functioning. It acts upon our cognitions by distorting the meanings that we assign to the events of our lives (Cervone & Shoda, 1999). Affect is stimulated by those distorted beliefs, by the painful stories we tell ourselves about the things we do and don't do, and by the things others do and the things we think they did. Beliefs and affect shape behaviors, just as behaviors shape beliefs and affect; and other people's responses to our behavior further contribute to the script pattern.

Every diagnostic category in the *DSM-IV-TR* (the *Diagnostic and Statistical Manual of Mental Disorders* published by the American Psychiatric Association, 2000) has script components. From the temporary discomfort of the adjustment disorders to the paralyzing patterns of obsessive compulsive disorders or the labyrinthine logic of the paranoid, script plays its part. This is not to deny, of course, the biochemical aspects of many psychiatric problems. Chemical imbalances and central nervous system malfunction are undeniably a part of the clinical picture for many clients, as are the tensions, stresses, and tragedies of their lives. But it is script that determines how physiological dysfunctions and external pressures will be experienced phenomenologically and how they will be reflected in the client's behaviors. Coyne (1999) speaks of "cumulative continuity" in his studies of depression. "An individual's experience with depression," he says, "channels him or her into an environment that reinforces the likelihood of future depression, thereby sustaining risk across the life course though the progressive accumulation of the consequences of depression" (pp. 376–377). In Coyne's view, the disorder itself is folded back into the script out of which the disordered behavior arises. The depressed individual creates depressing life experiences—either in reality, as a function of his or her impaired ability to maintain contact, or in fantasy, through his or her ongoing negative internal dialogue. Each of these events is experienced, understood, embellished, and remembered in script-consistent ways, and thus further reinforces the pattern. With each repetition, the scope of the script influence widens and more and more areas of functioning are affected. We would add to Coyne's description: non-self-created traumas, too, are folded back into script. It would be naïve to assume that *all* saddening (or frightening, or infuriating) experiences are brought about by script. Accidents can happen, jobs are lost during economic hard times, and terrorist attacks do kill; but everyone does not respond to such traumatic events in the same way, or remember them with the same intensity, or use them in the same way to reinforce old beliefs. It is in our response to and recollection of life events that script takes over, constricting our ability to recover from or rise above that which we cannot control.

As one becomes increasingly entangled in script, one's perspective becomes narrower and narrower. Life becomes a series of dreaded yet inevitable outcomes, and one tends to focus on those outcomes: on trying to ward off disaster and watching helplessly as the very effort to avoid the pain seems to make things worse. No matter how one tries to break out of the pattern, one repeats it over and over again. Freud (1920/1955) used the term *repetition compulsion* to describe the way in which his patients got themselves into the same sorts of painful situations again and again. To the outside observer, these behaviors do appear to be a kind of compulsive choosing to repeat a behavior that did not work well in the first place. From the inside, though, it does not feel like making the same choice over and over but, rather, that there is no choice to be made. One's responses and their consequences seem inevitable, unavoidable. Since the script is out of awareness, one cannot see the pattern or one's own part in creating it. The more one tries to understand, the more one searches for explanations and meaning in these experiences (explanations and meanings that must be consistent with the out-of-awareness script and must thus deny and distort one's perception of the actual events), the more one is likely to focus on an inner dialogue, further closing off contact with the world of people and things that might challenge the script. "Tragic and poorly articulated [script] narratives decrease the person's sensitivity to the interpersonal world by creating preoccupations with inner states and structures of which the person paradoxically remains unaware" (Gold, 1996, p. 42). It is the paradox of being focused upon that of which one must remain unaware that gives script its tenacity and its ability to spread into every aspect and every relationship of one's life.

This business of repression and contact distortion and script patterns creates a dismal picture. How tragic, that what begins as a creative means of protecting oneself from harm turns into something that is in itself harmful and causes damage in ever-increasing ways. Yet the very nature of script holds the seeds of its dissolution; since script must, by definition, be unaware, any increase in the client's awareness is script-destroying. Moreover, patterns of repression and contact distortion can serve as markers: they tell the therapist that script has been activated. "Pay attention!" these patterns announce. "Script alert! We just came close to something important!"

Relationship-focused integrative psychotherapists use the therapeutic relationship as the primary vehicle by means of which awareness can be enhanced and script dissolved. A broad range of interventions and techniques can be useful in helping clients to break out of script, and all are most effective in the context of a contactful relationship between therapist and client. To understand how they operate, how to choose among them, and why the therapeutic relationship is so central to their effectiveness, we must turn to a more detailed consideration of the role of relationship in human development.

## SUMMARY

All human learning and development are shaped by relationships. The earliest learnings, occurring in the context of child-caregiver relationships, result in schemas: ways of understanding and categorizing the world that are constantly being tested and updated. Schemas can be organized into scripts, and these scripts rigidify and limit one's ability to respond to others spontaneously and creatively. Scripts protect the individual from perceived harm or danger and are developed when one's relationships fail to provide needed support. Scripts are maintained because they provide predictability, identity, continuity, and stability; moreover, an individual's script system tends to be self-reinforcing.

Psychological defenses protect and maintain script. The primary defense mechanism is repression, which can be subdivided into denial (repression of thoughts), disavowal (repression of affect), and desensitization (repression of physical sensation). All of these forms of repression require loss of contact with oneself and with others. Introjection, a form of contact disruption that is of special interest to relationship-focused integrative psychotherapy, involves taking some aspect of another person into oneself and experiencing it as one's own.

The costs of script and the defenses that maintain it include internal conflict and dialogue; erosion of self-worth; loss of contact; an ever-narrowing and rigidified ability to interact with others; and, ultimately, the development of the kinds of symptoms and problems that bring people to psychotherapy.

# 3 CHAPTER | **Relationship and Human Development**

The person who seeks help through psychotherapy has a history, and that history contains the seeds of the challenges with which that person now is wrestling. The problems that bring people to therapy do not usually spring up overnight and are seldom suddenly thrust upon them by outside circumstances. People live and move within a stream of time, and their situation at any given moment is a product of who they have been and what they have learned throughout that stream of time. Therapists can easily overlook this dimension of their adult clients and treat them as if they were simply here-and-now beings dealing with here-and-now problems. But here-and-now problems are rooted in the experiences and learnings of then-and-there; if the problem of here-and-now is not to simply repeat itself in another way, another painful relationship, another depressive episode, then therapists and clients must deal with the then-and-there out of which here-and-now has grown.

The most significant and influential aspects of anyone's history are the relationships in which one has participated. From the work of Freud and his colleagues, through the many shifts and permutations that have shaped our profession, therapists, theorists, teachers, and researchers have emphasized the importance of relationship—both in the early stages of life and throughout adulthood—in giving meaning and validation to an individual. In this chapter, we look at how relationships support and shape our development, how they contribute to both health and dysfunction. In so doing, we set the scene for discussing how to use the therapeutic relationship, as well as therapeutic interventions within that relationship, as a vehicle for change and growth.

## THE EARLY EXPERIENCE OF RELATIONSHIP

We can never fully know the subjective world of the newborn infant. We cannot remember our own early infancy, and babies certainly cannot describe their phenomenology to us. Indeed, since the phenomenological experience of an infant is pre-verbal, and since we adults live in a world that is steeped in and surrounded by words, we might well be unable to make sense of infants' experiencing even if we could somehow get inside their minds. What we know about the psychology of infants is based on outside observation, on speculation, and on extrapolation from our own adult experiences.

This having been said, however, some general consensus seems to exist among child psychologists about what infants do experience during the first weeks and months of life. One of the most startling things about these infants is that they appear to be born as relationship-seeking and relationship-making sorts of creatures. Within hours of the moment of birth, babies respond differentially to other humans; they prefer looking at a stylized human face rather than an abstract design (Morton & Johnson, 1991; Johnson, Dzuirawiec, Ellis, & Morton, 1991), and they prefer their mother's voice to other people's voices (Querlu, Lefebre, Renard, Titran, Morillion, & Crepin, 1984). Mother, of course, is the most significant of all of the people in the infant's environment: Mother, whose heartbeat has sustained the infant through 9 months of intrauterine existence; Mother, whose voice has been heard (muffled, transmitted through a different set of elements) over and over again; Mother, whose warmth and touch are familiar even though different from the warm wet dark of before-birth. For the very new infant, Mother is both me and not-me. She is a part of who and what I am and without whom my existence would not be possible, yet she is now outside, appearing and disappearing, no longer an ever-present extension of myself.

The task of discovering the difference between what is a part of me and what is not is one of the earliest challenges that new infants face. Physically, they must learn which of the things in the perceptual world are parts of their own body (have you ever watched babies who have just discovered their own fingers?) and how to use those body parts. Psychologically, they must learn about living in relationship—that they are individuals, that there are other individuals in the world that they inhabit, and how to interconnect with them. This latter learning task has been called the process of *separation-individuation*, and it emerges out of very early contact between caretaker and infant. It is a primary building block in the development of a personality and the sense of self (Bowlby, 1969, 1973, 1980; Stern, 1985; Mahler, Pine, & Bergman, 1975).

The separation-individuation task might perhaps better be referred to as *separation-connection*, for neither separation nor connection is possible without the other. For the infant to experience him- or herself as a separate individual, there must be someone from whom to be separate. To experience connection— relationship—the infant must be an individual who can relate to other individuals. Relationship-focused integrative psychotherapists see the early separation-individuation process as a simultaneous growing apart from and reaching back toward the primary caretaker. They recognize the central importance of "the affective exchange between parent and child and . . . the simultaneity of connection and separation. Instead of opposite endpoints of a longitudinal trajectory, connection and separation form a tension, which requires the equal magnetism of both sides" (Benjamin, 1992, p. 49).

It was once thought that newborn babies experienced the world as a jumbled swirl of unrelated and disorganized sensations—William James's "blooming, buzzing confusion" (1890). Later observers have revised that belief; we now know that babies emerge into the world equipped with the ability to organize their perceptions. They see shapes, movement, and figures against background. Much earlier than was previously thought, they also see other people and distinguish them from mere objects. Whatever else there may be in a newborn's environment—the bright light of a hospital delivery room, the colors and textures of a bedroom, the odors and sounds of a kitchen—there is always at least one other human being. The presence of another person is the one universal element in the early experience of all humans, and these others are differentiated from the rest of the world very, very early. The infant is not alone. Other entities are in the world, entities that are "like me" in some fundamental way (Meltzoff, Gopnik, & Repacholi, 1999). The infant smile that earlier generations dismissed as "just a gas pain; the baby hasn't learned to smile yet" is probably not just a gas pain after all; while it may not carry the same sorts of meanings as the smile of an older person, it can nevertheless be a gesture of recognition and of relationship.

This awareness of an other is the basis for the infant's sense of self. Without an other who is like me but yet not me, I cannot develop my own selfhood. Others are more than psychological mirrors who reflect back to infants how they are seen by the people around them. Others provide the possibility of being; they provide the psychological boundaries with which infants collide and through which they come to know that they too have boundaries. "Without the existence of the other to serve as a foil for one's own reflection," says Agosta (1984), "awareness of the self is impossible . . . not only is the 'I' a part of the 'we,' but also . . . the 'we' is a component of the 'I' " (p. 44). And the importance of an other is not just a phenomenon of infancy; it continues throughout one's life. The self continues to grow, change, and be shaped by relationship experiences. Even though it is probably the most basic, the most fundamental set of schemas in one's mind (Goleman, 1985), the self is not static. Every significant person, every important relationship, leaves its imprint upon who we are and who we will become.

## Learning to Feel, Think, and Act

We have asserted that as infants learn to experience themselves more and more as separate individuals, they are able to be more and more in contact with others. Contact implies separation; entities that are not separate cannot make contact, because contact requires two distinct things that meet and acknowledge each other. Experiencing one's separateness is the flip side of connection and contact; each requires the other, and, without the other, each would be meaningless.

Contact and separation, coming together and moving apart, and sensing the presence of an other who is sometimes close and sometimes distant, affect every aspect of the infant's development. Probably the most primitive of those aspects is that of affect. The ebb and flow of chemicals in the body and the messages that those tides of chemical change send to the brain are the raw materials of emotion. Affect can be solitary; it begins as a simple positive or negative valence, an "I like/I don't like," and gradually differentiates into classes of pleasure or pain. For affect to become emotion, however, for pleasure/pain and like/don't-like to evolve into joy or fear or anger or sadness, there must be another person to resonate with one's own feelings. The emotional core of the self derives from our early experiences with others, with their reaction to our expressions of affect and with our perceptions of their emotional response to those expressions (Stolorow, 1992).

The notion that emotions are essentially a social phenomenon, developed out of relationship, is not difficult to accept. Emotions nearly always arise in the context of some social relationship, and they are most fully experienced when there is someone to share them with (or to hide them from). But what about thinking? Is our intellectual life also shaped by social relationships? The answer to that question is an unqualified "yes"; our very patterns of thought—our cognitive skills—grow out of our interaction with our environment, and the most salient elements in that environment are other people. The classes and categories into which we organize the world are taught to us by others; we know what a "dog" is, or a "house," or a "birthday," because someone taught us to use those terms. Language itself, without which thinking (as we adults understand and experience it) is not possible, is an inherently social phenomenon. The language we learn from the people around us determines how we think; people who speak Finnish or Urdu or Cantonese think differently and experience the world differently from English-speaking people. Clocksin (1998) asserts that intelligence cannot be considered apart from one's engagement with others, one's membership in a social group. The bridge between what is presented to us through sensory input and how we represent that input cognitively is constructed out of social consensus, as transmitted by the people from whom we learn to communicate. Social relationships lie at the heart of every word we utter and every thought we think.

To discuss thinking and feeling—cognition and emotion—as if they were two separate processes is, of course, a distortion of what really happens in human functioning. Our thoughts are inevitably undergirded and affected by our emotions, and our emotions are channeled and given meaning by our thoughts. Drawing a distinction between thoughts and feelings is a cognitive abstraction, itself made possible by linguistic convention. I would not be writing about cognitions and emotions unless I had learned those concepts from someone. Moreover, I would probably not have chosen to study them were those learnings not accompanied by some positive affective response. I have a noticeably different emotional reaction to the concepts of "differential calculus" or "carotid endartarectomy" than to "cognitive functioning," and I am unable to think about those—or any other—concepts without experiencing some emotional response. Emotions are a part of the background of whatever thoughts are foreground at any moment, just as cognitions form the background for every emotion we experience.

For the infant—again, this is no more than informed speculation, for we cannot ever truly know what happens inside that tiny head—affect and cognition are undifferentiated, a swirling stream of internal experience. Gradually, what was simply *lived* as an unquestioned, not-reflected-upon, ongoing "I am" begins to differentiate into different aspects, different kinds of internal experience; and these different experiences, reflected in behavior, are in turn responded to differently by the child's caregivers. "The child's conscious experience," note Stolorow and Atwood (1989), "becomes progressively *articulated* through the validating responsiveness of the early surround" (p. 368).

Given that thoughts and feelings are acquired in a relational context, it is inevitable that behaviors, too, are shaped through relationship. In fact, the influence of social relationships on behavior is quite easy to demonstrate. Behavioral psychologists have developed clear and convincing models of the effects of reinforcement: behaviors that are reinforced tend to be repeated; behaviors that are not reinforced tend to drop out. The most potent—and pervasive—reinforcers are social; a fleeting smile, a tiny gesture, a subtle change in voice tone from a significant person can have enormous effects on one's behaviors.

From conception to birth, through all of our waking hours (and, in dreams, through many sleeping hours as well), we are social creatures. Both our internal world and our external world are, in a very real sense, products of the relationships in which we participate. Each individual's psychological development is "best conceptualized in terms of the specific intersubjective contexts that shape the developmental process and that facilitate or obstruct the child's negotiation of critical developmental tasks and successful passage through developmental phases" (Atwood & Stolorow, 1984, p. 65). Those "intersubjective contexts" are created by the interplay among people, often child and caretaker, whose subjective worlds are different and separate but who, together, create an evolving reality that affects them both.

## The Development of Script

In chapter 2, we talked about script patterns—those out-of-awareness, self-perpetuating systems of thoughts, feelings, and behaviors that trap us into using the same old, out-of-date, and often dysfunctional responses over and over again. It should come as no surprise that such script patterns are acquired in a social context and are shaped by the quality of our relationships with others and by our attempts to sustain and improve those relationships.

The notion of script has been percolating around the psychological community for the better part of a century, although the term itself emerged in the mid-1900s. Freud's (1920/1955) phrase "repetition compulsion" captured much of what we would now call a *script pattern,* and Alfred Adler wrote similarly about "life style" (Ansbacher & Ansbacher, 1956). Eric Berne (1961, 1972) is most generally credited with bringing the word *script* into common usage; Fritz Perls, innovator of Gestalt therapy, described a self-fulfilling, repetitive pattern (1944) and later called this pattern a "life script" (Perls & Baumgardner, 1975). Recent psychoanalytic writers have referred to a developmentally preformed pattern as "unconscious fantasy" (Arlow, 1969b) and "schemata" (Arlow, 1969a; Slap, 1987). In psychoanalytic self-psychology, the term "self-system" is used to refer to recurring patterns of low self-esteem and self-defeating interactions (Basch, 1988) that are the result of "unconscious organizing principles" found in the "prereflexive unconscious" (Stolorow & Atwood, 1989).

Whatever they are called, the scripts we create have largely to do with our experience of needs and of how they are met. When infants experience a need, they instinctively reach out to the world around them and to the people in that world to satisfy the need. If they are hungry, they demand food. If they are lonely or bored, they cry for attention. As a need is met, it recedes into the background and a different need becomes foreground—and the infant again makes contact with the outside world in order to satisfy the new needs. This is natural behavior, an uninterrupted flow of shuttling between internal and external, between need-experienced and need-met. It is a series of *Gestalts:* indivisibly whole experiential patterns, involving cognitions, affect, behaviors, and physiological responses, cycling through time in an alternation of need and satisfaction that is as smooth and natural as the inhaling and exhaling of a sleeping baby.

In the course of growing up in a social environment, children soon learn that they are expected to modify this natural flow of experience. Sometimes when a child cries for attention, Mother does not come—or comes with a frown and a harsh voice, and the quality of the attention is not at all what the child wanted. Children are expected to share their toys with siblings, to empty their bladder only at certain times and in certain places, and to refrain from plucking bright-colored objects off the grocery shelves. They learn, through their early relationships, that some of their natural efforts to meet their needs are not acceptable. But needs and wants cannot simply be ignored: if the experience of need arousal is not satisfied or closed naturally, it must find an artificial closure that distracts from the discomfort of the unmet need. Children who learn not to cry for attention may amuse themselves with their toys or cover their head with a blanket; in time, they may even persuade themselves that they really want to play with the toys or hide under the blanket. The original need is driven underground, often in order to maintain relationship with some significant other person. Because the substitute solution is (at least temporarily) rewarding, it tends to be repeated; awareness of the original need retreats farther and farther underground. The artificial closure—the script pattern—begins to feel natural and even inevitable.

Crick and Dodge (quoted in Haines, Metalsky, Cardamone, & Joiner, 1999) talk about how a child's very early script patterns become elaborated over time. As the child grows and practices each set of responses (and remember, most if not all of this "practicing" is out of awareness), the patterns become both more efficient and more complex; they involve more and more perceptions and internal reactions, with increasingly subtle influences on other related concepts and relationships. The patterns also become "more rigid and resistant to change. . . . [They] begin to take on the qualities of personality characteristics in that they are stable and predictable across a wide range of situations" (pp. 72–73).

Script patterns, then, are born out of our life experiences. They become interpersonal strategies, ways of dealing with people. They are often transmitted from parents to children in early family interactions, and they affect all of the relationships in which we participate later in life. They "are guided by relatively enduring and complex mental representations . . . [and] may be generalized across family, marital, and friendship contexts" (Lyons-Ruth, 1995, p. 435). As shown in chapter 2, they are supported by beliefs about self, about others, about the nature and quality of life, and by the affect that surrounds those beliefs and is experienced when one of the beliefs is activated. The belief-affect combination leads to behaviors that are set, prescribed, and repetitious (even though they may feel natural and spontaneous). Those behaviors, in turn, set off predictable responses in others, responses that tend to perpetuate the behavior, reinforce the original beliefs, and justify the expression or containment of emotion.

Even when other people do not respond in ways that directly reinforce our script, we tend to interpret their responses to fit the pattern. Says Warner (1997), "Of course, there is no such thing as one's 'real' experience, only an actively constructed account of one's life situation, grounded within one's social and cultural milieu" (p. 132). A child, acting out newly forming responses, organizes the whole world into patterns, or schema; the schema string together and make sense of otherwise unrelated events. If a new experience cannot be assimilated into this organization, it is distorted—not unlike Cinderella's wicked stepsisters cutting off their toes in order to force their feet into the glass slipper—or ignored altogether (Weinberger & Weiss, 1997).

Script has its origin in a need not met, and the experience of need-not-met lies at the core of every script pattern. Script is developed to compensate for and ease the discomfort of unmet needs. These needs, while not always centered on relationship, always have a relational component; they are shot through with relational experiences and expectations. Children's developing scripts are predictive, for script perpetuates the belief that one's needs will not be met, that people will not be there for one and will not (or cannot) give one what one really wants. Children's experiences in relationships are then selectively perceived and selectively remembered to confirm those expectations; and, to protect themselves from being disappointed again and again, they may begin to close themselves off, making their contact with others increasingly limited and superficial. Or, they may repeatedly look for that one perfect relationship that *will* meet their needs, and meet them perfectly—and be demanding and critical because each new relationship eventually falls short of what they so desperately want. Each time the script pattern is repeated, it becomes more ingrained and rigid, and the script-bound person's relationships become more brittle, more shallow, and less satisfying to either of the participants. Instead of separation contributing to contact with others, and contact with others contributing to the processes of individuation and connection, the pattern has been reversed: separation now reduces the possibility of contact, and what pseudocontact there is reinforces and perpetuates internal distortions, defensiveness, fragmentation, and isolation.

## A Continuing Developmental Need

Most of the research and theorizing about how one learns to become an individual, connected yet separate, has focused on early developmental stages: the processes by means of which an infant, or a small child, builds a sense of self in relationship to others. But the importance of relationship does not end with childhood. We continue to experience the need for relationship at every stage of development, just as we continue to build and elaborate our sense of self throughout our lives. The need for relatedness with others is never outgrown. It is a basic biological fact, wired in, part of the psychological equipment that we are born with. We can no more turn it off than a cat can decide not to purr or a fish can stop breathing through its gills (Mitchell, 1993).

Orange (1995) asserts that relating to others, coming to know ourselves through that relatedness and coming to know the others through our experience of self, is necessary throughout life in order to maintain a continuous and positive self-concept. It is not "immature" to depend upon others, nor is it "mature" to deny such dependence. Rather, the natural and healthy state of humans is *inter*dependence, being a part of a continuously shifting and evolving stream of relationships. Whether at 9 months, or 9 years, or 90 years, it is only through such relationships that we can truly be individuals, knowing and celebrating ourselves even as we recognize and celebrate others.

## THE CONCEPT OF RELATIONAL NEEDS

People experience a wide variety of needs, and different psychological theorists have stressed different aspects of those needs. Maslow (1987) introduced the notion of a *need hierarchy,* in which awareness of some needs is deferred until needs lower on the hierarchy are satisfied: the need for respect and recognition, for instance, is not usually foreground for a person who is starving or whose personal safety is in jeopardy. Psychotherapists tend to be less interested in physiological needs—air, water, food—than in emotional needs. As relationship-focused integrative psychotherapists, we see all emotional needs as rooted in relationship. We have also noticed that people experience some needs that deal specifically with the quality of the relationships in which they find themselves. These relational needs are unique to interpersonal contact, and we believe that they are the essential elements that enhance one's sense of self-in-relationship. When these needs are not met, relationships are damaged and one's overall quality of life is impaired.

## A Paradigm Shift

Understanding human needs in terms of relationship—as emerging from relationship and reaching out to relationship—represents a basic shift in the way psychologists conceptualize human functioning. In the graduate schools of the 1950s and 1960s, students were taught to analyze the structures and systems that organized each individual. Needs—if they were conceptualized at all—were thought to be elaborations of basic physiological drives. People interacted with each other, wittingly or unwittingly reinforcing each other, on the basis of those drives and the responses that were learned in trying to satisfy them. Human society was seen as a collection of individuals colliding or cooperating as each attempted to take care of him- or herself. The human mind (again, if it was mentioned at all) was the product of evolving, innately derived patterns, only secondarily influenced by transactions with others.

By the 1980s, the view of the psychological self had begun to change radically. "Mind has been redefined from a set of predetermined structures emerging from inside an individual organism to transactional patterns and internal structures derived from an interactive, interpersonal field" (Mitchell, 1988, p. 17). Today, while we still recognize that a relationship involves individuals, we also assert that individuals are formed by their relationships. We *need* relationships, relationships with specifiable characteristics, to survive.

Freud, working without the benefit of these new understandings of the importance of human-to-human connection, talked about the *libido,* the life force, as being basically pleasure seeking. He thought that all of our behaviors, internal and external, could be traced back to a need to experience pleasant sensations and avoid painful ones. Almost a century later, we are beginning to realize that it is not primarily physical pleasure that people seek, but relationship. The most satisfying experiences of life are those that involve relationship. Even painful relationships exert their pull: marriage partners stay together even when they no longer like each other; children lie to protect their abusive parents. The need for relationships, as well as the needs experienced within those relationships, is a primary motivating experience in human behavior, in and of itself.

Emotions are squarely at the center of relationship. The sense of being in relationship *is* a kind of emotion, a feeling of connectedness and belonging. It may be positively valenced, in which case we enjoy the company of the other person, look forward to being together, enjoy pleasing and being pleased by each other, and feel sad or angry or frightened by the prospect of separation. Or the valence may be negative: we dread seeing the other person, dislike him, fear what he may do or say in our presence. Of course, most relationships are mixed, with good moments and bad, pleasure and pain, satisfaction and exasperation. Good or bad, however, there is always emotion in relationship. Here is another of those circular, two-directional influences: emotion is always present in relationship, and relationship is always present in emotion. Emotion (in contrast to sheer affect) is relational, transactional in its nature. My emotion requires a *you* to respond and resonate to that emotion, so that I, in turn, can respond to what I experience coming from you. Emotion without that kind of resonance (and remember that the responding other can exist in fantasy as well as in reality) is stunted and short-lived, just as relationship without emotion is shallow and transitory.

Not surprisingly, the emotional intensity of a relational need grows as the need remains unsatisfied. The relational need-not-met is often initially experienced as emptiness, a kind of nagging loneliness; behaviorally, it may be manifested through intolerance or frustration, through anger or aggression, or in closing down and withdrawing contact. Over time, unmet relational needs can result in loss of energy or hope and can show up in script beliefs such as "Nobody is there for me" or "What's the use of anything?" Such script beliefs are a cognitive defense against awareness of the unmet need and the feelings that arise when it is not responded to.

One further quality of relational needs (and the feelings associated with them) must be re-emphasized: these needs and feelings do not end with childhood. They are present throughout the entire life cycle, from early infancy through old age. They are a part of the background of every human relationship, emerging into awareness as longings or desires and receding again to background when they have been acknowledged and/or satisfied. The biological imperative for relationship and the kinds of needs that are manifested within relationships are as much a part of adulthood as of any other developmental stage. Although we may learn to disguise relational needs, or to compensate for their not being met, we never outgrow them. Relational needs are lifelong.

## Eight Primary Relational Needs

There are probably as many different ways of describing relational needs as there are people in relationship; humans are remarkably creative in how they relate to each other and talk about those relationships. In our work with clients and students and in our qualitative research into the nature of transference and of the characteristics of an effective therapeutic relationship, we have observed some needs emerging over and over again as people struggle to maintain or change their ways of being with others. We have come to believe that there are at least eight basic needs that must be dealt with in all relationships (Erskine & Trautmann 1996/1997). If these needs are met, the relationship will thrive and will support the growth and development of both partners.

If they are not met (in at least rudimentary ways and at least some of the time), the relationship will become toxic.

The first relational need is for *security.* In any relationship, one needs to feel secure. One needs to know that the relationship is a safe place to be who one really is, to show all of oneself without fear of losing the other person's respect and liking, without ridicule or humiliation. Relational security requires more than verbal reassurances. It is the visceral experience of having our vulnerabilities respected and protected, of having our needs and feelings accepted as human and natural, of knowing that we will not be attacked or humiliated if we make a mistake. It grows out of repeated experiences of sharing a new aspect of self and discovering that the relationship has survived, that both of us are still here and still okay.

Second is *valuing.* The need to be valued, cared about, and thought worthy is an obvious part of any relationship. Why would people want to be in relationship with someone who did not value, care about, or respect them? Valuing is a kind of validation: an affirmation that one is accepted, affirmed, and significant in the relationship; but valuing, as a relational need, goes even beyond a general sort of caring about. It has to do with the acknowledgment of one's psychological process, one's internal workings. Not just *what* one does, but *why* one does it, is the key to this sort of valuing. When I am valued in a relationship, I know that my partner expects and believes that whatever I do must have a reason, a reason that makes sense to me. I know that my partner cares about and trusts me and wants to understand the sense making of my behavior, my emotions, my hopes, fears, dreams, and fantasies. My partner accepts my relational needs as legitimate, experiences my affect as significant and important to him or her, and knows that whatever I may do or say serves (or is intended to serve) a significant psychological function.

*Acceptance* is third on our list of relational needs. It refers to being loved, respected, *let in* to the other person's life—and not just any other person; we're talking about a reliable, stable, and protective person, a person from whom one can draw strength, and whom one can let in and love and respect in return. This kind of acceptance allows one to feel protected and cared for by someone whose caring and protection are meaningful, reliable, and dependable. Toddlers who move out to explore their world but must frequently return to make sure that their caretaker is there, solid and supporting, exemplify the need for this sort of acceptance. Similarly, an adult client can move into frightening or dangerous internal territory, exploring thoughts and feelings and memories long buried and closed to awareness, with the support and acceptance of a dependable therapist.

We asserted earlier that each of the basic relational needs must be dealt with (i.e., acknowledged, if not actually satisfied) in a relationship if it is to be healthy and sustained. The need for acceptance from a dependable and protective other is perhaps an exception, in that adults appear to be able to sustain relationships with dependent children—who are neither protective nor particularly reliable—over long periods of time. Even in the case of a child with developmental delays, with whom one never achieves the kind of adult-

adult relationship that characterizes most healthy interactions between parents and their grown children, there can still be close and lasting relationships. Note, however, that persons who sustain this sort of relationship with a child are perhaps most needful of acceptance from dependable and strong others elsewhere in their lives.

The need for *mutuality* is the need to be with someone who has walked in one's shoes, who understands what one is experiencing because that person has experienced something similar, in real life or, at least, in imagination. Part of this need arises from the natural desire to not have to explain everything fully, to be understood without words; part of it has to do with being able to believe that the other person really does understand and accept and value: if you've been there, too, then of course you know what it's like for me. Mutuality gives depth to acceptance and valuing; if you've had the same experience, then you really do know how I'm feeling and your acceptance means you accept who I really am and not just who I pretend to be. How often we hear someone say, "If you knew what I was really like, you wouldn't want to be around me." Underlying that sort of remark wails a need for mutuality, a desperate longing for someone who *does* know, who *has* been there, and who still wants to maintain the relationship.

Fifth on our list is the need for *self-definition*. Self-definition in a relationship involves experiencing and expressing one's own uniqueness and having the other person acknowledge and value that uniqueness. It is the complement of the need for mutuality: the need to be unique, as contrasted with the need for shared perceptions and experiences. One needs one's relationship partners to acknowledge one's differentness, one's disagreements, and even one's irritation or anger when these emerge as a facet of one's individuality. When this happens, each partner can grow and change with full support from the other. It's that separation-individuation thing again: by supporting a partner's unique individuality, one strengthens the commonality in the relationship as well.

Next is *making an impact*. An essential part of all meaningful relationships is one's ability to have an impact on the other person: to be able to change the other's thinking, to make the person act a different way, and/or to create an emotional response in that person—and not only to cause these effects in the other but to be able to see the effects, to know that something has happened to the other person in response to one's input. We can all remember asking a question or making a comment to someone and getting no response, or sharing some strong feeling and finding no corresponding feeling in the other person. It is an uncomfortable experience, and it leaves us wondering if we really have a relationship with that person—or if we really want to have one.

In any relationship, one needs to *have the other initiate* some of the time. A relationship in which the same person must always make the initial approach, always take the first step, will eventually become dissatisfying if not painful for that person. We need our significant others to reach out to us in a way that acknowledges and validates our importance to them, that demonstrates their desire to be involved with us.

Finally, people in a relationship have the need to *express caring*. In any positive relationship, the participants experience affection, esteem, and appreciation for each other. In close relationships, the partners experience love and commitment. Expressing these feelings is a relational need; not doing so requires that one push aside and deny the internal experience—just like denying or trying to ignore any other need—and also avoids self-definition within the relationship. Part of who I am with you is how I feel about you; if I am to be fully contactful, fully in relationship, I must be able to express those affectionate feelings.

And what about the need to *be* cared about and loved? One feels loved—*is* loved—in a relationship in which all eight of the other needs are met, at least some of the time, and are acknowledged when they cannot actually be met.

Throughout our lives, we experience the need for relationship and we experience relational needs within our relationships. To the extent that these needs are met, our relationships are likely to be healthy and growth producing. When they are not met, our relationships wither, and become superficial and even less capable of satisfying our needs. Let us turn now to a consideration of how, specifically, relationship and relational needs affect development.

## DEVELOPMENT AND HEALTHY RELATIONSHIPS

### Physical Development

As we consider the whole idea of "child development," the most obvious thing that comes to mind is physical development. Children grow taller and heavier. The proportions of their bodies change. The structure of the central nervous system becomes more elaborated, the nerves themselves more capable of efficiently delivering messages to and from the brain. Not surprisingly, a child's experience in relationship affects even these most basic physiological processes.

Very early in an individual's life, the absence of contactful relationship with other humans leads to a condition known as *failure to thrive,* in which the child literally begins to dwindle; weight loss, susceptibility to disease, emotional withdrawal, and even death can result. Less dramatic but equally important is the role of relationship in a child's development of body sense. Knowing where one's own body ends and the outside world begins and recognizing the signals that one's body sends are critical learning tasks for the infant. Says Mitchell (1992), "Bodily experience only becomes known in necessarily social experience with others, and the very terms and categories through which it becomes known are shaped by linguistic and social experience" (p. 4). Just as a child's physical body grows best when the child experiences frequent, positively valenced *physical* contact with others, so that child's internal sense of his or her growing physical body requires *psychological* contact with others. Given such contact, the child can enjoy his or her body rather than being ashamed of it, can *be* that body rather than just using it as a tool to negotiate the world.

The infant-caregiver system regulates and organizes the new baby's experience of his or her internal states (Stern, 1985; Stolorow, 1992). Am I hungry? Sad? Nervous? Excited? Do I want to stretch? Sleep? Scream? The newborn infant acts so as to satisfy physical needs, with no intervening cognitive activity. As infants gain cognitive skills, they use them to modulate the connection between felt need and need-meeting behavior. The modulation works in both directions; cognitions affect both one's behavior and one's experience of the internal stimulus. A warm, contactful relationship with the caregiver allows the child's cognitive modulation to enhance and elaborate her phenomenological experience, so that she can sort, categorize, and label different kinds of experiences and learn new strategies of interaction between internal and external worlds.

## Behavioral Competence

The attempts of infants to interact with the world, to reach out for what they need and reject that which is unwanted, are primitive and unelaborated. One of the major developmental tasks is to hone those skills, to learn how to navigate both physical and social environments. Individuals learn to delay gratification, to go around barriers, to do *this* in order to accomplish *that*—the thousands of micro- and macro-skills that allow them to engage the world with competence and efficiency. These skills are, in large part, acquired through social interaction. Even the notion of acting "so as to" is a socially acquired concept; intentional behavior requires that one see oneself as "separate from a mind-independent world upon which one can act" (Olson & Askington, 1999, p. 2), and that sense of individuality and intentionality is gained through interacting with others and through watching others' interactions. In a healthy social environment, the child's acquisition of new skills is applauded and rewarded. Attempts to meet relational needs are supported; caregivers resonate to the child's expressions of relational need with corresponding affective responses. Infants come equipped with the ability to elicit such responses—babies are magnets for smiles and strokes; and, in a positive relational system, those innate abilities can develop into greater and greater sensitivity to both one's own needs and those of others and into increasing competence in dealing with those needs.

## Personality Development

*Personality*—the outward expression of the unique organization of emotions, beliefs, attitudes, expectations, attractions, and avoidances that characterizes each of us—emerges out of relationship. Through feedback from others, one's personality structure is confirmed and elaborated (Frank, 1991). If that feedback comes in the context of a loving and contactful relationship, it will be experienced as supportive (even though the content of the feedback may be critical) and will contribute to a positive sense of self. Some writers (Mitchell, 1988) assert that the self *is* the complex set of interlocking meanings that one creates as one moves through time, learning from and contributing to relationships. As individuals interact with their environment, and particularly with their social environment, they construct and tell themselves stories that connect and make sense of their experiences. These personal narratives (Clocksin, 1998) are the stuff out of which one's identity emerges. Relationship experiences are the building blocks with which people create themselves.

Eric Berne (1963) used the term *strokes* to refer to units of contact between individuals. Strokes can be conditional ("You did a good job putting away your toys") or unconditional ("I love you just because you're you"); they can be positive ("Mmmm, what a good boy!") or negative ("It was very naughty of you to bite your sister"). Most of the psychological meaning of a stroke is carried in its nonverbal component, rather than in its words (think of all the different ways one could say "What are you doing?" and all the messages, positive and negative, that could be sent with those words) and it is this psychological meaning that has the greatest impact upon the child's developing personality. And not just the child's. Individuals respond to strokes at any age, and their presence or absence, their positive or negative flavor, has an impact on the self-structure of adults as well as of children. Everyone needs a mix of strokes—positive and negative, conditional and unconditional—to provide contact and maintain relationships and to give them feedback about the effects of their behaviors. However, the effect of *stroke deprivation* is probably greatest in childhood, before the person has had time to build up a "stroke reserve" or to learn techniques of self-stroking that can be used as temporary relief when social strokes are absent. The opposite of stroke deprivation—that is, a social environment rich in contactful strokes from a variety of sources and carrying a variety of content—will make a greater contribution to a child's well-being the earlier it can be established and maintained.

An essential ingredient for a healthy and spontaneous sense of self is the ability to love, and this ability obviously grows out of relationships. Being able to love another person requires that we be separate from that other and that, at the same time, we recognize that other as a person like ourselves. Loving one's mother, one's spouse, or one's friend is very different from loving a favorite chair or a hot fudge sundae. Loving some other requires a kind of tension between moving toward (in order to be close) and moving away (in order to truly know the other as different from ourselves); it is the separation-connection issue again. Says Benjamin (1992), "To the extent that mother herself is placed outside [of oneself] she can be loved; separation is then truly the other side of connection to the other" (p. 53). Separation and connection, approaching and retreating, me and you—contact and relationship are learned by being in contact and by making relationship. We learn to love by loving and being loved, and our sense of self is shaped by that experience.

In sum, who we are to others, as well as who we are to ourselves, grows out of our relationships. Literally everything we learn in the course of our growing and becoming has a relational source and/or relational implications. "Even when the activity is solitary and is not relationally dominated, an empathic resonance with others is a necessary ingredient and backdrop for a fully vitalized sense of self" (Fosshage, 1992, p. 31). When our relationships are honest, contactful, and generally supportive, we will learn to value ourselves and to value others, to interact skillfully, and to pass on our relational skills and values to the next generation.

## DEVELOPMENT AND UNHEALTHY RELATIONSHIPS

This heading is somewhat misleading, in that all relationships have some less-than-desirable moments, with less-than-desirable consequences. Each person in a relationship is a unique individual, with unique needs, wants, beliefs, and behaviors, and sometimes these characteristics collide: what I want with you is different from what you want with me, and vice versa. Even the caretakers of young infants are not always able to respond to those infants in an optimal way. People get tired, cranky, and/or confused; they may not know how to provide what the infant needs or may be too preoccupied to even notice that the infant needs something. Nobody has a perfect childhood, in which all relationships are completely satisfying; indeed, a childhood in which all needs were met, completely and immediately, would not prepare us to survive in a less-than-perfect world. Nevertheless, the inevitable unmet needs of infancy and childhood create opportunities for script conclusions, decisions, and strategies that will later inhibit spontaneous and contactful dealings with others. Everyone has such experiences; no one comes to adulthood unscathed.

Relationships that involve more than two people are even more complex than the dyadic relationship between child and caretaker, and the potential for conflict is even greater. Children need to experience such relationships and to cope with their challenges; but, again, there may be costs for such learning. In a two-parent family, a child will sometimes get different messages from different caretakers and experience the different ways in which those caretakers meet— and fail to meet—the child's needs. Each parent sees the child in different ways and mirrors that image back to the child, with necessarily confusing effects on the child's developing sense of self. Says Mitchell (1992), "It is precisely because the mother's child is somewhat different from the father's child that conflict between different organizations of self is so universally generated" (p. 5).

The earlier that relational problems arise, the more serious their consequences. Dogs and cats often "lick into shape" their newborn, and this licking appears to be necessary for the baby animal's physical well-being. While humans seldom actually lick their babies, they do hold, cuddle, and stroke them; and human babies need this physical contact in order to bond with the mother. Without such physical bonding, there is no opportunity to develop the visceral core that is the foundation on which all experiences of self and others are based. The child's ability to recognize and express affect will be distorted, as will be that child's developing cognitive processes. These distortions, in turn, contribute to further problems in relationship, further loss of contact with self and others, and further development of script as a last-resort means of survival.

## Psychological Consequences of Relationship Deficit

Psychological difficulties, Wachtel (1990) reminds us, are never strictly an individual matter: "Every neurosis requires accomplices" (p. 435). Dysfunctional parent-child relationships are the breeding ground for dysfunctional adults. Two specific consequences of early relational deficit are the development of repression and the laying down of a life script.

**Repression**   In chapter 2, we discussed how people deal with unwanted thoughts and feelings by repressing them—pushing them out of awareness—so that they need not be experienced. The process of repression begins very early in life and is closely tied to one's relationship experiences. When an infant's primitive expression of affect is not met with an attuned response, a response in which the adult's own affect resonates to what the child is expressing, the infant has no way of integrating that affective experience. Because the needed response from the other is absent or does not fit with what the child is feeling, the child learns that his or her affect is somehow "wrong," something he or she should not feel or express. The result is a lifelong inner conflict, for whenever this particular affect arises as a natural response to some situation, it feels wrong, "childish," shameful. The forbidden affective response is experienced as hurtful to both the child's own internal sense of self ("something is wrong with me because I feel this way") and that child's relationships with others ("I mustn't let them know how I feel"). The inevitable result is repression—a growing habit of emotional disavowal and denial.

Repression and the whole array of defenses built upon it are often used by the child not only as an out-of-awareness means of protecting him- or herself from a "forbidden" affect but also to protect the child's caretakers. Because the child's affective expression is ignored, mismatched, or actively rejected, the child concludes that his or her emotions are unwelcome or even dangerous to the caretaker. Rather than risk harming that important other, the child first suppresses and eventually represses the affective response.

**Script Beliefs and Behaviors**   When a child is unsuccessful in attempts to satisfy relational needs, that is, when those attempts are not responded to by a caring and contactful other, the child is likely to conclude that the attempt at satisfaction, and even the need itself, are unacceptable. Not only the child's feelings but also the child's needs and the thoughts that accompany them must be rejected. Again and again, some aspect of internal experiencing must be split off and isolated, denied access to awareness. At the same time that these patterns of repression are developing, the child is also stamping in fixed beliefs about self (things like "my feelings are bad" or "I ask for too much"), about others ("they don't understand me" or "they don't care about me"), and the quality of life ("life is hard" or "things usually turn out badly"). As shown in chapter 2, such beliefs are a part of an overall script pattern, justifying (necessitating) script-bound behaviors, which in turn elicit relational responses that further reinforce the beliefs (Erskine & Zalcman, 1979/1997; Erskine & Moursund, 1988/1998).

Stolorow (1992) refers to these kinds of fixated script beliefs as "invariant organizing principles." Usually acquired in childhood, they are the scaffolding upon which subsequent beliefs and expectations are erected. They are pervasive, subtly distorting all subsequent experiences and eroding social contact. In their milder manifestations, they make it difficult for the child-growing-to-adulthood to form the kinds of relationships that will nurture her and support her growth as an individual. In more serious form, when the early relational deprivation has been intense and/or persistent, these beliefs can lead to serious psychopathology.

The influence of script does not end with its impact upon the script-bound individual. It spreads horizontally, tainting relationships and encouraging the development of interlocking scripts in the others with whom the script-bound person interacts. It also spreads vertically from one generation to the next, to the degree that a script-bound parent is unable to provide an emotionally contactful environment for his or her children.

## TRAUMA AND ITS CONSEQUENCES

As we have said, no child has a perfectly healthy environment in which to grow up. Everyone has experienced relational needs that went unattended to, and everyone has experienced disapproval of their expression of a relational need—since caretakers are human, they make human mistakes and express human weaknesses, and those mistakes and weaknesses often collide with the relational needs of the children in their care. Such collisions, especially if they happen more than once, may contribute to the development of script, but they do not constitute actual abuse. Painful but not necessarily traumatizing, they are the stubbed toes and skinned knees of psychological development.

Trauma, in contrast, is created by extreme and often prolonged relational deprivation. No longer a matter of stubbed toes and skinned knees, trauma creates the psychological equivalent of broken bones and festering wounds. Haines and colleagues (1999), in a discussion of the development of attributional style, talk about the "consistency, chronicity, and intensity" of relational problems. The more consistent, chronic, and intense the deficit, the more likely the child is to develop negative and unhealthy attributions. We believe that these same factors define trauma: trauma occurs when relational needs are ignored or their expression punished, consistently, chronically, and/or in situations of emotional intensity, and when there is no stable and protective relationship to mitigate the impact of the experience.

### Acute Trauma

An acute trauma is related to a specific event or series of events. Something bad happens; someone is abused or injured, terrified or humiliated. The experience and the feelings it engenders are intense and painful. Yet it is not the event itself—the physical abuse, the automobile accident, the schoolyard taunting—that creates the most lasting damage. More significant than the trauma itself is the absence of a healing and supportive relationship following the traumatic experience (Erskine, 1994/1997d). It is this absence that transforms the experience from a painful, one-time incident to a script-forming trauma.

Several factors contribute to this transformation. One of these has to do with the way in which memories are created and stored in the brain. The memory of an event is not simply a mini-movie that can be replayed on demand. Memory comes in many modalities: verbal, auditory, visual, emotional, and physiolgical. Following a traumatic event, one is likely to be in emotional turmoil, and those intense emotions tend to interfere with the ability to describe, clearly and logically, what has just happened. If nobody is there for the traumatized person to talk to, no one who will help that person to think about and verbalize what has happened, a verbal description will neither be created nor remembered. The memory of the event will be largely emotional, with only fuzzy or distorted cognitive content. There may be patches of visual or auditory memory as well—a blurred, angry face; the sound of breaking glass—but there is likely to be no coherent story that makes sense of the whole thing. Writes Freyd (1996), ". . . [M]emory for never-discussed events is likely to be qualitatively different from memory for events that have been discussed. This difference will be greater when the sensory, continuous memories for the events were not recoded internally in anticipation of verbal sharing. Thus, if an event is experienced but never recoded into shareable formats, it is more likely to be stored in codes that are continuous, sensory, and dynamic" (p. 111). In the absence of a relationship in which the traumatic event can be described, discussed, and dissected, the memory of that event is likely to involve raw feelings with little or no meaning attached. When the memory is stimulated, the person will experience the pain or the terror, often without conscious knowledge of what those emotions are attached to; without such knowledge, there is no way to understand or cope with one's distress.

Humans are meaning-seeking creatures; we always want to know *why*. This is certainly true of trauma. "Why *me?*" is one of the most common responses to any sort of human tragedy. In the absence of an obvious reason (and there is seldom any obvious or logical reason for trauma), individuals manufacture something to fill in the blank space, to provide a reason for the unreasonable. The nature of that manufactured reason is strongly affected by the ongoing relationships that are in place at the time of and following the event. Consider a child who is in a serious auto accident; the child hears the crash, is hurt, sees blood, and watches as people rush around and shout at each other. The experience is painful and frightening. But if a parent is there to hold him, help him to talk about his pain and fear, and assure him that he will be all right and that it is not his fault, the effects of the experience will be relatively short-lived. If, in contrast, the parent, too, is injured and unavailable and nobody is there for the child, he will fill in the gaps in his understanding with meanings constructed from his fantasy: "I caused it to happen"; "Life is dangerous"; "My parents will die." These sorts of meanings are too terrible to be borne, and so the self-protective, repressive, script-forming process begins: *If I made it happen, then that part of me is bad and must be buried away, split off from the rest of my conscious self. If my fear of losing my parents is so painful, I better not feel the fear at all—bury the feelings and never let them out. Anything that awful should not be remembered at all—slice off the memory and store it where it can never be recovered.*

Finally—and perhaps most important in the transformation of negative experience into script—the victim feels a sense of betrayal during and after a traumatic event. The event itself is a kind of betrayal, by a perpetrator of abuse or simply by the world in general; the absence of a supportive and nurturing relationship is another betrayal, a betrayal by those who were supposed to be there and provide care and safety. This is especially true in childhood, for children have not yet fully developed their self-protective skills and need the protection of caretakers. One's parents are supposed to keep bad things from happening, or—if they can't do that—at least know that something bad did happen and try to make it better. Lister (1981), describing abused children whose nonabusing parent chose to ignore the ongoing abuse, reports on ". . . the child's wish for her parents (or the uninvolved parent) to know, to intuit what has happened. The parents' failure to elicit some report of the trauma was perceived as an act of hostility by both of my patients" (p. 874). Not only was the abuse itself traumatic, but now the child's caretaker-protectors have turned on him as well.

Abuse by a parent or by some other trusted caretaker is the worst betrayal of all. Because the abuser has been trusted, the victim is exquisitely vulnerable. The essence of trust is that we drop our guard, allow ourselves to be vulnerable to the trusted other. Especially in the case of a child, the relationship with the abuser (or with someone who colludes with the abuser by refusing to recognize the abuse) may be necessary to survival: how does a small child survive without a parent? "When the betrayer is someone on whom we are dependent," writes Freyd (1996), "the very mechanisms that normally protect us—a sensitivity to cheating and the pain that motivates us to change things so that we will no longer be in danger—become a problem. We must block the awareness of the betrayal, forget it, in order to ensure that we behave in ways that maintain the relationship on which we are dependent" (p. 74).

Trauma in childhood, unmitigated by a healing relational experience following the trauma, is psychologically damaging. Repeated trauma, again without a healing relationship, is even more damaging. The younger the child and the more intense the traumatic experience, the greater is the need for psychological support and the more serious the emotional consequences when that support is not available.

Adults, too, can suffer serious consequences when they are relationship-deprived following trauma; What are those consequences? If a traumatized person cannot access a contactful, supportive, and reparative relationship, the traumatic experience cannot be assimilated, worked through and integrated into the person's emotional and cognitive memory banks. The unmet need for protection and the longing for empathy and nurturing following the trauma cannot be acknowledged or validated satisfactorily. The absence of acknowledgment and validation, in turn, initiates the process of isolating the experience from awareness and, in more extreme situations, may lead to isolating aspects of self from awareness as well (Erskine, 1994/1997d). Freyd (1996) writes, "With dissociations between different memory stores for the same event and the blockage of information about current reality to some processing units, a firm foundation for assessing reality using all available internal sources of knowl-edge cannot be laid. . . . This lack of integration is likely to produce alterations in consciousness, dissociated states, and problems such as depersonalization—feeling detached from one's own body" (pp. 165–166). A self-protective script develops, often accompanied by withdrawal—not only from the traumatizing persons but also from those who did not respond to the post-trauma emotional needs. The punishing and/or neglectful people may be introjected—their *negative* parts taken into the victim's own personality—so that they can be more easily managed, and the *good* parts left outside as characteristics of the other person, so that there is someone there with whom to maintain at least a rudimentary relationship.

Blocking out those aspects of self that are capable of feeling pain, barring them from awareness, creates a split in the personality, an "I" that does not know all of the aspects of self. A split may also form as a result of blaming oneself for the traumatic event(s) and then pushing out of awareness the *bad* part that caused the bad thing(s) to happen. Both of these kinds of split can be a consequence of trauma when it is unmitigated by a healing relationship. The splitting process may occur quickly, or it may be gradual, completing itself over the weeks and months following the traumatic event. Thus, the psycho-logical consequences of trauma are often not visible immediately after the trauma, and even the victim is seldom if ever aware of how he or she is pro-tecting him- or herself. The split-off parts and the mechanism that keeps them split off are like a poison capsule, hidden away deep inside, leaking a tiny bit at a time (just enough to distort and destroy relationships and leave the per-son with a nagging sense of something wrong, something missing), and even-tually bursting open with the kinds of symptoms that diagnosticians know as "post-traumatic stress disorder" and are experienced by the victim as debili-tating emotional pain.

## Cumulative Trauma

The abrupt and identifiable painful events of one's life are not the only expe-riences that can be traumatic. Even more debilitating, in some ways, are the ordinary, commonplace, over-and-over-again little discounts and hurts that are not even recognized as traumatic at the time they occur. Berne (1961) differ-entiated between *traumatic neurosis,* caused by a specific trauma on a specific date, and *psychoneurosis,* emerging from an ongoing series of traumas occur-ring from month to month over a long period of time. Khan (1963), who coined the term *cumulative trauma* to describe the effect of repetitive negative events, recognized that here, too, relationship failure is the primary agent. Speaking of small children, he writes, "Cumulative trauma is the result of the breaches in the mother's role as a protective shield over the whole course of the child's development, from infancy to adolescence" (p. 290).

Even though it can lead to the same sorts of script patterns that are typical in cases of acute trauma, cumulative trauma is initially developed in a different way. Rather than protecting oneself from the pain of a specific incident, the person must deal with a slow but constant accumulation of tiny, almost insignificant criticisms, neglects, and hurts. Over time, the person comes to accept this pattern as simply a part of the way he/she/others/life has to be. Like the slow drip of calcium-laden water that builds over the years into a stalactite or stalagmite, the drip of cumulative trauma results in the slow building up of script beliefs in the cavern of one's unconscious. There is nothing to point to later in life, no way to say "that is what happened to me, and this is how I reacted." The life occurences are not traumatic—perhaps not even noticed—at the time or in the context in which they happen; or, if they are noticed, they are easier to forget or to discount than a single event, since each repetition provides another opportunity to develop the repression (Terr, 1991). They lead to script-building consequences only cumulatively and are recognized (if one is able to figure out the pattern and understand its influence) only in retrospect (Khan, 1963; Lourie, 1996; Erskine, Moursund, & Trautmann, 1999).

Perhaps the most common source of cumulative trauma is simple neglect. The caretakers do not abuse or punish; they simply fail to respond. They do not support and resonate with the child's expression of affect; they do not acknowledge the child's relational needs. Lourie (1996) defines cumulative trauma as "the totality of the psychological failures, or misattunements, that a child endures from infancy through adolescence and beyond" (p. 277). These failures are not necessarily—or even usually—the result of deliberate and conscious choices on the part of caretakers. They are more often caused by parental ignorance, fatigue, or preoccupation with other concerns; or the parents may be tangled in script patterns of their own that are incompatible with meeting the child's needs. The child, however, is unlikely to understand adult preoccupation or fatigue or life script and may well fantasize intentionality when none is present. "Mom has no time for me; I'm not important enough." "Dad doesn't even look at me; he must be really mad at something I did." Such fantasies, over time, take on the characteristics of an acutal, historical event and add to the toxicity of the cumulative trauma pattern.

Weinberger and Weiss (1997) point out that, in some forms of cumulative trauma, the child may not even be given the opportunity to formulate or express relational needs. "An infant need not have its affective expression ignored or rejected to be thwarted in its development. The environment may simply provide no opportunity for such expression. This occurs in situations of deprivation. The affective expression is not walled off; it simply never gets articulated in the first place" (p. 36).

Children whose relational needs are not acknowledged and validated have no social mirror in which to view themselves. Cumulative trauma robs children of the opportunity to discover and create themselves as unique individuals within a web of social relationships. "A severe consequence of cumulative trauma," says Lourie (1996), "is the loss of trust in and knowledge of self resulting from the vast assortment of parental misattunements . . . that the child endures" (p. 277). These children come to believe that, at their core, they are inadequate and unlovable; they hide this belief from others—and from themselves—and the result is an inability to form a lasting and satisfying intimate relationship. They may withdraw from the company of others or may chain themselves on a treadmill of endless and superficial social activities; they may constantly demand attention and caretaking; or they may make themselves over-responsible for the needs of those around them. All of these behaviors serve to distract them from a basic sense of loneliness and inadequacy. These behaviors do not satisfy relational needs—and, over the long run, actually prevent truly satisfying those needs—but they quiet the needs for a time, dulling the pain and giving temporary relief.

Does this sound like a pattern we have talked about before? It is the template upon which script is constructed: erroneous, pervasive, and self-perpetuating beliefs that inhibit spontaneity and erode the ability to form and maintain relationships. Moreover, the kinds of script patterns that grow out of cumulative trauma are often more difficult to deal with therapeutically than those caused by acute trauma, because their onset is so gradual and their cause so difficult to pinpoint. "I didn't have a bad childhood," says the client. "I had plenty of food, good clothes, a room of my own. Mom and Dad seldom punished me. Nothing bad ever happened." With no describable causal event to help clients make sense of their feelings, recipients of cumulative trauma are likely to blame themselves for their unhappiness, their sense of emptiness and depression further bolstering the negative self-image that lies at the heart of their script.

## SUMMARY

The earliest learnings of the human infant involve connection and individuation: learning how to be a unique and separate individual in ongoing relationship with other individuals. The need for relationship is most obvious in infancy and childhood, but this need continues throughout life. Healthy and contactful relationships nurture psychological growth, fostering one's ability to think, to express feelings, and to experience oneself as a valuable member of a social group.

All people experience relational needs: the need for particular kinds of behaviors and responses from the other person with whom they are in relationship. Among the most important of these relational needs are those for security, for valuing, for acceptance, for mutuality, for self-definition, to make an impact, for the other to initiate, and to express love.

In the absence of relationships in which relational needs are acknowledged, self-protective script patterns are developed. This is particularly evident when there is trauma. Whether the unmet relational needs are experienced following an acute trauma, or whether the unmet needs themselves create a cumulative trauma, the result is an emptiness that the child fills in with memories of previous experiences or with self-generated fantasy. This is done cognitively, with beliefs that tie together and make sense of the experience, and emotionally, by splitting off and burying out of awareness the source and nature of the pain and/or by introjecting the person(s) who is (are) the source of the pain. The result is a life script: a system of rigid beliefs that predict how one's life will be and prescribe the behaviors needed to cope with that life, of repetitive feelings that echo the pain and loneliness of the original trauma, of automatic and seldom-questioned behaviors growing out of the beliefs and feelings, and of selective perceptions and memories that reinforce the other components.

# 4 CHAPTER | **Healing the Hurts**

We have spent some time discussing the ways in which humans grow and develop and how relationship failures can interfere with that growth and development. Now, we turn to the ways in which psychotherapy can deal with the problems that occur when development has been diverted from its optimal course.

## A SET OF INTERLOCKING SYSTEMS

Just as each aspect of human functioning affects all the others during the course of development, so must each aspect be taken into account as we, as therapists, attempt to heal the hurts of people who come to us for help. The human experience is an interlocking system in which each subsystem interacts with all the others. Changes in one subsystem reverberate through the whole; problems in one subsystem can show up as malfunctions in another. The psychological "subsystems" include cognition, emotion, behavior, and physiology (and each of these can be further subdivided); all must be considered as we work with clients. Consider, for example, a client who presents with symptoms of major depression. He has trouble sleeping, has no appetite, has stopped interacting with his friends. He feels sad and hopeless and has had thoughts of taking his own life. He constantly obsesses about his situation, telling himself that he is stupid (for not being able to figure out what to do), lazy (for not doing whatever that something might be), and quite possibly crazy to boot. His self-critical thoughts support his depressed feelings, and the feelings justify and stimulate the thoughts. Thinking and feeling as he does, it is no wonder that his sleeping and his appetite have been affected or that he is no longer able to enjoy social activities; the lack of adequate sleep and nourishment and his social isolation contribute to his feelings of sadness and hopelessness and to his thinking that something is wrong with him. Change could begin anywhere: with his self-critical thoughts, with his feelings of sadness and anxiety, with his self-defeating behaviors, or with his patterns of eating and sleeping. Change in any of these areas would invite change in all the others; and failure to change any one of them would ultimately undermine changes already accomplished in the others. We can focus on thoughts, feelings, behavior, or physiology at the beginning of treatment, and the choice of a focus is usually determined by our assessment of where the client is most open to contact. Later on, we will help him to work with those facets that he has closed down, where he does not make contact; at first, though, we will invite him to start where he is most comfortable. But, whatever the starting point, all of the other facets must eventually be addressed. Not to do so leaves the system lopsided, precludes full contact and awareness in all dimensions, and risks allowing the cycle of change to be reversed again, with the system reverting back to its earlier dysfunction.

## Cognition and Emotion

Cognitive functioning is perhaps the most usual starting point in psychotherapy. The client has had to think about his problems and decide that he needs help in order to get himself into our office. He is used to talking about things, relating incidents, and dealing with events in a linear, narrative way. We hope that he will be thinking clearly enough with us to be able to describe what is wrong, what he wants to change, and what he has already tried to do about it. Taking care of the preliminary "housekeeping" details of psychotherapy requires thinking: discussing scheduling, fees, insurance coverage, and confidentiality; filling out forms; getting whatever general information the therapist needs in order to have a sense of what is going on. Handling these details invites the client into a cognitive mode; it suggests that, whatever else may happen in therapy, client and therapist are going to think together about how to deal with the situation at hand.

Simply "thinking together" can be curative in and of itself. The client has been thinking alone or with people who—for whatever reason—have been unable to help and who may have even contributed to his pain. Being able to discuss things with someone who is not a part of the problem and who is trained to help people sort through the details of their lives and make sense of the confusion can relieve anxiety and instill a sense of hope. The therapist has been here before, has dealt with other folks who are in the same kind of pain. She understands. Moreover, she does not condemn the client, or scold him, or act as if she thinks him stupid or selfish or silly.

*Stupid, selfish, silly*—these are the self-critical clubs with which many clients beat themselves. "I should be able to solve this on my own," they tell themselves. "Something's wrong with me because I can't. People who have to see a shrink are really messed up. Maybe I'm actually crazy. Maybe I expect too much. I'm probably just plain dumb even to imagine that anything can help. . . ." The litany goes on and on, as the client adds to his distress by blaming himself for being distressed in the first place. This sense of shame and self-blame is one of the things that interferes with his ability to think clearly and problem solve effectively: it is a good example of how emotions and cognitions interlock. "I can't figure this out" (cognition) leads to feelings of anxiety or despair; the negative emotion, in turn, further degrades his cognitive capabilities.

Shame and self-blame are not, of course, the only sort of negative thoughts and feelings that clients bring to the therapy process. Indeed, it is usually some other, highly painful emotional experience that finally persuades most clients to seek help. They may be depressed, constantly anxious, unreasonably angry, or a host of combinations and variations of these sorts of feelings. Their feelings, they report, are interfering with their ability to maintain relationships, to work, to play, to enjoy themselves. They want the therapist to make those feelings go away so that they can get on with their lives.

While we generally begin with the psychological function within which the client works most easily, we do not stay there. A useful rule of thumb for therapists is that clients are likely to need to focus, fairly soon in the course of treatment, on the aspect of their experience that they talk least about. Clients who present with problems involving affect—who look emotionally upset and report that their primary problem has to do with feelings—are likely not to be thinking clearly about their situation and probably need help learning to do so. Conversely, clients who begin their work in "thinking mode," talking about causes, effects, contributing factors, and the like (not necessarily, of course, in those terms) are apt to be out of touch with their feelings and unaware of how those feelings affect their problem solving, their creativity, and their relationships. These clients need help to recognize their own (and others') emotional responses, to reclaim the feeling part of themselves and integrate it into their overall functioning.

Henry A., a computer systems programmer, was a competent, professionally successful man. He had two children, a fine job and a silver BMW, and played squash at the local gym every Tuesday night. He also had just been left by his wife, who said he was "a robot" and that unless he changed she would divorce him. He didn't want to lose her and came to therapy to figure out how to make the changes she was demanding. That *figure out* part is significant: *figuring out* is what Henry was good at, and it was what was driving his wife wild. She wanted him to stop analyzing and thinking things through, and just let go and "be himself." But Henry did not know how to "be himself," because he did not know who "himself" was. Quite early in life, he had decided that, in his family, showing your feelings got you ignored, or teased, or worse. In that family, the best thing to be was big and tough; next best was quiet and smart. Henry did not have the physical equipment to be big and tough, so he opted for quiet and smart. He learned to ignore his feelings and to hide them when they could not be ignored. He learned to be a problem solver, and he learned how to use his wits to get what he wanted. What's more, he understood all this—he just didn't know what to do about it. Therapy that continued to help him use his well-developed cognitive skills might provide him with further insights about how his problems had developed but would not be likely to yield the kind of change that Henry was looking for. Rather, his therapist needed to help him re-discover his long-repressed affective responses, to learn to recognize his feelings, and to allow others to see and respond to them.

Loretta B., in contrast, had no trouble feeling her feelings or sharing them with others. Her life was one long soap opera of emotional crises. In therapy sessions, she cried and screamed and pounded her chair as she talked about what she would like to do to her unfaithful boyfriend. She, too, wanted to make changes that would result in more satisfying connections with others— she had been in one abusive relationship after another—but, unlike Henry, she had no idea how she had contributed to her romantic disasters. After the first stormy session, Loretta's therapist realized that encouraging Loretta to express her feelings would not be useful at this point. Loretta needed, instead, to set her emotions aside for the moment and *think* about her behaviors and their consequences, about her wants and needs and what she did to try to meet them, and why it wasn't working.

Henry, the thinker, needed to learn how to integrate his feelings with his thinking. He needed to "lose his mind and come to his senses," as Perls (1969a) put it. Loretta, the emotional, needed to learn to think and, particularly, to think about the function of her emotions. She needed to curb the superficial tempest of affect in order to develop her ability to problem solve and plan ahead, to anticipate how others would respond to her, and, ultimately, to reclaim the authentic feelings now hidden beneath her histrionic display. Henry and Loretta are each at an extreme of the thinking/feeling dichotomy—few clients display so one-sided a set of learned behaviors as they did—but the principle holds for those nearer the middle of the continuum as well. While respecting a client's choice of a starting point, the point at which he is most open to contact, the therapist must bear in mind that he will probably need more help with the facet he is *not* using than with what he chooses to use. Before the end of treatment, he will almost certainly need to circle back to where he started and deal with his preferred style as well. But that is for later, when much of the repressed material has emerged and more of the whole self is available. By then, the quality of the affect, the cognition, or the physical responses that he began with will have changed as a result of work in other modalities, and all will be more easily integrated into a full and authentic blending of affect, cognition, behavior, and physiology.

Affect and cognition interact not only in the here and now of daily activitiy but in memory as well. Accurate memories are a blend of thoughts, feelings, and physical reactions. All of these may not have been put into words, but they were present at the time the memory was laid down and now form the foundation on which that memory rests. The cognitive aspects of a memory are often the most easy to bring into awareness, since talking about a memory—translating it into language—requires cognitive activity. The associated emotions may be harder to recall, but they are always there: had there been no emotions involved, the incident would probably not have been stored in memory at all. Affective intensity is, in fact, one of the major factors in the choice of which experiences will be remembered. You can easily test that assertion for yourself by thinking of two or three things that you remember from childhood. Chances are very good that each of those things was associated with some strong emotion, either pleasant or unpleasant.

Even though emotion is an integral element in every remembered experience, a client may not consciously recall those emotions when discussing the memory. He may not have recognized and consciously encoded his feelings at the time, or he may have made an out-of-awareness decision to forget (repress) them because they seemed unpleasant or dangerous. With the loss of emotional significance, he is likely to lose cognitive awareness of the memory as well; the whole experience fades into unawareness. Such cognitive loss of memories often holds the key to understanding script decisions, and retrieving those decisions and replacing them with ones that work better can be important tasks of therapy. The more a client is able to recognize his emotions in the here and now, the better will be his access to his feelings in the past; reclaiming those feelings helps him, in turn, to think about his experiences and thus reconstruct the whole incident. "Affect," says Stone (1996), "provides us with a golden thread to trace the labyrinths of memory" (p. 31). Helping a "thinking" client to learn how to feel can be as important as helping emotionally labile clients to learn how to stop and think.

## Behavior and Physiology

Without changes in external behavior, internal changes are likely to be short-lived. We need to act on our insights and our reclaimed feelings, using them to guide us in reaching out to the world to meet our needs and to make contact with others. Again, the causality is two-way: changes in thinking and feeling can lead to changes in behavior, and changes in behavior can change what we think and how we feel. When the initial changes are internal, it is important to talk with the client about how those changes are likely to make a difference in his life, how others will know that he has changed, or how he wants to use those internal changes to help him reach his goals. Questions like this encourage clients to experiment with new behaviors that will, in turn, support their gains in thinking and feeling.

Therapists working with depressed clients know that depressive symptoms often lift when the clients become more active: behaviors such as regular exercise, healthy eating, and spending time with friends can lessen the feelings of sadness and hopelessness that come with depression and can change the way depressed persons think about themselves and others. Encouraging clients to make changes in their behaviors and suggesting "experiments" in behavior change for them to try out during the session or later at home can help reverse the downward spiral of script-bound behavior. Changes in behavior lead to changes in internal experiencing; and those changes, in turn, make it possible to solidify and improve upon the behavioral changes. Other people's responses to the new behaviors often challenge script beliefs; the whole script system can begin to shift. Long-buried memories creep into awareness; long-forbidden feelings begin to emerge; contact with others increases as contact with self is enhanced. What began as an artificial "just try it out and see what happens" can become a natural part of clients' everyday behavioral repertoire. Their blind adherence to familiar life script patterns is disrupted, and their old defenses are not as effective as they used to be.

Physiological changes, too, are a part of the overall pattern of healing. Just as many physical ailments are caused—or at least exacerbated—by psychological dysfunction, so those physical ailments are eased when the psychological problem is dealt with. Our bodies are the battleground for conflicts among thoughts, feelings, and behaviors; those conflicts are reflected in all sorts of physical distress, from headaches to backaches and from asthma to ulcers. And the reverse? It should come as no surprise that changes in physiology can also lead to changes in other facets of human functioning. Perls, Hefferline, and Goodman (1951) assert that repression—keeping thoughts and feelings out of awareness—is always accompanied by some sort of muscular holding in, and it is this holding in that is translated into physical symptoms. Relaxing the tension invites the repressed material back into awareness and opens the door to script change. Massage therapists tell us that their clients often report a surge of emotion as tight muscles loosen and relax: the feelings, and often memories as well, move into awareness as the body lets go. Physical change can pave the way for psychological change, and vice versa.

All of this brings us back to our earlier assertion: all of the facets of human functioning must be taken into account in the healing process. We are likely to begin our work in the modality in which the client is most open to contact; and work in that area is likely to affect all of the others. But we must make sure that each system is attended to, that contact is achieved within and among all of the facets of the client's being, if integration is to be accomplished and healing is to last. Otherwise, we risk simply replacing one overused and rigid pattern with another. "The goal of all forms of psychotherapy," says Rossi (1990), is "facilitating the many pathways of mind-body information flow" (p. 357). When all of the pathways are working, cognitions, affect, behavior, and physiology each inform and support all of the others, and each is available for contact with the external world. Contact, internal and external, is both the goal of therapy and the means of achieving that goal; it leads to integration of the personality and decommissioning of the script system. The therapeutic relationship, managed well, enhances clients' ability to initiate and sustain contact with self, with the therapist, and with the other significant people in their lives. We shall return, later in this chapter, to the notion of developing contact in each of the major facets of functioning; first, though, let us look more generally at the connection between relationship and healing.

# THE ROLE OF RELATIONSHIP IN THE HEALING PROCESS

Greenberg and Mitchell (1983) distinguish among three different groups of theorists who focus on relationships and their influence on human functioning. The first of these groups consists of theorists who posit that the need for relationship is a biological given, "wired in" genetically, and whose interest lies primarily in how different sorts of relationships develop and maintain themselves. Theorists in the second group, which Greenberg and Mitchell call the "relatedness by intent" camp, focus on the object—the other—of relationships: what others do and the effects of their behavior on the person with whom they are interacting. The third group is most interested in the developing, relating self and how it is constructed through experiences with others. These focuses, of course, are not mutually exclusive but are rather a matter of emphasis. Relationship-focused integrative psychotherapy concerns itself with all of them: the self, the other with whom the self is in relationship, and the nature of the interaction between them. All are of critical importance in the client's life, in the etiology of the client's distress and in the relief of that distress.

People know themselves through their relationships with others. Their psychological ease or dis-ease arises through relationships and plays itself out in relationships. As agents of the healing process, psychotherapists enter into relationship with clients; that relationship is a microcosm of all of the other real and fantasized relationships that the clients have known. The kind of relationship that therapists create, and the skill with which they use it, will be the primary determinant of the sucess or failure of the therapeutic enterprise. "Mind and self come into being through communication with others," says Jack (1991). "One cannot heal the self in isolation" (p. 205).

## Therapist Use of Self

Speaking the client's language and respecting his relational needs—both current and developmental—are helpful in understanding what his life is like and how he experiences his world. Sands (1997) reminds us, though, that this kind of understanding, by itself, is too narrowly focused on the client. To truly enter into a therapeutic relationship, we must also be concerned with *our* response to that other person—to "understanding the patient as he or she resides in *us*" (p. 664). A therapeutic relationship, like any other relationship, requires involvement on the part of each participant. Each one learns of him- or herself through knowing the other person, and each learns of the other through experiencing his or her own response to that other.

The first task in psychotherapy is getting acquainted. And more than just acquainted—getting to know what it's like to live inside that client's skin, and view the world through his eyes. We achieve that kind of knowing through relationship: as we make contact with a client, we allow ourselves to imagine *being* that client, to think his thoughts, feel his feelings, hope his hopes, and dream his dreams. Consider the following scenario. My client sits down, crosses his legs, shifts uncomfortably in his chair. He looks at me through eyes that are just beginning to moisten, and his lip trembles slightly as he says "I don't know what to do." I allow my body to feel that shifting discomfort and my eyes to moisten in response to that discomfort. I imagine the sensation of a trembling lip, and I think about what it would be like—and has been like—to truly not know what to do. I find in myself those ways of experiencing that are similar to what I see in him, and I explore that part of myself; the questions I ask him and the observations I make are formed out of my self-exploration. I learn to know my client through knowing the part of myself that is similar to him.

Knowing and understanding one's client are important. They pave the way for healing. The therapist's understanding, in itself, though, is not what builds the healing relationship. A technician can understand; given the explosive growth of cybernetics, the day may soon come when even a machine can understand. But a machine, or a technician, is not a therapist: it does not enter into a living relationship with its client. "Understanding that heals requires a *mutually experienced* emotional connection between patient and analyst" (Orange, 1995, p. 4; italics ours). To create a healing relationship and move from technician to therapist, we must be "able and willing to enter the patient's suffering and share the painful history, able and willing to 'undergo the situation' with the other" (Orange, 1995, p. 5).

## How Relationship Heals

Asserting that relationship is an essential element of psychotherapy and that the therapist must be willing to share the client's experience authentically is all very well. But why? What is there about the therapeutic relationship that is so important? How does relationship heal? Relationship-focused integrative psychotherapists believe that the therapeutic relationship exerts a healing influence in several ways. One of these has to do with the acccuracy of the therapist's empathic response and the keenness of her attunement to the client. By allowing herself to be involved, to feel genuinely, the therapist finds in herself the reflection of the client's inner experience, and can respond to the client out of that inner knowing. Stolorow (1992), discussing the therapeutic process, says that the impact of interventions with a client "lies not only in the insights they convey, but also in the extent to which they demonsrate the analyst's attunement to the patient's affective states and developmental longings" (p. 164). His observation is valid not only for a relationship-focused therapy, but for other therapeutic approaches as well: not only are therapists' insights more acute and their interventions more appropriate because of the genuineness of their involvement with clients, but clients sense therapists' genuineness and experience themselves as understood and cared about.

A second benefit of participating in a genuine relationship with clients is that in the context of that relationship we can provide a model of the sort of process in which we would like the client to engage. The therapist is aware of how she feels and what she is thinking about in this relationship; she shuttles readily between her internal experience of self, and her awareness of what the client is doing and saying. "As I listen to what you are telling me, I'm beginning to get angry too," she might say. "In fact, I'm surprised at how angry I feel!" Or, "Even when you haven't done anything wrong, or would not have been able to change the situation your son was in, you still feel guilty. And the more you talk about that sense of guilt, the more distance I sense between us. It's like you sink into yourself, and I can't reach out and find you. Do you feel that distance, too?" By her own example, the therapist invites the client into a new sort of internal/external awareness, into examining both his phenomenological experience (including emotions, memories, fantasies, needs, hopes, and fears) and the way this experience is shaping the ongoing relationship. The therapist is able, says Snyder (1994), "to model and facilitate the capacity . . . to enter one's own life world and to do this . . . on a level that includes keen attention to our embodied emotions, the continual formation of meanings, and the capacity to constitute and interpret experience in a way different than we habitually or reflexively do" (p. 90).

In chapter 3, we talked a great deal about individuation and connection, and how children develop a sense of self out of their relationships with their caretakers. This sort of self-knowing is also facilitated by a therapeutic relationship. Intimacy in relationship requires and fosters self awareness. As the client is gently invited into closer and closer psychological contact with the therapist, so he is also invited into deeper and broader contact with himself. Self-awareness leads to more full relational contact, and the relational contact in turn supports the next step in self-exploration.

There is yet another aspect of the therapeutic relationship, one that is difficult to put into words because it is so deeply visceral that it goes beyond language. Relationship creates an *in-between,* a space that is neither client nor therapist but partakes of them both. Bromberg (1998) calls it "a twilight space in which the impossible becomes possible; a space [where] each one awakens to its own 'truth' " (p. 16). It is a numinous ground within which we can experience moments of transcending self, of an almost mystical sort of *being-with*—what Maslow (1987) referred to as a "peak experience." The client exposes his vulnerabilities to another person, a stable and trustworthy person, in a psychologically out-of-time-and-dimension interaction, and discovers that the world does not end. He is not scolded, ridiculed, or punished; the therapist does not recoil; the relationship is still there. Such an amazing experience allows him to go beyond, for a few moments, the limitations of his life script, to borrow from the therapist the courage and protection needed to explore the unexplorable and to face the terror of his darkest side. With the therapist's support, the client can re-examine his ways of being with and thinking about others and about himself. With the therapist's genuine respect and caring, he can begin to change some of those ways of being with and thinking about. The therapeutic process, as Mitchell (1992) puts it, is "a struggle to find and be oneself in the process of atonement and reconciliation in relation to others, both actual others and others as internal presences" (p. 15). The potency of the therapeutic relationship—as well as the mystery of the in-between—provides a kind of psychological absolution that makes atonement and reconciliation possible.

Finally, authentic, contactful relationship, emerging from the increasing willingness of both client and therapist to be open and honest with each other, usually feels good. The experience of genuine contact with another person can be pleasurable, frustrating, comfortable, scary, or exciting—and it is what being fully human is all about. It is enjoyable to be with a partner "from whom one knows how to elicit a response, but whose responses are not entirely predictable" (Benjamin, 1992, p. 46). Such encounters not only reinforce the client's own efforts to grow and change but also are simply valuable for what they are, in and of themselves.

## Transference and Countertransference

We cannot talk about the therapeutic relationship and the genuineness with which each participant enters into that relationship without dealing with the concept of *transference*. But "transference" is an elusive sort of thing; its definition has evolved and changed so much that the whole idea has gotten rather slippery and hard to pin down. Originally, as Freud (1912/1958a) used the term, transference referred to the displacement onto the therapist of feelings and thoughts originally experienced in previous relationships. The therapist was supposed to present a "blank screen" to the client (exactly the opposite of the sort of entering into relationship that we've been talking about) so as to facilitate this transference of feelings. Once the transference was established, it could be analyzed and destructured, so that archaic feelings and beliefs no longer affected the client's present functioning. *Countertransference*, in this view, was the mirror image of transference: it was the thoughts and feelings of the therapist, left over from old relationships and transferred onto the client (Racker, 1968). Countertransference was thought to interfere with the therapist's ability to do her job properly, and one of the goals of the "training analysis" required of all psychoanalysts was to root out the sources of countertransference so that it would not contaminate the psychoanalytic process.

More recently, many therapists have begun to understand that the division of relationship responses into "old, left over from previous relationships" and "current, appropriate to the here and now" is at best an artificial one (Erskine, 1991/1997b). People are who they are because of their previous relationships; the self is formed out of our ways of being with others throughout life. One can no more divest oneself of the influence of old relationships than one can shed one's skin or excise one's personality. Transference and countertransference involve the whole of the client's and the therapist's inevitable feelings about and responses to each other. To do away with them would be to become machine-like in one's interactions and to have no human relationship at all. Tansey and Burke (1989) say that ". . . therapy is a radically mutual process fully involving two individuals who exert a mutual and ongoing influence upon one another" (pp. 3–4). That "mutual and ongoing influence" grows out of transference and countertransference. Transference on the part of the client may indeed signal old relationship baggage that he could well do without; but it also is the fuel that allows him to sort through and evaluate that old baggage. And countertransference, far from being antithetical to good therapy, is the very stuff that makes good therapy possible.

Elaine D., a client with whom I (J. M.) worked for many months, was a rumpled-looking young woman who seemed to attract trouble like a magnet. Things never seemed to turn out well for her; whatever she did ended up badly—through no apparent fault of her own. As she described her disappointments, week after week, I began to feel myself growing irritated with her. I didn't understand my annoyance and tried to mask it (from her and from myself) by being sympathetic and supportive. Not surprisingly, this strategy failed; my irritability grew rather than lessened, and her tales of woe grew correspondingly more lengthy and detailed. Finally, with supervision, I realized that a good share of my irritation had to do with Elaine's resemblance to my daughter, who as a teenager had expected me to rescue her from a series of self-created disasters; I was continually torn between exasperation and guilt as I tried to be a "good mother" through those years. Once I realized the connection, I could look at both the similarities and the differences between Elaine and my daughter and could also see how my own over-responsibility was the source of my uncomfortable feelings. Bringing all of this to awareness and allowing myself to feel it all during the sessions with Elaine provided me with a much richer base from which to interact with her—I could share both my frustration and my genuine affection for her in a way that was authentic and trustworthy. In response, Elaine became more willing to talk about her resentment toward me (I was, to nobody's surprise, somewhat like her own mother) and, eventually, to break through the pattern of self-sabotage that was her script-evolved way of expressing that resentment.

Historically, transference and countertransference have played quite different roles in psychotherapy. Transference—the client's feelings toward the therapist—has been used as an avenue into issues and expectations of which the client is unaware. In fact, the "analysis of the transference," as Freud described it (1912/1958a, 1915/1958b), was originally thought to be the primary task of therapy. Freud talked about analyzing and working through transference issues; in relationship-focused integrative psychotherapy, we talk about breaking through script patterns and replacing old script beliefs, feelings, and behaviors with full internal and external contact. Most of the psychoanalytically oriented psychotherapies have similar goals, though their terminology is different. And most now recognize that here-and-now responses to the therapist blend with then-and-there relationship patterns and that not everything the client feels toward the therapist must be transferential, in Freud's sense of the word (Greenson, 1967). Nevertheless, those feelings are still regarded as important signals about old relationships and the unresolved issues stemming from them.

More current views of countertransference, though, are radically different from those of the early analysts. Using countertransference therapeutically, instead of trying to stamp it out, represents a major shift in our understanding of the process of psychotherapy and of the therapist's role in that process. "Rather than viewing countertransference as a hindrance to the analytic work that should be kept in check or overcome and that should, in any event, be kept to a minimum, most analysts today recognize the ubiquity of analysts' feelings and fantasies regarding patients and hope to utilize their own reactions as a means to understand their patients better" (Aron, 1991, p. 32). Stone (1996), too, supports this view: "While at one point the countertransference may have been viewed primarily as error to be corrected, it has more and more been recongized as a necessary component of the human interaction involved in psychotherapy" (p. 29).

Therapists, like clients, are human; they enter into the therapeutic relationship as real people, and they inevitably have feelings about the clients with whom they work. Those feelings are bound to be affected by how they have experienced other people in the past. Rather than trying to override their feelings, their random thoughts, and their fears and fantasies when with a client, relationship-focused therapists use them as a rich substrate into which they can dip, emerging with a more complete sense of who this client is and how they (and others as well) respond to him. Think of the line of images you see when you look into one of those mirror-facing-mirror arrangements in a clothing store fitting room: an image of you, looking at an image of you, looking at an image of you. . . . Just so, the therapist looks at herself, looking at the client, who is looking at the therapist, who is looking at the client—an infinite regress, completing itself in the whole symphony of thoughts, feelings, impressions, and inclinations that therapist and client experience in this relationship. The therapist's thoughts, feelings, impressions, and inclinations—growing out of past relationships and blending into this current one, all fully available to awareness—help her to make accurate clinical assessments and to plan effective interventions. Even more important, as she expresses who she is and what she feels toward the client, she is able to invite him into an authentic relationship, a relationship that supports and promotes his own movement toward authenticity.

## A Two-Edged Sword

As with any other powerful force, the therapeutic relationship can be misused. Too great an involvement on the part of the therapist, or an involvement that primarily seeks to benefit herself rather than the client, is not in the client's best interest (Modell, 1991). If the therapist is too intensely involved in her relationship with her client, she may lose her ability to stand back and look at the larger picture of what is going on in that client's life. She may begin, unconsciously, to encourage the client to become dependent or to do things to please her or stay in relationship with her, rather than to facilitate his growth. Nor is a therapist-client relationship likely to be helpful if the therapist's feelings and hypotheses about the client are muddied by unresolved relational issues from the past. Those sorts of responses are more likely to interrupt and distort contact than to enhance it. In other words, both over-involvement and out-of-awareness countertransference (these two usually overlap) are likely to make the therapist more invested in her own feelings and needs than in those of the client.

"There is no question, in my mind," says Bacal (1997), "that the analyst's subjectivity may constitute *both* the greatest obstacle to understanding the patient and the most useful device for doing so, and that it is essential that we are always aware which of the two is predominating" (p. 673). Participation in postgraduate training, ongoing supervision, case discussion groups, and individual peer consultation are helpful in monitoring the quality and intensity of our involvement with clients. It is always possible, though, to mislead a colleague or a consultant by telling only part of the story, withholding whatever might be embarassing or make us look bad. There is no substitute, in the long run, for a regular review of all of our cases (it is amazing how easy it can be to "forget" to review the very case that is most problematical in terms of our personal involvement) and a rigorous self-examination of our feelings, beliefs, wants, and needs with regard to each of our clients.

## RELATIONSHIP AND THE FACETS OF GROWTH AND CHANGE

We have seen how life script patterns grow out of old relationships, particularly those that have involved some sort of trauma and/or some prolonged disruption of contact. Core script beliefs about people—about how they are going to behave toward us and about what we must do to get along with them (or even to survive in their presence)—must inevitably have been formed on the basis of our interactions with the people we have known throughout our lives. Participating in a different sort of relationship, in which one is understood, valued, and respected, gives the script-bound client an opportunity to experience something very different from neglect and abuse.

### Relationship and Cognition

In relationship-focused integrative psychotherapy, the differences between the therapeutic relationship and the script-generating relationships of the client's past are not allowed to simply slide by, experienced but not explicitly discussed. Instead, verbalized, they become a means of dealing with some of the cognitive aspects of the client's script. An important part of the therapist's job is to help the client to notice the quality of the therapeutic relationship, to challenge his beliefs about "the way it was is the way it always has to be," and to support him in the risky business of changing those beliefs.

Therapists do not urge clients to throw out *all* of the things they have learned over the years, of course. To discard all of one's past learnings simply because they came out of some distressing relationship would be as rigid and maladaptive as hanging on to all of them. Instead, effective therapists attempt to create a therapeutic milieu in which clients can think about what they believe and feel—think clearly, critically, and constructively, adding the experiences of this new relationship to what they have learned in older ones. Andrews (1991) talks about how all thought processes need to bring together the old and the new: "Optimal change occurs when new thinking incorporates the most valuable principles from earlier conceptualizations, redefining them so that they become ingredients in a more inclusive paradigm" (p. 232). This is what cognitive integration is all about: keeping the concepts, procedures, and hypotheses that still make sense and expanding and updating them by adding in new learnings. Thesis, antithesis, synthesis—Hegel (1812–1816/1976) probably did not realize it, but he developed a concise and accurate model of the way in which cognitive growth occurs in relationship-focused psychotherapy.

## Relationship and Affect

The therapeutic relationship also impacts the client's affective processes— perhaps even more than his cognitive functioning. Affect surrounds and underlies cognition; it gives flavor and dimensionality to what would otherwise be sterile, linear, and machinelike. "Cognition is to affect," says Stone (1996), "as words are to music" (p. 23). The music of the therapeutic relationship allows it to be experienced in the client's heart as well as in his head. It invites the client to join in a duet rather than singing alone, a duet in which the therapist follows and harmonizes with him, adding some new improvisations now and then, but always supporting the client's melody line. Because they are making this music together, they can sing the sad, scared, and angry songs as well as the sweet ones—the songs that were far too upsetting for the client to sing alone.

Painful experiences create painful memories, and it only makes sense that people try to avoid that kind of pain. Repressing a memory, in order to not feel its pain, may seem like a reasonable strategy. But repressed memories never have a chance to lose their painful emotional charge; the feelings lurk, out of awareness, ready to bite and sting whenever they can escape into consciousness. Worse, many painful memories seem to grow in intensity over time; it is as if they thrive in the darkness, becoming even more monstrous and terrifying. To shrink them back to size, draw out the poison and "de-fang" the experience, they must be recalled and faced; the interchange of the therapeutic relationship ensures that the client need not face them alone.

Colleen, a client who had survived significant childhood abuse and who initially came to therapy because of painful flashbacks, talked about the relief she experienced through this process. "My memories used to be like 3-D movies, only I wasn't just watching them, I was in them. But every time I worked through one, it turned into just a photograph. I didn't forget what happened, but I could paste it into an album and then shut the book." Within the safety and support of the therapeutic relationship, Colleen was able to stop running away from her memories, to turn around and confront them, and to recover the parts of herself that had been taken over by them. Only then could they be assimilated into her whole personality. Each memory became simply another historical event that no longer had the power to re-create the fear, pain, or humiliation that was experienced at the time the memory was laid down.

The emotional connection created within a supportive therapeutic relationship invites and encourages the client to explore painful memories and the feelings that attach to them. In so doing, the client moves toward what Stolorow (1992) describes as the fundamental goal of psychotherapy: "the unfolding, illumination, and transformation of the patient's subjective world" (p. 159). For many clients, that subjective world is a dark maze of must-not-think-abouts that can only be negotiated with care and dread. The therapist offers to help the client explore the maze, offers to accompany him—may even bring a lantern!—so that together they can venture into the shadows, connect the long-blocked pathways, and open the dungeon to light and air and freedom.

## Relationship and Behavior

Subjective changes are likely to be short-lived if clients do not also change how they act. What better place could there be for practicing new behaviors, new ways of being with others, than a relationship in which the function and underlying intent of everything one does is valued and respected, even if the behaviors themselves are clumsy or hard to understand? The relational need for safety is never so strongly felt as when we are about to try out a behavior that has been punished or laughed at in the past, and the therapeutic relationship provides that safety. "I'll be here with you," says the psychotherapist—often without words. "I won't be repulsed, or horrified, or think you're silly. Even when I don't know why you're doing what you do or saying what you say, I'll stick around to find out because I know that there's an important reason for it. And I'm not going to stop caring about you just because you didn't get it right the first time."

New ways of behaving in a relationship create new emotional experiences and emotional memories. New emotions require new ways of thinking about what has happened. New thoughts and feelings support further experimenting with new behaviors. It is that mutual causality again; changes in one aspect invite changes in all the others. Life scripts demand that nothing new and different—nothing that would upset the system's homeostatic balance—be done, thought, or felt. Participating in a contact-inviting therapeutic relationship *is* new and different and *does* shake up the system; with every new behavior tried out, every newly expressed thought or feeling, the life script becomes more open to change.

## ACCESSIBILITY

Students of learning have recognized for years that there are many different kinds of "knowing." Chamberlain (1990) distinguishes *declarative* knowledge (knowing that something happened) from *procedural* knowledge (knowing how to do something). Stein and Young (1997) point out the distinction between *explicit* learning (the things we know and remember when we learned them) and *implicit* learning (the things we know but do not know where or when they were acquired); these are also known as *semantic* versus *episodic* memories. You may remember learning to read or being helped to balance on that new two-wheel bike; that is an explicit or episodic memory. Explicit memories can be affective (that time in school when you were so proud because the teacher put your drawing up on the bulletin board) or cognitive (you know how to access the Internet, and you remember figuring it out). Pleasant or unpleasant, they are there, they happened, and you know about it. Implicit knowledge, in contrast, seems to have no origin. Even though you know you must have learned it sometime—and may even be able to remember times before you learned it—you still feel somehow as if the learning has always been there. Learning to walk and learning to talk are easy examples that most of us share.

Out-of-awareness patterns, knowings, and memories form yet another category: different from things we know but cannot remember acquiring, these are the things we know but do not know that we know. Only in retrospect can we say "Oh, I knew that all along; I just didn't think of it before." Included here are the things we have learned to do, to think, and to feel without realizing that we are doing, thinking, or feeling them. Mary, for example, learned to take care of other people as a way of making up for not getting taken care of herself, but if you ask her about it, she will probably not even understand what you are talking about. She will say that she does not do that; she gets pleasure out of helping others; she gets plenty of attention for herself. Or Bob, who changes the subject adroitly whenever the current topic of conversation becomes uncomfortable—Bob acknowledges that he does it, sort of, but does not recognize how often it happens or where he learned to do it.

Knowing but not knowing that we know; feeling but not knowing that we feel; behaving but not recognizing that we behave—it is a strange, almost *Twilight Zone* area of human functioning. Adaptive forgetting, says Freyd (1996), is a matter of inhibiting information rather than discarding it entirely. We may not know that we know, but the knowledge can be retrieved; it is not completely lost. The package has not been thrown away but is stored off in a closet, and we have forgotten where it is—or even that we ever had it. Such closets are areas with which psychotherapists are very familiar, for they are where life script patterns are found. Many of these script patterns were acquired very early in life and may have been laid down at a different rate of speed or through a different sort of process than the things of which we are now consciously aware. Weaker stimuli may have been processed implicitly, and stronger ones explicitly (Stein & Young, 1997). Things that we experienced in one state of consciousness may not be available to awareness when we are in a different state (Terr, 1994). And, of course, there is always repression—purposeful (though not conscious) forcing some memory or knowlege out of explicit awareness in order to avoid psychologial distress. Nathanson (1996) believes that distress, itself, can relegate some learnings to the limbo of known-but-not-known: "[J]ust as one affect may bring something into consciousness, another may push the triggering event and its accompanying affect into a special compartment that makes it difficult to access or retrieve" (p. 3).

The concept of ego states provides another way of understanding this curious split between what we know that we know and what we know without knowing. Berne (1961) described three basic states of the ego: the *archaeopsyche*, which consists of all of the patterns of thinking, feeling, and relating to the world that we have used in previous developmental stages; the *exteropsyche*, composed of the thought/feeling/relating patterns we have introjected from others; and the *neopsyche*, the patterns that we consciously create and use in our here-and-now lives. There are subdivisions within these main ego states, of course: we have introjected different patterns from different people; and we certainly have behaved, thought, and felt differently at different times in our lives. But the general contours are there—the old, archaeopsychic ways of being, usually tracing back to childhood (thus, the familiar designation of these patterns as "Child" ego states); the introjected-from-others patterns (and the others have most often been parents or other early caretakers, so these ego states are known colloquially as "Parent" ego states); and the age-appropriate, present-time-focused patterns of feeling, problem solving, and relating to people, known as the "Adult" ego state.

The boundaries between the different ego states may be more or less permeable; rigid and impermeable boundaries keep one ego state from awareness of the others, so that knowledge, expectations, or emotional responses held in one may be implicit—or totally out of awareness—to another. Although psychologically healthy individuals will spend most or all of their time operating out of an Adult ego (using Berne's terminology), these individuals may draw upon the experiences, the beliefs, and the affective expression of other ego states. Conversely, to the degree that people are trapped in a given state of the ego (usually parent or child), unable to shift into other states or to access information from those other states, their awareness of and contact with self and with the world around them will be constricted and their ability to function in the world severely limited.

Watkins and Watkins (1990) do not suggest the tripartite division (into parent, child, and adult) that Berne has outlined but do describe a similar sort of function: "We conceptualize personality structure as being a multiplicity organized into various patterns of ego states, and we define an ego state as a body of behaviors and experiences bound together by some common principle and separated from other such entities by boundaries that are more or less permeable" (p. 404).

Script-bound people live their lives on the basis of rules, expectations, and emotional responses that have their roots in ego states (or substates) that are not accessible to conscious awareness. Such individuals are often unaware of these rules, expectations, and responses, much less of their origins; they use them but do not know that they do so. The experience of the original decision, of forming the original expectation, of developing the original belief, has been hidden away, outgrown or overshadowed or actively repressed by their current psychic organization. The hidden ego state pattern, though unaccessible to awareness, is nevertheless still affecting the way they live their lives. Until that hidden pattern can be accessed, the old learnings and decisions are protected from being updated, discarded if they are no longer needed or changed to fit the changing circumstances of the person's life.

## Working with the Out-of-Awareness

The challenge for the client in psychotherapy is contact. *Internal contact* refers to contact with all of one's ego states—access to the memories, learnings, decisions, feelings, beliefs, and patterns that were developed at some time in the past but are no longer available to conscious awareness. *External contact* refers to contact in relationship with the other people in one's world. Explicit, episodic memory is relatively easy to work with therapeutically; the client knows what happened and with whom it happened and can deal logically with the consequences of the experience. Implicit learnings are more problematic, since the origins of the learned pattern are lost to awareness; but, at least, the client knows something about the problem, something of the pattern that needs to be changed. But how can clients access ego states of which they are unaware, decisions they do not remember making, or beliefs they do not know they hold?

There are two general ways in which out-of-awareness patterns can be used. We can work to effect changes in what *is* available, trusting that change in one part of the system will bring about changes in all the others. Or we can focus on helping the client to bring to awareness that which has been hidden— to make the previously inaccessible information accessible. Interestingly, these two approaches often merge; bringing about a change in one aspect of functioning (one that is in awareness and, thus, amenable to change) can stimulate hidden memories, feelings, behaviors, and beliefs so that what was once inaccessible is now accessible. Sometimes simply bringing a pattern to awareness is enough to start a process of change that will continue on its own; sometimes clients need help to bring about such changes; and sometimes awareness of one pattern leads to the realization that some other learning, even more deeply buried, lies at the root of the problem.

Accessibility, then, is the key—access to that which needs to be changed and access to the means of changing it. This book, as well as the relationship-focused integrative psychotherapy out of which the book has grown, is based on the premise that the primary purpose of a therapeutic relationship is to foster the kind of contact that leads to accessibility. In the context of a full and authentic relationship with a supportive, skillful therapist, accessibility expands; that is, behaviors can change, memories can be stimulated, old patterns can emerge into awareness, and new possibilities can open.

In the chapters to follow, we discuss how therapists can help clients to move into an accessible state, a state in which behaviors, beliefs, and feelings are most open to awareness and to change. We look at the ways in which change can most readily be accomplished, once the needed information is accessible. Finally, we discuss closing the work—the work of an individual session and the work of the whole course of therapy. Through it all, we consider the two primary dimensions of the therapist's craft: (a) the ability to create and maintain a contactful therapeutic relationship, and (b) the specific skill and techniques that may be utilized in the context of that relationship. We begin by looking more closely at the nature of the therapeutic relationship and how it can be developed and nurtured.

## SUMMARY

To work effectively with clients, a therapist needs to consider all of the major interlocking systems of human functioning—thoughts, feelings, behaviors, and physiology—and how they interact. All of these interactions take place in the context of relationship, and relationship is the critical factor governing psychological change.

Therapists attempt to know their clients from the inside, temporarily experiencing the world as the client does. This level of attunement facilitates the client's self-knowing. The therapist's self-awareness also provides a model for similar self-awareness on the part of the client. Together, therapist and client create an "in-between" that is a place of growth and healing.

Transference and countertransference are integral aspects of the therapeutic relationship. Both involve a blending of responses learned in old relationships, as well as responses unique to the present. Recognizing transference responses can help both client and therapist bring life script patterns to awareness; countertransference, too, can help the therapist recognize those patterns and their effects on others.

The therapeutic relationship, skillfully managed, can have a positive impact on client's cognition, emotions, and behavior. This is accomplished in part by developing increasing accessibility in the client: he learns to access his previously hidden thoughts and feelings and to share those internal experiences with the therapist. In so doing, he may move into various states of the ego, some introjected from past significant others and some connected to earlier developmental stages. Accessing these ego states can also lead to increased self-awareness. Bringing hidden patterns to awareness allows them to be changed; changing one aspect of a psychological system requires that all of the other, interlocking elements also change. Such changes can, in turn, lead to dissolving a life script, reducing distress, and recovering the ability to form and maintain healthy relationships.

# Creating a Therapeutic Relationship

# CHAPTER 5

Psychotherapy involves both art and science. The "art" side has to do with those aspects of psychotherapy that cannot quite be captured in words, cannot be specified in a list of techniques and procedures. Therapeutic artistry comes into play, more than anywhere else, in creating and maintaining a therapeutic relationship, a relationship that is purposeful and professional on the one hand, and personal and involved on the other. As has been emphasized in previous chapters, we believe that developing and maintaining such a relationship is the single most important factor in successful psychotherapy. Current research appears to bear out this belief: Horvath (2001), reporting on a meta-analysis of 90 independent clinical investigations, concludes that "it is likely that a little over half of the beneficial effects of psychotherapy accounted for in previous meta-analyses are linked to the quality of the alliance" (p. 366)—that is, to the therapeutic relationship.

Horvath goes on to discuss a number of therapist variables that appear to be related to an effective therapeutic alliance: communication skills, experience and training, personality and intrapersonal process, and collaboration with the client. There *are* things that can be specified about creating and utilizing a good therapeutic relationship, and many of these things can be taught directly. Some of them have primarily to do with attitude: the "unconditional positive regard" that Rogers (1951) talked about, and a sense of one's own purpose and competence. Others have to do with techniques, the interventions one learns how to make in a therapy session.

In recent years, there has been an increasing emphasis in the psychothera-peutic literature on matching therapeutic technique and client dysfunction. Some clients, with some sorts of problems and dynamics and script patterns, will respond better to one approach; others will do better with a different approach. Bornstein and Bowen (1995) say that ". . . the clearest way to describe an integrated approach to working with the dependent psychotherapy patient is to begin by describing therapeutic techniques that affect specific aspects of the dependent person's functioning" (p. 528). The same could be said of the "resistant" client, or of the "trauma survivor," or of any number of other concerns and problems that clients bring to therapy.

More important than client-specific techniques, though, are the things that effective therapists do with *all* clients. These are the skills of relationship man-agement: how to create and cultivate the kind of relationship environment in which the client will experience both safety and challenge, and in which our other, more specific techniques will be most useful. In other words, both general skills, skills and behaviors that are helpful with all clients, and client-specific techniques, techniques that are helpful to some clients but less so to others, are valuable. And both sorts of skills, general and client-specific, are wrapped in and nourished by the therapist's art—her unique, unvoiced, and unvoicable way of *being with* another person.

General versus specific; art versus science—both are, in fact, false dichotomies. In the rich complexity of the world of psychotherapy, they are all necessary. Norcross (1995), speaking of the distinction between general and specific techniques, says "Psychotherapy will prosper by avoiding the dual extremes of specific effects and of common factors and by endorsing the Aris-totelian median" (p. 503). More simply put, we must not embrace either posi-tion exclusively but, rather, must garner that which is to be learned from each. "Adapting or tailoring the therapy relationship to specific patient needs and characteristics," concludes the Steering Committee of the APA Division 29 Task Force (2001), "enhances the effectiveness of treatment" (p. 495). This also applies to the tension between therapy-as-art and therapy-as-science: neither extreme will be as useful as a middle position that recognizes the value of both.

When we, as therapists, use both our artistry and our learned skills for the client's benefit, we find that each potentiates the other. Our technically based interventions become warm and three-dimensional because they come from an involved and caring person. Our warmth and caring can be channeled into a purposive treatment plan by the appropriate use of technical skills. The most effective therapy, then, arises out of the interaction between who we are in the therapeutic relationship and the specific strategies we use in that relationship. "The value of a clinical intervention," say Mahoney and Norcross (1993), "is inextricably bound to the relational context in which it is applied" (p. 423). Without the support and protection of a carefully maintained therapeutic rela-tionship, the most ingenious and appropriate intervention can be experienced by the client as threatening, condescending, or irrelevant. In contrast, a good therapeutic relationship increases both the power of an intervention and the client's willingness to be affected by it. Even in short-term, time-limited therapy, the quality of the therapeutic relationship is a critical factor in the effectiveness of treatment.

As we have seen, most clients come to therapy feeling "stuck." They are mired in patterns of thinking and feeling and behaving that are not working any more, but they see no alternative. Often the very thing that most needs to change is the thing of which they are least aware. Logic alone—pointing things out, giving advice, nagging or criticizing—does not help; if it did, the client's outside-of-therapy relationships would have taken care of the problem. The encounter with a therapist who does something different—who asks questions or offers interpretations or suggests experiments in the context of a particular way-of-being-with—is what shakes up the old patterns, creating a kind of clash between the way the world has always been (and, as far as the client can see, must always be) and what is actually experienced (Gold, 1996). Experiencing this clash is a little like discovering that what you thought was north is really south, or that what you believed happened yesterday is in fact scheduled for tomorrow, or that the experience you have been terrified of is actually enjoyable: it requires a shift in your whole way of looking at and responding to the world.

Shifting a familiar pattern is not easy. Script patterns provide (among other things) a way of organizing the world. The organization may not be comfortable, and it may not bring one the things one really wants; but at least it's familiar, dependable, and predictable. It follows that our task as therapists, if we are to have an impact on the client's script, must include breaking into the old way of experiencing the world so that new ideas and feelings can be entertained. In creating a relationship different from those that the client has experienced before, we do exactly that: the old beliefs don't fit what's happening here, the predicted patterns don't occur, the old understandings don't work. The client may deny the reality of his here-and-now experiencing—he will probably do so more than once before he finally allows himself to believe that what he feels in this therapeutic setting is real. Once he accepts that reality, his only alternative is to re-examine his old rules and expectations. That re-examination, in turn, can lead to a new set of organizing principles that are incompatible with the script patterns that have been governing his life (Rowe, 1999).

Simply experiencing—participating in—the therapeutic relationship can go a long way toward moving the client out of his stuckness into new ways of being with himself and with others. The experience will be even more powerful if it is made explicit. "What did you think when I said . . . ?" or "What was it like for you when we were talking about . . . ?" are questions that encourage clients not only to experience the relationship but also to be consciously aware of that experience. In chapter 6, we discuss this sort of therapeutic inquiry at greater length. But it is not only the client who needs to be sensitive to what is happening in the relationship. Conscious awareness of the relationship experience is even more important for the therapist. She needs to notice what is going on, not only in the client, but also in herself and in the interaction between them. "The interviewer's own affective and emotional life has to be available to consciousness simply to aid in the process of sifting the data and identifying the sources of the affects that are found [in the client]" (Stone, 1996, p. 30). Knowing what she is experiencing and where that experience comes from helps the therapist to know what is her own "stuff" and what is coming from the client. When that distinction is clear and solid, her own internal process provides some of her best cues as to what her clients need.

Relationship-focused integrative psychotherapists do not generally believe that simply maintaining a client in a therapeutic relationship, allowing him to experience it, is the optimum treatment strategy. Rather, we agree with Gehrie (1999): "The relationship is not the treatment, but *the relationship makes the treatment possible* if it is properly managed" (p. 87; italics ours). In the following paragraphs, we look closely at this strange thing called a "therapeutic relationship": its characteristics, how it is maintained, and how it is built upon both art and science, upon personal involvement and technical skill.

## DEVELOPING THERAPEUTIC PERSONHOOD

Becoming skilled as therapists requires that we learn something new about being with another person: that we learn how to use ourselves, *ourselves in relationship*, so as to provide a growing and healing experience for our clients. It requires that we learn to use techniques that will transform our behavior from that of a friend, or a colleague, or simply an interested listener into that of an effective professional. But the term "techniques" sounds so cold, so calculating and manipulative! How can we be genuine and real in a relationship and still use "techniques"? This dilemma resolves itself when we learn to integrate our techniques into our honest caring and interest. What started as a technique becomes a facet of who we are and what we are about. Technique + genuine caring = therapeutic personhood; and therapeutic personhood is what makes therapy work. Says Gold (1996), "The 'presence' of the therapist . . . is defined as the therapist being with the patient in the most fully human, authentic, unique, and open way possible" (p. 78). Elsewhere (Erskine, Moursund, & Trautmann, 1999), we have described this sort of personhood as "contactfulness combined with therapeutic intent and therapeutic competence" (p. 97). Being a therapeutic person requires not only that one be aware of and open to one's own feelings and needs; it also requires that one's most salient feeling/need be a concern for the client's welfare, and that this concern find its expression with competence and skill.

### Observing from Within

Being both authentic and skillful helps the therapist to observe herself, her client, and the way they are together. Instead of standing back and "looking at" or "listening to" the client, she observes and listens *with* him. She explores not just the client's experience but the experience of client-with-therapist—and of therapist-with-client as well. She is interested in what the client thinks and feels, how she herself thinks and feels, how the client thinks and feels in response to her thoughts and feelings, and how she thinks and feels in response to him. Gehrie (1999), describing the development of his own therapeutic personhood, says that he and his colleagues had to "adopt a technique that emphasized emotional availability, because to do otherwise made empathy impossible. Either we stood 'outside' the patient's experience and examined it, or we stood more 'inside' it and acknowledged our part in the creation of it" (p. 85). It's the *in-between* again—the notion of a therapeutic space in which each participant, therapist and client, has a part in the creation of what the other is thinking and feeling and doing. Client and therapist bear a mutual responsibility for whatever happens during their time together. Acknowledging, examining, and cherishing that mutuality is contact-making and awareness-enhancing—for therapist as well as for client.

What does it mean to *listen with* rather than *listening to?* How do therapists enter the "intersubjective field" (Atwood & Stolorow, 1984) and observe what is happening from *inside* the therapeutic interaction? An important part of this skill is that the therapist constantly reminds herself that she is not a neutral observer. She is not watching things unfold within the client, like a spectator in a theater: she herself is part of the drama. The client is thinking, feeling, and behaving differently than he would if the therapist were not with him; and the therapist's thoughts and feelings (about the client, and about herself) are affected by the client's being with her. One of the most important things for a therapist to remember is that her perceptions of the client are shaped by her own internal experience. "What I essentially have *heard*," says Socor (1989) "are the client's words played on my sound system. . . . I may not purport to have heard the client's truth—only my translation of it. . . . My very act of translation (i.e., the way I hear the 'truth' and what I ask about it) will shape the emerging narrative. I cannot claim 'abstinence'" (p. 108).

When we observe from within, we learn to realize our own responsibility in shaping what happens from moment to moment in the therapy session. We recognize how we help determine what the client tells us and how he is responding to our interventions. Acknowledging that we are partly responsible for what the client says and does—that we are co-creators of the therapeutic drama—not only provides a more accurate understanding of what is going on in the therapy session but also helps us to avoid being judgmental: *Do I not like what the client is doing right now? Do I experience him as resistant, as overly dependent, as thinking when he should be feeling, or emotional when he needs to think? If so, then I must look at how I am helping to make that happen. I may or may not choose to tell him what I have discovered about myself and my experiencing, but if I do tell him, I will make it clear that both of us are creating this process, and that both of us need to deal with it together.* This suggests another benefit of observing from within, rather than from outside: it allows us to explore the nature of the contact between therapist and client. Exploring the ways in which therapist and client make, distort, or break contact with each other generally enhances that contact; and enhancing *interpersonal* contact encourages and supports enhanced *intrapersonal* contact and awareness.

One last advantage of observing from within the relationship has to do with the therapist's emotional availability, and this brings us back to the notion of therapeutic personhood. When the therapist sits outside and looks *at,* she is likely to intellectualize and analyze and to put her own feelings to one side. If she does feel something about what is happening, she labels it as a response to what the client is doing, and adds that piece of data to her analysis. The client becomes an object to be understood, manipulated, and repaired; the therapeutic relationship becomes irrelevant or disappears altogether. Looking *at* is emotionally distancing. In contrast, observing from within brings the therapist's own uniquely personal responses into the relationship-forming process. Because she is being real with herself, her authenticity permeates her interactions with the client and makes true relationship possible. The client needs that authenticity, that emotional availability. The therapist's personhood, her willingness to be involved in the process, creates a context in which the client can dare to risk experiencing that which has been unavailable until now. Observing from within, allowing oneself to be truly a part of the ongoing process, keeps one present for the client, available as a whole person. The client does not have to do it all alone: we are together through whatever will happen on this journey that we are taking.

## Self-Awareness

Staying within the field and taking responsibility for our part in creating it requires that we be self-aware. We can hardly hold ourselves accountable for doing something if we do not know that we are doing it. Many young therapists, beginning to learn their craft, try to submerge themselves in the client's experience, to be completely focused on what it is like to live inside that client's skin. To the extent that they succeed, they lose themselves—and the loss of self means that the client is again alone. The very thing that these novice therapists think will be most helpful turns out to be quite unhelpful, for it is relationship damaging. Moreover, when we try to ignore our own feelings and responses in order to focus on the client, we become less and less sensitive to our own behavior and its effect on that client. How can we understand one half of an interaction without knowing something about the other half? It is like trying to understand the movements of a dancer without being able to see what his partner is doing. Responses that make perfect sense as part of an interaction between two people can be utterly incomprehensible when seen as solitary behavior.

The therapeutic exchange takes place in an interpersonal space created by and belonging to both client and therapist. Even though the interpersonal space of therapy belongs to both participants, though, it is the therapist's responsibility to make that space therapeutic. She does so, first and foremost, by attending—attending with her ears, with her eyes, and with her heart. She attends not only to the client but to herself—first to her responses to the client but also to whatever emerges from her own ongoing needs and fantasies. She places her awareness of her own thoughts and feelings in the context of her commitment to the client's welfare, and in this context she decides what she will share with the client and what she will keep to herself. She notices how the client responds to her, and how she experiences that response. She demands of herself no less self-awareness than she hopes for in her client.

Of course, the search for self-awareness cannot become the therapist's only, or even her primary, focus during the therapeutic hour. Her first concern is to enter the inner and outer world that the client is telling her about. The therapist's attention to self is in service of her attention to the client. To the degree that the therapist's focus on her internal experience enhances her understanding of the client—of what he is saying, doing, and feeling—it will further the development of a healing therapeutic relationship. If it repeatedly interferes with attending to the client, it will detract from that relationship. The therapist's attention shuttles between self and other, between what-is-happening-in-here and what-is-happening-over-there. The client, perhaps with less skill and less awareness, is doing the same thing. Both patterns of attention—that of client and that of therapist—are ingredients in the relationship; neither can be ignored because each is only understandable in the context of the other.

One of the major factors to be taken into account in understanding the interweaving of causality between client and therapist is the sensitivity that clients display with regard to what their therapist says and does. Often without awareness, they respond to the most minimal shifts in voice tone, expression, or posture. Says Frank (1997), "Not only deliberate interventions, but virtually *all* of the analyst's activity, even inactivity, is expressive and continuously communicates meaning to the patient" (p. 286). Sometimes the meaning communicated is not at all what the therapist intended; sometimes the client will misinterpret the therapist's behaviors, and sometimes he will read accurately what the therapist would have preferred to keep to herself. Whatever meaning he makes, though, the therapist's best chance of exploring and understanding it with him lies in her noticing the stimuli to which he is responding— and those stimuli come, in significant part, from the therapist herself.

It may seem somewhat paradoxical that, in order to know what goes on inside the client, we must look within ourselves. Yet, as we shall discover in our discussion of empathy later in this chapter, our own ability to resonate with the client provides our best cue as to what he is thinking and feeling. "The person who is at home with the subjective stirrings of his or her own inner being tends to be sensitive to the inner felt world of others and is not afraid of responding from this awareness" (Barrett-Lennard, 1997, p. 111). Sensitivity to client and sensitivity to self work together; as self-examination and self-awareness become almost automatic parts of one's therapeutic behavior, one finds oneself increasingly able to read the nonverbal messages the client is sending.

Our internal response to the client may be useful in three ways, according to Bacal (1997): as a reaction to what is going on in the client, as a reflection of what is going on in the client, or as a mixture of both (p. 678). When our internal experience *reflects* what is going on in the client, we can sample that experience and use it to understand what the client's internal world is really like. When we *react to* the client, and take note of that reaction, we understand better the effects the client may have on others and what his social experiences are likely to have been. Most often, we will have both, reaction and reflection. The importance of distinguishing between the two cannot be overstated. Imagine, for example, a therapist who experiences a sense of frustration, mixed with deep sadness, as she listens to her client's story. If the frustration is a reflection of the client's frustration, and the sadness is her own reaction to his pain, she will be moved to intervene in one way; if the sadness is what she feels coming from the client and she is frustrated by his inability to move beyond it, she is likely to formulate a very different intervention. If she gets it wrong, if she mistakes her own emotional response for a reflection of the client's feelings, her intervention is very likely to be off the mark and unhelpful.

Frank (1997) recommends not only that the therapist be self-aware, but that she be willing to share that self-awareness with her client. Doing so allows both therapist and client access to whatever creativity, past experience, and insights the therapist may find within herself. Frank suggests that therapists cultivate a "willingness to be known" and goes on to say that "such an attitude empowers the work, allowing the therapist to respond with personal as well as professional resources—common sense, personal experience, wisdom—rather than through strict adherence to a clinical methodology, which, of course, continues to inform the analyst's role" (p. 309). Notice that Frank does not advise us to simply present the client with a monologue describing our own internal state. Our sense of what is clinically appropriate—helpful to the client—is always a factor in determining what we choose to share. Again, it is the combination of therapeutic skill and personal involvement, of objectivity and subjectivity, that creates a unique therapeutic environment, a kind of interpersonal greenhouse in which the client's tender new awarenesses are invited to grow and flourish.

## Process Exploration

Since the therapeutic relationship is so critical to the client's experience, it only makes sense that that relationship should be a focus of therapeutic dialogue during the therapy session. Of course there will be discussion of the client's concerns, about what brought him to treatment, what has happened to him in the past, and how those experiences have shaped his life. But there will also be inquiry about what is happening between client and therapist and about how the client is affected by the relationship that is being created in this therapeutic space. There is no substitute for this sort of here-and-now exploration. Descriptions of past events may be informative, but such past events are static, history, no longer open to change. The client's present experience is alive, constantly changing and shifting: new vistas open up; feelings and connections wink in and out of awareness; he goes down a familiar path and suddenly finds something he never noticed before. The therapy session becomes a kind of laboratory, with the client's ways of making and breaking contact, of being open and of hiding behind silence or subterfuge, right in front of him, ready to explore in all of its kaleidoscopic complexity.

The therapist's task is to further that exploration, wherever it may lead. She does so by encouraging the client to look inside, to attend to his ongoing thoughts, feelings, hopes, fears, needs, and expectations as he talks with her. She helps him to notice the connections between what he experiences here, in the therapy hour, and what he has experienced elsewhere in his life. She invites him to stay with those parts of his experience that he ordinarily brushes past or pushes away. And she herself is genuinely involved in that exploration, with her own human feelings and thoughts available to her and—when she makes the therapeutic choice to share them—to her client. The therapist uses herself like a spotlight in a dark room, highlighting what the client tells her (in words and nonverbally), and pointing ahead toward spaces that have been dim and unknowable for him. As Atwood and Stolorow (1984) remind us, everything that the client discovers about how he is, here with the therapist, is also a discovery about who he is in the external world; and every discovery about how he is and has been in his daily life will help him understand what is happening with him now, with the therapist. Each intervention that "successfully illuminates for the patient his unconscious past simultaneously crystallizes an illusive present—the novelty of the therapist as an understanding presence. Perceptions of self and other are perforce transformed and reshaped to allow for the new experience" (p. 60).

## SYMMETRY AND ASYMMETRY

As we talk about the unique relationship between client and therapist, a new paradox begins to emerge: the paradox of *symmetry*. We have asserted over and over that the therapist must be fully and personally involved in the therapeutic relationship, willing to be affected by the client and to acknowledge the client's impact on her, just as the client is open to the therapist's impact. There is a symmetry here, an *I-thou* quality (Buber, 1958), in which each person in the relationship gives to and takes from the other.

However, in another very important sense, the relationship between client and therapist is far from symmetrical. Client and therapist are not "equal"; the whole purpose of the therapeutic encounter is to benefit the client. The client comes to therapy to be helped; the therapist's task is to provide that help. How, then, can we create a relationship that is both symmetrical (i.e., two people, both genuinely involved in the process) and asymmetrical (with differences in focus, in power, in the nature of their investment)?

To sort out the dimensions of this dilemma, we need to look at involvement and symmetry simultaneously. Figure 5.1 shows a diagram of how these two variables (much simplified, of course) might come together in a relationship. Let us consider each in turn.

The best examples of relationships that are both *symmetrical and involved* are good marriages and close friendships, in which both participants are open, caring, and willing to be vulnerable to each other; in which each expects to

**Figure 5.1** | Symmetry and Involvement in Relationships

Symmetry

| | High | Low |
|---|---|---|
| High | Symmetrical, Involved | Asymmetrical, Involved |
| Low | Symmetrical, Detached | Asymmetrical, Detached |

Involvement

both give to and take from; and in which neither has more power, more status, or stronger influence. A *symmetrical and detached* relationship has that same sense of equality—both parties expect pretty much the same thing from each other—but, from an emotional standpoint, their expectations are very low. For example, I see a colleague at professional meetings; I know his name, and he knows mine; we are courteous to each other but have no particular interest in pursuing a close relationship.

A third sort of relationship, *asymmetrical and detached,* might exist between a lawyer and client or a doctor and patient: there is a shared expectation that the relationship exists for the primary benefit of the client or patient, that the lawyer's or doctor's job is to assist the client or patient; but the two participants have little or no emotional involvement with each other. For the final combination, *asymmetrical and involved,* we turn back to a family example, the relationship between parent and child. Here, there is emotional involvement, vulnerability, and caring on the part of both. While the relationship clearly provides benefits for each, there is also a shared expectation that it is the parent's job to care for the child and not the other way around. (Interestingly, over the lifespan of a parent-child relationship, the direction of the asymmetry often gradually shifts, finally reaching a point at which the now-adult child is caring for the aging parent.)

Of these four kinds of relationships, the one that best approximates psychotherapy is the last, the relationship between parent and child. Therapist and client are emotionally open to each other, each genuinely caring about the other's welfare. But there is a clear and mutual expectation that the purpose of the relationship is to assist the client in meeting his needs. When the client is particularly vulnerable or regressed, the therapist may function much like a good parent, supporting the client's exploration, protecting him from self-harm, applauding his success. As the client begins to move out of his life script, into less-painful patterns of being with self and others, less and less quasi-parental functioning is demanded of the therapist—not unlike the parent's changing role as a child grows to adulthood.

## Therapeutic Intent

There is no doubt that parents are emotionally involved with their children, vulnerable to their children's pain. Yet good parents know how to be involved and still provide the kinds of things children need: clear limits, support, generosity tempered by good judgment. Good parents do not expect their children to take care of them emotionally; a commitment to effective parenting precludes using one's children as emotional caretakers. Good therapists do the same sorts of things, setting limits, providing support, using good judgment in their decisions about how much to give of themselves. Their commitment to their therapeutic function prevents good therapists from using clients to further their own emotional well-being. They do not expect their clients to do this or that in order to please them; they do not want their clients to be so busy worrying about their therapists' feelings that they cannot fully explore their own. This commitment to the therapeutic process is known as *therapeutic intent*. Therapeutic intent allows one to be involved, real, and present in relationship with a client and, at the same time, to maintain the kind of asymmetry that will best promote his growth.

Modell (1991) points out that ". . . our body in its response to the patient's affects does not make a distinction between individuals in ordinary life and those within the therapeutic frame. We are all hard-wired to respond in a complementary, albeit idiosyncratic fashion . . ." (p. 18). Therapists do have emotional responses to clients; we do sometimes become upset, discouraged, angry, or saddened by what our clients tell us. That is part of being involved, part of our personhood—part of making a healing relationship. But we strive to use those emotional responses therapeutically, for the client's benefit. That is therapeutic intent. Therapy occurs within an asymmetrical relationship; in relationship-focused integrative psychotherapy, both the relationship and its asymmetry are essential. When we get it right—when we are able to be authentically involved in an appropriately asymmetrical relationship and to use our skills within that relationship—we can call ourselves therapists.

As the client learns that he can trust both the genuineness of the therapist's involvement, and her commitment to use that involvement for the client's benefit, he can talk more and more freely about his experiences. Lister (1981), speaking of clients who have experienced trauma, says, "To speak about what has happened and to share this information with another person are both emotionally laden acts with multiple consequences. Framing into words involves a departure from initial defenses, which may have altered the memory of the event itself—through suppression, repression, dissociation, or even psychotic disorganization. Coming to therapy solidifies a conscious sense of what has happened, or the reality of these events, or their pain and importance" (p. 874). In some sense, everyone has experienced trauma: the everyday vicissitudes of life, the relational hurts that are an inevitable part of growing up with caretakers who are also human, create some trauma for all of us. Whether one has only experienced these "garden variety" traumas or has passed through the major and tragic traumas that mark some individuals' history, talking about those experiences in the presence of someone who is involved and who acts out of therapeutic intent does help one to depart from defenses, to bring to awareness what has happened and how those events have affected one's way of being in the world—and with awareness comes the possibility of change.

Maintaining one's therapeutic intent is not without cost. Frank (1997) reminds us, "Because they involve self-revelations, each and every one of the analyst's communications, including interpretations and, especially, deeply resonant empathic responses, involve self-exposure and leave the analyst open to potential criticism and rejection" (p. 294). That openness to criticism and rejection is doubly risky because we *care* about being criticized or rejected. We *care* when the client fails to benefit from our work together. We *care* when he gets hurt or disappointed or suffers the consequences of some less-than-wise behavior on our part. We do not protect ourselves by being detached, putting on a veneer of phony "professionalism." Nor do we expect the client to hold back his criticism or rejection or to soften the story of his pain, so as not to hurt us— remember, this is an asymmetrical relationship, and the client is not here to take care of us. Instead, we encourage him to tell it all, including the parts that may be hard for us to hear. If it stings, we allow ourselves to feel the pain and to be aware of our responses to that pain. Always, our therapeutic intent is the guide to how those responses will be used in the therapeutic process.

## EMPATHY

Frank's comment about self-revelations, quoted in the preceding section, included a word that is perhaps the most common descriptor of what happens in psychotherapy: *empathy*. A therapist's empathic ability is her stock-in-trade; with it, she can understand the client, walk for a moment in his shoes, be truly with him as he does his therapeutic work. Without it, she is doomed to be a step behind, not quite there, not quite getting it. The skill of empathic understanding is a foundation stone for any other technique the therapist may use; it was one of Rogers's (1951) three necessary and sufficient conditions for therapeutic growth, and it is no less important today than it was half a century ago when Rogers was first formulating the client-centered approach. Clearly, this thing called *empathy* is worth looking at more closely.

Strangely, though, the more closely we look at the phenomenon of empathy, the more complicated it gets. Even defining the word is a rather difficult task. Everyone seems to agree that empathy has to do with being able to understand what the other person is experiencing; but, after that, things get rather slippery. From one perspective, empathy seems to be a basic human ability—if not inborn, then acquired very early in life. Small children are sensitive to the moods of others; if you have ever spent time in a nursery, you know that one crying infant can set off the whole room. Empathy is not difficult to achieve; everybody does it. Some people even seem to be hurtfully empathic, using their insight into others as a weapon. "Surely on the highway you have met that other driver who knows exactly what you want to do—change lanes, pass, or turn—and deftly, persistently prevents you from doing it. That is empathy without sympathy" (Shlien, 1997, p. 64). Although we tend to think of empathy as somehow good, it is in fact value-neutral. Like so many other powerful forces, it can be used for good or for ill. As therapists, we may use our empathic skills to encourage, support, and strengthen our clients; we also have the choice of using them to manipulate, coerce, and hurt (MacIsaac, 1997; Orange, 1995).

However it is used, empathy does have to do with one's knowing of another. For some theorists, this knowing is primarily focused on emotion: empathy is the ability to feel, or at least to know, what another person is feeling. For others, cognition is equally important; it is the totality of the other person's internal experience—thoughts, feelings, hopes, and fears—that is sensed through empathy. Orange (1995) sees empathy as going beyond even this sort of thoughts-and-feelings knowing. For her, empathy is a sensing of the other person's deep humanness—of what makes him real and alive and turns him from an object to be analyzed and dissected into a true *other*. "Empathy," she says, "is the knowledge that emerges from personal relation and creates the other as a subject" (p. 21). Empathy is what makes relationship possible; for, until there is an *other*, like myself but separate from me, there can be no relationship. Conversely, relationship is also the source of empathy, informing me about that other and making contact between us. In other words, empathy is both cause and effect, both that which creates relationship and that which is created by relationship.

We should not really be surprised by this duality, for empathy is a creature of the in-between: that numinous realm that defies our efforts to order and quantify. Empathy is found at the border between art and skill; it partakes of both but is limited to neither. Like the nervous impulse that leaps across the synaptic gap, empathy leaps across the chasm that lies between two separate, skin-enclosed entities—perhaps even when one of those entities is not a person at all. "Empathy means, if anything, to glide with one's own feeling into the dynamic structure of an object, a pillar, or a crystal or the branch of a tree, or even an animal or man, and as it were, to trace it from within" (Buber, 1958, p. 97).

## Aspects of Empathy

"Trace" is an active verb, and Martin Buber's poetic description suggests that to be empathic is to actively seek out a sense of the client's world. Indeed, this is one way in which empathic understanding is achieved: inquiring about what the client is thinking, feeling, and sensing. Yet it is not the only way. Those readers who have seen films or videos of Carl Rogers (surely one of the great masters of empathic understanding) working with clients may remember that

Rogers very seldom asked a question in his sessions. He simply received the information that the client chose to share, added his own reaction to that information and to the way in which the client presented it, and gave the result back to the client. Over a series of such transactions, with the client correcting his perceptions and/or using them as a stimulus to further exploration, Rogers and his client together came to develop a growing awareness of the client's world.

Therapeutic empathy is a receptive, supportive, enfolding sort of phenomenon. It takes what the client gives, savors it, cherishes it, and gathers it together with everything else known and sensed about that client. Empathy is also an inquiring, hungering-for-more, moving-out-into-the-client activity. It forms hypotheses, asks questions to test those hypotheses, examines the answers, and extracts every possible bit of information from every response. Empathy can be based on analysis of what the client says, noting his non-verbal signals, thinking our way into understanding. It has also been described as an almost telepathic activity in which a sense of the client is acquired in a rather mysterious fashion, not (yet) amenable to scientific understanding. Empathy is most often thought of as a valuable thing, and to be empathized with is comforting; but, stripped of positive intent, it is value-neutral and can be used to help, to hurt, or to manipulate. Contradictory statements? Yes, and yet each is true. These descriptions mark the boundaries of empathic receiving and responding; they show us the range of activities involving empathy. The most effective empathic behaviors move along and within the whole range, combining aspects of each of the apparent contradictions. Empathy is both art and skill, both rational and mystical, both active and passive. Empathy has many aspects; and, as we develop our empathic skills, we need to remember to use them all.

Tropp and Stolorow (1997) recommend using different words to refer to different aspects of empathy. "We have characterized [therapeutic empathy] as an attitude of *sustained empathic inquiry,* an attitude that consistently seeks to comprehend the meaning of a patient's expressions from a perspective within, rather than outside, the patient's subjective frame of reference. We suggest the restriction of the concept of therapeutic empathy to refer to this distinctive investigatory stance and use some other term, such as *affective responsiveness,* to capture the 'powerful emotional bond between people' that Kohut believed can also produce therapeutic effects" (p. 281). Empathy, for these writers, is primarily a thinking activity, a matter of *comprehending.*

Most of those who talk about "empathy" do not make the distinction that Tropp and Stolorow suggest; they tend to lump together the intellectual (the intent to comprehend the client's world) and the affective (feeling as the client feels). In the real world of therapy, the two cannot be separated: without an internal emotional response, our "sustained inquiry" would be likely to miss the most important parts of the client's messages, and without that sustained inquiry we would have only limited data to stimulate our affective responsiveness. Both are essential; taken together, they create a whole that is greater than either of its parts. As with so many other complex skills, though, we learn to create the whole by looking at the parts; we separate them in order to understand them, even as we recognize that they must ultimately come together again to retain their true identity.

**Attending**   The most basic ingredient in the empathic process is attending: listening to what the client says, noticing what he does. This attending is *purposeful*—we are not simply watching a movie, waiting to see how it unfolds; we are sorting, comparing, and storing for future reference. Our intent is to know what it is like to be inside this skin, behind these eyes, to live in the context of the memories this history has provided and the beliefs these experiences have generated. We are fully and actively involved in the process.

In our attempt to understand in this way, we must take care not to make the client into some "out there" thing, totally separate and distinct from ourselves. We, too, are a part of the equation; our understanding of him is flavored by our own history and expectations. We listen from within. Our own responses are the guide we use to interpret and give meaning to what he says and does. This is *vicarious introspection*—taking into oneself what the client presents and then exploring that internal representation together with our own responses to it (Kohut, 1984); or, as Bacal (1997) puts it, "Empathy effectively constitutes a reading of the analyst's own affects and . . . when we 'empathize' we are always interpreting the effect on our subjectivity of what the patient feels, believes, or does" (p. 670). There is nothing new about this notion; we do it frequently in ordinary social interaction. "If I were you, I would think/feel/want/wonder . . ." is a common response between friends. As therapists, though, we are expected to go beyond this conversational sort of vicarious introspection, constantly sharpening our sensitivity to the nuances of what the client is telling us and to our own responses to the client's message.

According to Tansey and Burke (1989), "It is only by attending to the affective signals coming from within himself that the analyst is able to fathom their hidden meanings and to bring into his own consciousness what the patient is unconsciously communicating about himself through this inductive process" (p. 17). We know more about others and about our relationships with others than we are aware of. Attending to our small internal events, bringing them into awareness, will help us to make conscious (and useful) that which was previously out of awareness. As was mentioned earlier, attending to our own subjectivity also helps us to be clear about which part of our experience has been imported from the client and which is our own. Empathy always involves a certain amount of emotional contagion, but it must also include recognizing that the client is the primary source of the emotional experience (Agosta, 1984). Gelso and Hayes (2001) stress that "it is important that the therapist maintain healthy boundaries between self and patient . . . even though at times these boundaries can become blurred" (p. 421). Confusing the client's and the therapist's responses is one of the most common empathic errors: getting lost in the feelings we are taking on from the client or assuming that, because we are responding in a certain way, the client must be responding that way too. We must always remind ourselves that we are *not* this other person, that—even though we may know him very well and sympathize deeply with his situation—our responses are nevertheless ours and not his, just as his responses are his and not ours.

**Cognitive Understanding**   While affect is perhaps the most common focus of therapeutic empathy, it is not the only aspect of the client's functioning that we are interested in. Greenberg and Elliott (1997) point out that there are various "targets" for our empathic responding and that one very important target is the client's cognitive process. We want to understand *what* clients are thinking and, even more important, *how* they are thinking. We want to trace the way in which they order their thoughts, how they move from one topic to the next, what sorts of ideas they shy away from, and what associations they use to cover or protect themselves. Most of all, we are interested in the basic assumptions that they use to make meaning, to organize their world into familiar categories. These assumptions represent their basic guiding values, standards, or beliefs about self or others.

Empathizing with a cognitive focus requires the same sort of vicarious introspection as affective empathy. We take in the client's words, think about what they mean to us; we ask ourselves how we might come to think like this, where these ideas could have come from, what other beliefs we would need to hold in order to believe this, and how this belief might affect our other thoughts and ideas. Empathic sensitivity to both feeling and thinking involves resonating to the client's feelings and thoughts, finding the part of us that knows how to feel and think that way, adding in our own personal affective and cognitive responses, and then standing back and putting the whole experience into the context of the client's ongoing story.

**Contagion versus Distance**   Good empathic listening entails a kind of back-and-forth quality, an oscillation between attending to what is going on inside oneself and what is happening to the client. At one extreme of this oscillation is *emotional contagion,* being swept away in the client's experience; at the other extreme is an objective, analytic, noninvolved interpretation of that experience. The therapist moves along the continuum created by those two extremes, sometimes more involved in resonating internally to the client's experience and, at other times, more concerned with observing, figuring out, and noticing patterns and connections. Mostly, competent therapists find themselves operating somewhere in the middle range of the continuum: "Ordinary empathic listening entails neither total immersion in the patient's experience nor some kind of distant intellectual reflecting about the patient. It requires the maintenance of a certain degree of closeness . . . which enables the analyst to be receptive to affects, states, and moods in the patient so that he may *sense* within himself what the analysand is going through without actually experiencing the patient's experience *in full*" (Bacal, 1997, p. 676).

As Bacal so correctly informs us, empathic understanding does not require that we experience in full what the client experiences. To do so would be countertherapeutic, for it would leave us trapped in the same life script pattern as the client is in, with the same blind spots and the same lack of perspective. Moreover, it would mean that we would be forced to suffer the same emotional pain, with the same intensity, as the client experiences. Who would choose to be a therapist if it meant that kind of punishment? Instead, we sample the client's experience and, at the same time, maintain an awareness of self, using that awareness as a shield against being overwhelmed by what the client is going through. Again, this kind of psychic shielding is not unique to psychotherapy; we use it every time we make ourselves emotionally available to a friend in trouble. We sympathize with the friend and try to understand what he is going through, but we also keep a certain distance. "The reason all of us do not walk around perpetually being taken over by the affects broadcast by others in our environment," says Nathanson (1996), "is that we build what I call an 'empathic wall' that allows us to maintain our personal boundaries in society" (p. 14). Some of us build thicker "empathic walls" than others; some walls are so thick that very little empathy is possible, while others are far too thin and their owners far too vulnerable to emotional contagion. Needless to say, we therapists strive for a middle range, thick enough to protect ourselves from the intensity of the client's pain, yet thin enough for us to truly understand his experience. For Bacal (1997), *understanding* is the key to maintaining this middle range. By stepping back from the raw experience—the flood of feeling—and attempting to understand what is happening (to the client, and to ourselves as well), we can create a "certain psychical distance" that simultaneously protects and informs us (p. 681).

## Conveying Empathy

Thus far, we have been focusing on the receptive aspects of empathy: the ways in which a therapist comes to understand and—to a lesser degree—share in the client's experience. If empathy stopped there and only involved the therapist's internal knowing of the client, it would be of limited therapeutic value. Empathy comes alive in the therapy hour as the client becomes aware of the therapist's understanding and sharing. Our job as therapists is not only to understand but also to let the client know that we understand. Kohut is quoted by Warner (1997) as pointing out that "empathy is never by itself supportive or therapeutic. It is, however, a necessary precondition to being supportive or therapeutic. In other words, even if a mother's empathy is correct and accurate, even if her aims are affectionate, it is not her empathy that satisfies her child's . . . needs. Her actions, her responses to the child do this" (p. 130).

How does the therapist let the client know that she does understand? This is accomplished in a variety of ways. One of the most important of these is the therapist's spontaneous, nonverbal responses. As she listens to the client, and takes in what he is sharing with her, the therapist responds emotionally; that emotional response has physiological correlates that show up in her posture, facial expression, and respiration—therapists, like their clients, are constantly giving off signals about what is happening inside themselves. Clients read those signals (sometimes accurately, sometimes not), just as therapists read their clients' body language. The first answer to "How do we convey empathy?" then, is "automatically." We don't have to work at it; it simply happens. The therapist's body lets the client know what kind of impact he is having on her.

Body language is good for conveying emotional information; it is less useful for cognitive information. To convey thoughts and ideas, we most often turn to words. One of the first skills that beginning therapists are expected to acquire is that of paraphrasing: giving back to the client in one's own words what the client has just said. The most effective paraphrases are built upon empathy: they include not only the literal information the client has given but also reflect the therapist's awareness of the emotional context of the information, and her own response to that awareness. By giving such a paraphrase—assuming that it is accurate—the therapist does convey her understanding, does communicate empathy.

Other sorts of verbal responses, too, let clients know that the therapist is exploring with him, a partner in his discovery of self. Greenberg and Elliott (1997) discuss five forms of empathic responding. The first of these, *understanding,* is essentially the sort of paraphrasing we have been talking about; it includes sharing the therapist's sense of what the client is saying, and descriptions of her own responses or experiences that are similar to those of clients. The second, *evocation,* involves comments that take the client more and more deeply into his current experience. The therapist must be in some kind of synchrony in order to do this successfully. She begins with the client's current experience and helps him to enhance and intensify it; the success of her efforts will depend in large part on the accuracy of her understanding of the client's starting point.

Next on Greenberg and Elliott's list is *exploration,* going with the client into new areas of awareness. Again, one cannot help someone explore unless one is with him on the journey; in order to suggest where to look next, the therapist must be close enough to see what the client sees right now. Exploration and evocation require an emotional resonance to the client's experiencing, in order to both follow and lead him further into himself. *Conjecture,* the fourth form of empathic responding, involves the therapist sharing her hunches about what the client is experiencing. Many different explanations exist for these sorts of hunches; intuition, gut feeling, and subliminal perceptions are just a few. Wherever they come from, they are based on the therapist's sensed but not fully understood response to the client's behavior. The therapist is never completely certain of their accuracy—she does not know for sure that the client just experienced a momentary wave of sadness or that he was irritated by something she just said or distracted by thoughts of something quite unrelated to the therapeutic conversation. But she *senses* it, and she shares that sense with the client, not as a demonstration of her ability to read his mind but as a caringly curious "Did this just happen with you?"

The final item on the list is *interpretation,* and—to the authors' way of thinking—it should be surrounded by large signs reading "Danger!" and "Beware!" Interpretation involves pointing out patterns and relationships that the client has not yet noticed: that he gets frightened when he talks about his father, for instance, or that he seems to have the same sort of relationship with his children as he has with his students. One of the most obvious dangers in using interpretations is that they may not be correct. When an interpretation is off the mark, the client has the choice of rejecting it (and knowing that the therapist did not really understand) or accepting it (and denying the validity of his own experience). Neither of these is likely to enhance the therapeutic process.

Even when an interpretation is accurate, though, it may not be helpful. Errors in timing, or in judging how deeply a client is willing to look, will render the most accurate interpretation useless—or even harmful. On the other hand, an accurate interpretation, delivered at just the right moment and taking the client just the right distance into his blind spot, can be a most effective conveyor of empathic understanding. Putting together this kind of interpretation is a difficult challenge—thus the "Danger!" and "Beware!" signs.

Interpretations that are less than accurate or are given at the wrong moment can derail the course of therapy. With other expressions of empathy—paraphrases, conjectures, and the like—getting it wrong or making an error of timing is not so hurtful. As Orange (1995) points out, "Often our attempts will be inaccurate, but in the atmosphere of emotional safety provided by our very responsiveness, many patients can use what we offer as a kind of catalyst for their own emotional expression" (p. 128). By the very nature of things, our expressions of empathy cannot be perfectly accurate all of the time; we, and the client as well, are aiming at a moving target, trying to convey in a given moment of time an experience that is constantly changing. We will always be a little off, a little behind where the client is by the time we have finished our comment. Therapeutic errors are inevitable, and acknowledging those errors in a caring way is often highly therapeutic (Guistolese, 1997). If we are *partly* right, if our words and actions come close to the client's experience, his very attempts to refine our understanding will move him into greater awareness of the shifting, moving panorama of his internal landscape.

Empathic understanding and empathic responsiveness lie at the roots of the therapeutic relationship. The various skills of empathy undergird all of the many psychotherapies being practiced today. For some, empathy is a centerpiece, a primary agent of change and growth. For relationship-focused integrative psychotherapists, empathy provides a foundation upon which additional therapeutic activities are built. In one sense, these activities go beyond the traditional definitions of empathy; in another, they are enhancements and intensifications of the empathic process as it operates in a relational context. We have come to categorize these "beyond empathy" therapeutic ingredients as attunement, inquiry, and involvement. We examine them in chapter 6.

## SUMMARY

Good psychotherapy involves both general and specific factors; it is both an art and a science. Artistry and science potentiate each other, creating a series of relational experiences that challenge the client's script and help him to develop a new set of organizing principles with which to understand and deal with his world.

Psychotherapeutic interventions and techniques are most impactful when delivered in the context of an effective therapeutic relationship. To create and maintain such a relationship, the therapist must develop her therapeutic personhood, her ability to listen *with* the client rather than *to* the client, to observe from within the relationship rather than standing outside it. She must make herself emotionally available to the client. To do this, she must cultivate self-awareness.

Psychotherapy is an asymmetrical yet emotionally involved process. The element that distinguishes it from other similarly valenced relationships is therapeutic intent, the consistent commitment of the therapist to the client's welfare.

Empathy, the ability to feel with the client, builds the therapeutic relationship; the relationship, in turn, enhances empathic sensitivity. Empathy can be both active and passive, analytic and receptive. It involves attending, understanding, and some degree of emotional contagion. To have a therapeutic effect, empathy must be conveyed to the client, not simply experienced by the therapist.

# Beyond Empathy | CHAPTER 6

In a previous book, *Beyond Empathy: A Therapy of Contact-in-Relationship* (Erskine, Moursund, & Trautmann, 1999), we characterized the skill of inquiry and the qualities of attunement and involvement as central to effective psychotherapy. Empathy, as discussed in chapter 5, is the foundation for inquiry, attunement, and involvement. Each of the three, however, goes *beyond empathy* in some way—or, at least, beyond the definitions of empathy that one finds in the literature. It is likely that truly empathic therapists are also skilled inquirers, sensitively attuned to their clients and appropriately involved in the therapeutic process. If so, then attunement, inquiry, and involvement are not extensions of empathy so much as subdivisions: aspects or facets of the overall empathic frame within which change and growth are nurtured.

Whichever they are—extensions or subdivisions—attunement, inquiry, and involvement deserve our close attention. To the degree that we can provide them, our therapy is likely to be more effective and satisfying to both our clients and ourselves.

As is true for nearly every other effort to describe or define some important aspect of psychotherapy, discussing attunement, inquiry, or involvement alone requires an artificial and unrealistic teasing apart of what is essentially indivisible. Inquiry without attunement and involvement is sterile and inquisitorial; involvement and attunement without inquiry have no sense of direction or purpose. All three, moreover, are useful only when they are guided by what we have called *therapeutic intent:* a commitment that the client's growth and healing take priority over anything else that may happen in the therapy session.

## ATTUNEMENT

Attunement involves sensitizing oneself to the client and responding accordingly. Empathy, as we have seen, is a kind of "vicarious introspection" (Kohut, 1977), in which the therapist understands the client by finding something akin to the client's responses within herself. Attunement involves using both conscious and out-of-awareness synchronizing of therapist and client process, so that the therapist's interventions fit the ongoing, moment-to-moment needs and processes of the client. It is more than simply feeling what the client feels: it includes recognizing the client's experience and moving—cognitively, affectively, and physically—so as to complement that experience in a contact-enhancing way.

In this sense, attunement is not a subdivision of empathy but does extend the concept:

> Attunement goes beyond empathy: it is a process of communion and unity of interpersonal contact. It is a two-part process that begins with empathy—sensitive to and identifying with the other person's sensations, needs, or feelings; and includes the communication of that sensitivity to the other person. More than just understanding or vicarious introspection, attunement is a kinesthetic and emotional sensing of the other—knowing their rhythm, affect and experience by metaphorically being in their skin, and going beyond empathy to create a two-person experience of unbroken feeling connectedness by providing reciprocal affect and/or resonating response. (Erskine, 1998a, p. 236)

The attuned therapist leads by following. Her interventions often feel, to the client, more like confirmations than questions: they direct his attention to what he is ready to know but has not yet quite realized. She anticipates and observes the effects of her behavior on the client; she decenters from her own experience in order to focus on the client's process. Yet she also is aware of her own internal responses, her thoughts, feelings, and associations. She is *multitasking,* simultaneously following both the client and herself, as well as noting the intricate interactions between self and other. She communicates this synchrony; with body language and voice tone as much as (or more than) with words, she weaves a fabric of understanding and concern and, at the same time, conveys her belief in the client's ability to grow and change. "I know where you are," she seems to be saying, "and we will travel from there together."

To the degree that the therapist is attuned to the client and conveys that attunement, the client feels respected. "This therapist not only understands me—she's really *with* me! Maybe the things I'm thinking/feeling/doing/wanting aren't so hopeless after all." Attunement conveys interest, as well: one of the ways we know if people care about us is by their interest, understanding, and involvement; their close attention to our story; and their acknowledgment of our needs and wants.

Respect and interest, in turn, create a climate of safety. The therapist who respects me won't turn on me, laugh at me, be disgusted by me. She is interested enough to take the time and make the effort to understand, all the way through, what I am trying to say; she won't leap to the wrong conclusions and steer me in a wrong direction. It's okay to be here, okay to be who I am, okay to (maybe, just a little) let the defenses down and peek at the things I really haven't wanted to see.

A client who feels respected and secure in the presence of his therapist can get on with the primary aim of therapy: reclaiming that which has been closed off, healing that which has been fragmented, making both internal and external contact where contact has been interrupted. Attunement reaches beyond the client's concern with an immediate problem, down into the hopes and fears and beliefs that keep the problem from being fully solved. Attunement encourages the client to come to grips with those deep hopes, fears, and beliefs, to explore them and update them in the light of more recent learnings. And attunement provides a constant invitation to contact, a gentle but firm and dependable "I'm here" when the client is feeling overwhelmed and hopeless.

We note one last benefit of attunement: when the therapist does get it wrong and makes that inevitable error, her previous level of attunement will ease the process of re-synchronizing and re-establishing a climate of trust. The general level of attunement sensitizes the therapist to the client's reaction to having been missed and allows her to catch her error quickly, acknowledge it, and request clarification. Acknowledging and apologizing for an error are usually, in fact, another demonstration of attunement; when the therapist goes off the track, what the client most needs and wants is that she admit it, apologize, and re-establish contact (Guistalese, 1997).

Attunement comes in many varieties, for there are many aspects of the client's experience with which to be in tune. We have found it convenient to attend particularly to five areas of attunement: affective, cognitive, developmental, rhythmic, and relational (i.e., attunement to relational needs). We consider each in turn.

## Affective Attunement

Most therapists are trained to be aware of, and even encourage, clients' affect. We learn to be comfortable with our clients' tears, anger, fear, and (strangely, often the most difficult for us) joy. We help clients to deepen their affect (or heighten it, depending on whose vocabulary is being used) and to access emotional responses that they had previously closed off and hidden from others and even from themselves. Our ability to respond empathically helps clients to do this affective work. We have talked a lot about empathy already; so what does *affective attunement* add?

In an empathetic response, the therapist feels what the client is feeling. She metaphorically crawls inside the client's skin and shares the client's affective experience. The affectively attuned therapist goes beyond empathy, meeting the client's affect with her own personal and genuine affective response (Erskine, Moursund, & Trautmann, 1999).

Moreover, affective attunement requires that the therapist attend not only to the emotion itself but also to the message being sent by the emotional display. Emotion is a two-person phenomenon; it is a way of communicating with others who are present physically or in fantasy. Attunement—being in resonance with the client—allows us to distinguish between, for example, tears that plead "please take care of me and make things better" and tears that say "I'm ashamed to be so upset about this" and to respond appropriately.

An attuned response, by the way, is really a three-stage phenomenon, although the stages may follow each other so rapidly that they are difficult to distinguish. The first stage of an attuned response is that of noticing, recognizing, and empathizing with the client's affect: the client's eyes fill with tears, for example, and the therapist recognizes and sympathizes with the client's sadness. The second stage involves the therapist's internal reaction: perhaps first one of vicariously feeling the client's emotion, or a less intense echo of it, and then moving to her uniquely personal response to that emotion. Recognizing that the client is sad, the therapist finds herself feeling compassionate, wishing she could make things better, and at the same time glad that the client's sadness is finally breaking through the defensive barrier that has kept him stuck and miserable for so long. Finally, the third stage of the therapist's response is what she communicates to the client. She may simply reflect that the client looks sad, or she may share some of her own feelings—or she may simply wait quietly or hold out her hand in a gesture of comfort.

Affective attunement is achieved in a variety of ways. The first of these is simply attending to the cues that signal an emotional response in our clients. It is easy to get so caught up in the content of the client's story or in our eagerness to find a solution to his problem, that we fail to notice the tiny facial, gestural, or voice tone changes that often accompany a feeling response. It is equally easy to attend just to the display of affect and ignore the message that the emotion is sending. When we make either of these errors, the usual result is that the affect goes underground: the client either decides that it was inappropriate (because we didn't validate it) or that we are insensitive and therefore not safe to be emotionally vulnerable with. Not only is the current opportunity lost, but we may have to prove ourselves all over again before regaining our clients' trust.

Lee (1998) has suggested that emotional tuning in between two individuals involves one person unconsciously imitating the other's facial expression and in so doing setting up a similar affective response in oneself. Affectively attuned therapists probably do some of this sort of unconscious imitation, but the imitation quickly gives way to a more authentic and personal response to what has been sensed in the client. Tuning in to oneself is as important as tuning in to the client; internal contact combines with external contact to take affective attunement an important step beyond empathy.

Some internal responses to someone else's feelings, of course, may not be therapeutic. Partners who become enraged at each other or parents who are either overcritical or overprotective of their children may be observing the other person's emotion quite accurately and responding to it quite authentically—and

**Figure 6.1** | Reciprocal Responses and Actions Demonstrating Affective Attunement

| Client's Emotion | Reciprocal Affective Response | Reciprocal Action |
|---|---|---|
| Sadness | Compassion | Silence; facial expression; words of acceptance or comfort |
| Anger | Respect; openness to be impacted | Take client seriously; be impacted |
| Fear | Sense of wishing to protect | Activate clinical skills that assist client to deal with fear |
| Joy | Pleasure; share the feeling | Express pleasure (not to exceed that of client) |

hurting the other person in doing so. For affective attunement to be therapeutically useful, it must be combined with therapeutic intent and with clinical competence. Therapeutic intent keeps us focused on the client's welfare, and competence helps us to understand what sorts of things the client may need from us at any given moment and how to create a response to that need. Together, therapeutic intent and clinical competence provide a framework for our internal response to the client, ensuring (in most cases) that that response will be helpful—or at least not destructive.

Each general class of affect seems to call for a certain kind of reciprocal response, whether the responder be a therapist or someone else in close relationship to the "sender" of the emotional message (see Figure 6.1). Sadness, for example, requires compassion—not a gushy, "oh you poor thing" sort of sympathy but a genuine sorrow that the other person is in pain. Anger involves a request to be taken seriously: the attuned therapist will attend, will be respectful, will not make light of or try to diffuse or explain things away. Anger is a serious thing; and, to take it seriously, the therapist must see the world from the perspective of the angry client and allow herself to be impacted by his anger. It is not necessary that she too feel angry, but it is certainly unhelpful (and relationally destructive) to be amused by or frightened of what the client is experiencing.

The most appropriately attuned therapeutic response to a client's fear is a sense of protectiveness. This does not mean that the therapist acts to protect the client—in most cases, such behavior would get in the way of the client's working through his fear—but, rather, that the impulse to protect is stirred in her. The impulse to protect stems from the therapist's sensitivity to the nuances of the client's feelings. Taking those feelings seriously, she is roused to activate her clinical skills, to figure out what sort of intervention will be most useful in helping the client deal with his fear; her efforts also convey to him that she is contact-available, that she has received and is responding to his message.

We have talked about the three most common uncomfortable affects; what about the pleasant ones? How do we appropriately attune ourselves to a client's feelings of happiness, joy, or triumph? Here, the answer is simple: share them. Feel the joy ourselves—but slightly less intensely than the client does. It is the client's joy, not ours; the client leads and we follow (Erskine, 1998b).

## Cognitive Attunement

Humans are thinking creatures. How we experience our world is largely determined by how we think about it, by what meanings we make of it. A given event can be experienced as amusing, frightening, boring, or exciting; watch people emerging from a carnival "fun house" and you will see variants of all of those reactions. Our emotions do affect how we think, to be sure, but equally strong is the effect of our thoughts on how we feel. Cognitions, says Lee (1998), interact with affects so as to magnify or attenuate the affective processes (p. 145). We can talk ourselves out of experiencing a strong emotion ("I just won't think about it; it really isn't so bad; I'll feel better in the morning") or, as Ellis and the rational emotive therapists (Ellis, 1997) are fond of pointing out, we can "awfulize" a situation and make ourselves feel intensely bad about it.

Cognitive attunement involves understanding and temporarily borrowing the process by which a client makes meaning—not only as those meanings affect his emotions but as they affect his whole way of making internal and external contact. How does he "sort out" his world? How clearly does he distinguish between his various perceptions, suppositions, and memories? How does he go about solving problems—or avoiding them? What are the rules that determine what he allows himself to think about, and what is forbidden ground? In *Beyond Empathy: A Therapy of Contact-in-Relationship* (Erskine, Moursund, & Trautmann, 1999), we described cognitive attunement in this way:

> Cognitive attunement is more than simply attending to content. It is not the same as "understanding the client's cognitions" because it goes beyond simple understanding. It involves attending to the client's logic, to the process of stringing ideas together, to the kinds of reasoning that the client uses in order to create meaning out of raw experience. It's about *what* the client is thinking; but more importantly, about *how* the client is thinking it. As we attune to the client's cognitions, we enter the client's cognitive space, moving into a kind of resonance with the client and using our own thoughts and responses as a sounding board to amplify the tiny cues that the client is giving. We bring the client's words and nonverbal expressions into ourselves; take on their meanings, implications, connections; experience this way of thinking ourselves in a kind of internal "as if." (p. 54)

Just as affective attunement requires a kind of alternation between attending to the client's affect and attending to our own affective response, so cognitive attunement requires that we alternate between the client's way of thinking and our own. We adopt the client's thought process, as closely as we are able, in order to see the world through his eyes, experience its events as he does, discover what it is like to live with his blind spots and his defenses. However, we cannot allow ourselves to stay in that place; it is the contrast between his cognitive process and our own that allows us to note those distortions and defenses. Without such a contrast, we would be as blind to his process as he is, and as unable to imagine any other way of thinking. We move back and forth, thinking about the client's frame of reference, then thinking within that frame of reference, then thinking about what it was like to be within it.

Because we are attuned to the client's cognitive process, we can better understand and respond to what he is trying to tell us. Indeed, sometimes we will understand even before he spells it out: thinking in the same way, we often know where he is going and what conclusions he may reach. With the trust and the sense of safety that comes from being understood in this way, the client is increasingly open to pushing the boundaries, both by exploring new areas on his own and through our invitations and suggestions that he review a memory, consider a possibility, or examine an interaction.

Sometimes, of course, we will be wrong. Cognitive attunement can never be perfect; we can never fully enter into another person's stream of thought. We must constantly remind ourselves that our understanding of the client's cognitive world is a hypothesis, not a fact, and that our trying on of his meaning-making process is an experiment that requires validation from the client himself before it can be fully trusted. If we do get it wrong, the most important thing we can do is acknowledge our error and ask the client to help us get back on track. Sometimes these sorts of error-and-correction sequences are extraordinarily helpful: they signal our therapist's willingness to respect the client's wisdom and to admit our own fallibility, and they invite the client into a process of shared exploration in which he and we each make a uniquely valuable contribution (Guistolese, 1997).

## Developmental Attunement

"In all therapies, including psychoanalysis and psychodrama," write James and Goulding (1998), regression occurs whether it is planned by the therapist or client or whether it is spontaneous" (p. 16). Regression has been defined in a variety of ways; for our purposes, we define it as a return to patterns of thinking, feeling, and/or behaving that were present for the client at an earlier time in his life. It occurs not only in psychotherapy but in daily life: whenever we find ourselves responding as we did in a previous developmental period, we have regressed. Regression is a common phenomenon; it occurs most often under stress but may also be observed during states of childlike joy or excitement.

Psychotherapeutically, regression is of interest when it represents a fall-back to old patterns of dealing with the world, patterns that were learned earlier in life and remain available to us when our current strategies are not working. The therapist may invite a client to regress ("take yourself back to a time when . . .") in order to facilitate discovering what those old patterns are and how they relate to the client's current difficulties. Other therapeutic regressions may be spontaneous, a response to the "safe emergency" (Perls, 1973) of the therapy session. The client may be aware that he has regressed and, indeed, be actively cooperating in achieving and maintaining the regression, or may be quite unaware of it. In either case, it is important that the therapist be attuned to the level of regression and respond accordingly. We refer to this sort of attunement as *developmental attunement* because it requires sensitivity to the developmental level to which the client has returned, cognitively or emotionally or behaviorally.

Depending upon one's theory of psychotherapy, regression may be seen as useful, as irrelevant, or as an impediment to achieving the client's goals. Therapists who take a strict behavioral or cognitive behavioral position are likely to discourage regression, seeing it as interfering with the client's ability to evaluate, problem solve, and follow through on a plan for change. Others, more psychodynamically oriented, believe that regression is useful in that it allows clients to access defended memories and experience otherwise forbidden affect. We believe that the value of regression depends upon when and how it occurs and how the therapist chooses to use it. Contact is the key here: a regression in which contact between client and therapist is lost (usually because the therapist is still responding to a here-and-now adult client rather than to a psychologically younger person) is likely to interfere with the therapeutic process. In contrast, the client who experiences the therapist's contactfulness throughout a regression is likely to feel deeply understood. Developmental attunement helps us to maintain contact with a regressed client, and either invite him back to a more here-and-now appropriate level of functioning or support his continuing regressive experience.

Recognizing that a client has regressed and identifying the level to which that regression has taken him are essential for maintaining contact. Using adult language with and expecting adult responses from someone who is experiencing the world the way a 4- or 8- or 12-year-old does, is not likely to enhance the client's sense of connectedness or trust. Children, like adults, yearn to be understood; the phenomenological child that is the product of a client's regression wants to be seen and heard and respected, not ignored or missed altogether. How, then, can we recognize and identify a client's level of regression? How can we keep ourselves developmentally attuned?

Obviously, in order to attune oneself to a client's developmental level, one must have a sense of what that level is. Eric Berne (1961) has suggested four ways in which a therapist can assess the client's developmental level of functioning. The first of these is the *client's own phenomenology*. We may ask the client how old he is feeling at this moment, or the client may spontaneously report a regression: "I feel like a five-year-old," or "I'm scared, just like when my Dad used to come home drunk." A second aid to identifying regression and maintaining developmental attunement is the therapist's awareness of the *client's unique developmental history*. If we know that the client was raped when she was in high school, or that he was sent to live with his grandmother when he was 10 years old, it can help us to interpret the meaning of verbal and nonverbal communications and of the developmental level from which they spring. We can also call upon our general *understanding of child development* to relate the client's current behavior to behaviors typical of a younger stage; and it behooves us to have a good knowledge of the typical stages and phases through which young children move. This is particularly important when the client is regressing to a relatively early stage of life and his ability (and desire) to communicate verbally may be limited.

Probably the most important set of guidelines, though, comes from our own intuitive, *emotional response* to the client's behavior. How old does the client *feel* to us? What sort of younger person seems to be looking out of his eyes? If we put to one side the adult body in front of us, what seems to be the most natural way of responding to what he is doing and saying? We are often able to pick up tiny cues, cues of which we are consciously unaware, from the nonverbal behavior of our clients; such cues can aggregate out of our awareness and make themselves known as a general hunch about how to respond most effectively. Spending time with children—learning to interact with them at their level and sensitizing ourselves to our own reactions to them—is a good way to hone our ability to attune in this way.

Developmental attunement, if it is to be useful, must be communicated. You may know that your client is, at this moment, seeing the world and responding to it as he did when he was a toddler; but this knowledge will be of little use unless the client feels your understanding and your support. At the same time, the client also needs to know that you are aware of the adult, here-and-now self who is also participating in the process. Maintaining attunement with a regressed client requires a kind of therapeutic "double vision," an ability to recognize and acknowledge both the regressed-to-childhood (or adolescence, or young adulthood) person and the self-observing adult. Both are present, both require contact, and both play an important part in the client's growth.

One of the most potent ways to maintain developmental attunement is to use the client's own language and language patterns. As he regresses, his vocabulary is likely to shift too; the developmentally attuned therapist shifts with him. If the therapist senses that the client is moving into the psychological world of a 6-year-old, she talks to him as she would to a 6-year-old. Her own body language is keyed to his: not imitating it, but responding to it as an adult responds physically to a child. The therapist can facilitate a client's regression by encouraging childlike gestures and movements; conversely, she can invite him out of the regression by requesting that he assume a more adult posture and by using adult language and phrasing in her responses to him.

We have found, over years of working with clients, that therapeutic regression is a powerful tool in enhancing contact with self and, eventually, with others as well. It is useful in overcoming the unconscious defenses that prevent full awareness of thoughts, feelings, and memories. We have more to say about this in chapter 9, when we talk about specific therapeutic interventions. For now, though, suffice it to say that developmental attunement is the single most vital factor in developing and therapeutically facilitating a client's regression. Without developmental attunement, regressions are likely to be short-lived and therapeutically sterile; with it, they can lead to the corrective emotional experience that lies at the heart of a relationship-focused integrative psychotherapy.

## Rhythmic Attunement

In a sense, it is odd to give rhythmic attunement a special section of its own, since attuning to the client's rhythm is an essential aspect of cognitive, affective, and developmental attunement. When we are out of synch with the client's rhythm and timing, he will not experience us as being attuned in any other way. But there are some particularly interesting aspects of rhythmic attunement, and dealing with it as a separate topic is one way to make sure we talk about those aspects.

The term "rhythmic attunement" really defines itself: being sensitive to and responding within the client's rhythmic patterns. Rhythm is one of the primary ways in which people, out of awareness, assess the quality of their contact with each other. When two people are rhythmically attuned, their transactions mesh together easily. Their silences are comfortable; there is no competition for who will speak when. Even when they interrupt each other, it is as if one of them is stimulated by the other's thought, and the interruption does not jar or derail their process. In contrast, when they are not attuned rhythmically, their conversation is jerky and their silences strained. Neither is likely to feel at ease with the other, though they often cannot explain their discomfort.

In ordinary conversations, each person is responsible for adapting to the other's rhythm, maintaining a pacing and style that is comfortable for both. In therapy, the primary responsibility for attunement falls to the therapist. The therapist must attune to the client, not the other way around; expecting the client to match the therapist's rhythm will force him into an artificial way of speaking, thinking, and feeling that will interefere with his work. Tuning in to and matching a client's rhythm requires, first, that the therapist attend to that rhythm and how it may differ from her own. Does the client use long pauses to collect his thoughts, and is the therapist impatient with those pauses? Or does he jump from idea to idea, illustrating his words with quick gestures and appearing uneasy if the therapist speaks slowly or has to search for words?

We can relatively easily (at least in theory) slow ourselves down to attune to the rhythm of a client who is processing his experience more slowly than we ordinarily do. Speeding ourselves up to match a rhythmically rapid client is more difficult: how can we think and feel faster, without losing important information? Rather than try to push ourselves to keep up and risk distorting or disrupting contact with ourselves and/or the client, it is best for us to acknowledge the differences and openly request time to digest what the client has been telling us: "You are moving through these ideas very quickly, and I don't want to miss anything. Give me a moment to think about what you've been telling me. . . ."

While individuals do develop their own unique rhythms, some general rhythmic patterns seem to hold for nearly everyone. Most of these involve slowing down rather than speeding up. A major goal of therapy is to attend to what has been overlooked and to explore what has been defended against, and this generally requires that we move more slowly than usual; indeed, racing along from one association to the next is a way to *not* notice things and *not* feel one's feelings. One of the paradoxes of our work is that slowing down is likely to speed up the therapeutic process, while going too fast is likely to slow the client's overall progress.

Affective work, in general, proceeds at a slower pace than cognitive work. It is not that we experience emotions more slowly than we think—quite the contrary; emotions spring up quickly and can shift and move with lightning speed. A loud, unexpected noise can create an immediate startle-scare feeling; it takes no time at all to experience tenderness and love when we look at our infant grandchild; but putting those feelings into words can be a slow and laborious process. Talking about feelings requires translation from a global, wordless experience, mediated primarily through body chemistry, to a linear, verbal process. Moreover, many clients have trained themselves to *not* attend to their feelings, and they accomplish this by rushing past them, moving on to a new thought. Giving such clients permission to slow down, so that they can feel and think and talk about their internal experience, will further their ability to make and maintain full contact with themselves and with others.

Developmental level—regression—also affects one's rhythm, and developmentally attuned therapists recognize that as clients move to younger and younger psychological levels, their rhythms tend to slow. Indeed, a slowing of rhythm may be a major indicator that the client is regressing. Just as we tend to talk more slowly to a young child, the therapist needs to attune herself to the slower rhythm of the client who is at this moment experiencing the world from a younger, less verbally sophisticated place.

Reviewing what we already know is easier than exploring what is unknown; clients who exhibit a quite rapid pace when sharing well-rehearsed material are likely to slow down as they begin to explore new thoughts and previously walled-off emotions. Just as if they were feeling their way around a dark and unfamiliar (and often frightening) room, they need to take time to find out what is there and to examine it fully. They need time to integrate the new with the old, to figure out how their discoveries fit with the familiar and comfortable parts of themselves that they have known about all along.

For all of these reasons, errors in rhythmic attunement are much more likely to involve going too fast rather than going too slowly. As therapists, we pride ourselves on being quick to understand, being good at putting things together; we have been rewarded throughout our schooling for coming up with right answers quickly. Now we need to put that skill to one side, slow ourselves down, and slip gently into the client's rhythm of speaking and moving. When we do so, the client is likely to feel joined, met, in contact. Our matched rhythms will create a sense of moving together; the need for lengthy explanations will decrease; the client will feel protected by our willingness to be together in his way.

Rhythmic attunement extends beyond the sort of transaction-by-transaction rhythms that we have been discussing. People differ in the length of time they are comfortable in spending on one topic, one idea, before moving on to the next. They differ in the amount of "warm-up" time they need at the beginning of a session before moving into full contact with themselves and with the thera-pist. There are even differences in rhythm over much longer periods of time: clients often differ in the length of time they need between sessions to process their work. Some do best with shorter sessions, more frequently spaced; others prefer longer sessions at greater intervals. The weekly, 50-minute session is con-venient for the therapist, but it may not match the client's rhythm (Efron, Lukens, & Lukens, 1990). If a client would benefit by changing the length or frequency of his sessions, it is advisable to do so; when such changes are not pos-sible, the therapist can at least acknowledge the client's need. If the therapist lets the client know that she recognize his preferred rhythm, and shares her reasons for not adapting to that preference, the absence of attunement here will be less jarring.

As noted at the beginning of this section, rhythmic attunement flows through all of the other aspects of attunement. For the client to experience cognitive, developmental, or affective attunement, the therapist must be oper-ating within that client's rhythm—his rhythm is a part of his cognition, his affect, and his developmental level.

Verbal and nonverbal messages sent by the therapist are like the instru-mental voices of a symphony. When one or more of those voices is off tempo, the whole performance sounds wrong. Moreover, just as listeners respond to one piece of music or another depending on the state or mood they find them-selves in, so the clients will respond differently to different therapist "sym-phonies" depending on their own state—dealing with affect or cognition, regressed or not, energized or fatigued, and so on. It is no accident that a musi-cal metaphor like this fits with the notion of "*attune*ment." Hearing all of the nuances of the client's melody and rhythm, and responding from and with the harmony of one's whole therapeutic orchestra, verbally and nonverbally, is what attunement is all about.

## Attunement to Relational Needs

In chapter 3, we introduced the notion of relational needs: those needs that arise in the context of a relationship. When I need something from you, some particular kind of response or behavior, I am experiencing a relational need. Not surprisingly, clients have relational needs in therapy, needs to which they want their therapist to respond. Some of these needs can be met by the thera-pist, and some can—or should—not. Whether or not the therapist chooses to meet her client's relational need, she must still acknowledge and respect it; to do so, she must be attuned to the way in which that need comes up for and is expressed by the client.

Therapists, too, of course, experience relational needs, and sometimes we find ourselves needing/wanting something from our clients. If we didn't, our relationship would be sterile and superficial: choosing to be contactful and real in our therapeutic relationships guarantees that we will sometimes have feel-ings about our clients, emotional reactions to them, and will want them to think and feel and behave toward us in certain ways. However, being attuned to and responding appropriately to *their* relational needs will often require that we put our own wants and needs to one side. Callaghan, Naugle, and Folette (1996) warn us that even when the therapist is expressing appropriate feelings, the client may misunderstand or misinterpret what is said. "Therapists must be able to express their reactions and feelings in their interactions with clients while being sensitive to how this impacts the individual clients with whom they work" (p. 387). Attuning to the client's view of us, being sensitive to what he is needing from us at a given moment, helps us to make sound decisions about sharing our own inner experience.

The client's needs come first. If sharing her own feelings will serve the client's interest, the therapist may choose to do so. If decentering from her needs and wants, and focusing on the client, is the most growth-enhancing choice, that is the choice the therapist should make. Note, though, that focusing on the client's needs is not the same as trying to meet those needs. Whether or not to act so as to actually meet a client's relational need will be determined by a host of factors. The client's developmental history, the availability of other social support in his life and the way in which he uses that support, the nature of the need itself, the point in treatment at which the need is expressed, the way in which it is expressed—all of these enter into the therapist's clinical judgment about what sort of intervention will best serve the client's interests. Let us review the eight major relational needs described in chapter 3, looking at how each need might arise and manifest itself in the therapy session and exploring some of the therapist responses that may be helpful.

**Security**    The need for security in relationship is the most basic of all relational needs. The client needs to know that his therapist is trustworthy and competent and has his best interests at heart; but beyond that he needs the visceral experience of having his physical and emotional vulnerabilities protected. He needs to know that he will be neither humiliated nor pathologized as he begins to reveal his most secret thoughts and feelings. The need for relational security is most likely to be foreground at the outset of treatment, when the client may be ambivalent about the whole process and does not yet know much about this therapist in whom he is expected to confide. Once the therapist has established herself as worthy of the client's trust, the security need tends to recede into the background. It will arise again if the therapist makes a mistake or if old issues around trust and safety are being explored. Rather than being expressed directly, the client's need for security is most often signaled by his drawing back from contact: coming late for sessions or canceling them altogether; becoming quiet or talking about superficial matters; misunderstanding or accusing or blaming the therapist for things that happen both in and out of session.

A client's security needs must always be attended to, for little substantive work can be accomplished if the client does not feel safe in the therapeutic relationship. However, direct reassurances will be of little value. "I want this to be a safe place for you to work" or "I will never do anything to hurt you" can be mere empty words to a client who is feeling unsafe. Acknowledging the client's concern—along with our own desire to allay his fears and our recognition that words alone will not suffice—is generally helpful. Even more important is attuning and responding appropriately to all of his other relational needs: over time, this is the behavior that will demonstrate that the relationship is, indeed, safe for him.

**Valuing**   The client's need for valuing, you will recall from chapter 3, has to do with valuing the significance and function of his psychological processes—the *why* of what he does and says, more than the actual behavior. This sort of valuing is conveyed through the therapist's contactful presence, and through her respectful attention to and interest in the client's phenomenology. Rather than focusing on the client's external behaviors, the therapist talks about those behaviors in the context of the client's ongoing experience within himself and in relationship to others—including the therapist herself. Her conviction that every behavior—every response—serves an understandable and important function allows her to inquire with no hint of criticism or judgment. If the client doesn't seem to make sense, if his behavior seems hurtful or silly, then the therapist (and quite probably the client as well) have simply not yet understood it fully.

While all clients need to feel valued by their therapists, the need for valuing emerges most intensely in the context of shame. Feeling shame about something he has shared, about some part of himself that he has exposed, the client's ability to value himself is undermined; not valuing himself, he imagines that nobody else can value him either. He withdraws, huddles inside himself—or moves into an exaggerated, whistling-in-the-dark sort of pseudoconfidence. Acknowledging and normalizing his need, and the sense of shame that precipitated it, will help him to re-establish contact. Once contact is re-established, he will be more receptive to the therapist's verbal and nonverbal indications that he is indeed valued and respected.

A client who does not experience being valued in his outside-of-therapy relationships may become overly dependent upon the therapist's valuing. He may demand frequent evaluations of his behavior and progress in therapy or may compliment the therapist in the hope of getting some positive stroke in return. Verbal reassurances are generally less than helpful for these clients, since they tend to reinforce the client's dependency; acknowledging the need, engaging the client in exploring its significance, and helping him to find other relationships in which it can be met, is usually a better strategy.

**Acceptance by a Dependable Other**   "The degree to which an individual looks to someone and hopes that he or she is reliable, consistent, and dependable is directly proportional to the quest for intrapsychic protection, safe expression, containment, or beneficial insight" (Erskine, 1998a, p. 239) The need for acceptance by a dependable other is closely related to the need for relational security, but it goes farther: it has to do with our experience not only of the other person's competence but of her genuine willingness to understand and to help. It has to do with being allowed to make the other person special to us, without having to be ashamed of how we feel toward her. When clients experience this need, they want to be with someone from whom they can draw strength, guidance, or wisdom and who will not criticize or belittle them for wanting that kind of support.

The need for this sort of acceptance is sometimes manifested through idealization of the therapist—she is wonderful, she's different from anyone else in my life, I think about her all the time . . . Such idealization is a normal and natural stage through which many clients pass; it is an out-of-awareness request for protection and support, and its function should be respected and valued just as we respect and value every other aspect of the client's behavior.

When the need for acceptance by a dependable therapist is foreground for a client, it is not particularly helpful for the therapist to express her own uncertainty or concerns. At this moment, the client needs her strength, her reliability; he needs her to be a kind of good parent who can be depended upon to care for him with wisdom and skill. "As an example of the crucialness of responding," comments Lee (1998), "when a therapist detects a client's fear, yet responds to this fear in an anxious way, the client experiences the therapist's exacerbating response as unempathic" (p. 130). Although the therapist in this example accurately notes the client's fear, she allows herself to be contaminated by it: she allows her affective attunement to outweigh her attunement to relational needs and thus misses the client's need that she be able to contain his fear rather than share it.

**Mutuality**  Experienced in the therapy session, mutuality is the need to be with a therapist who has shared one's experiences: She *really* understands, because she has been there herself, and her acceptance is based on that understanding. Moreover, the client who feels a mutuality with the therapist can experience a sense of "I'm okay, and what I do/think/feel is okay, in part because this person I trust has done/thought/felt the same sort of thing." Clients for whom the need for mutuality is foreground may want their therapist to have had (and dealt with) the same sorts of problems that they have, or to have shared a similar childhood history. The need for mutuality may be expressed through direct questions ("Do you have children too?" "Have you ever lost a job, like I just did?") or through probing comments ("I'm not sure anybody can understand this unless they've been abused themselves." "Straight people don't know what it's like to be gay.")

While a therapist cannot possibly know firsthand everything her clients have gone through, she has had (in reality or in fantasy) similar experiences. When she senses the need for mutuality in a client, it can be useful to talk about herself, her thoughts or feelings or experiences that parallel the client's experience in some way. Meeting the need for mutuality, then, requires a degree of self-revealing; each therapist must decide for herself, on the basis of her personal comfort level as well as of her sense of what will be helpful to the client, how much self-revelation she is willing to provide. To the degree that she does choose to self-reveal, it is essential to acknowledge that she can never know completely what it was/is like for this client, because he is the only person who lives inside of his skin.

Asking personal questions of the therapist is not always a signal that the client is experiencing a need for mutuality. Sometimes this sort of question is used as a smoke screen, a way for the client to avoid dealing with his own painful issues. Even when the mutuality need is foreground, it may not always be in the client's best interest to meet that need; the client may be trying to use his relationship with the therapist as a substitute for satisfying relationships outside of therapy. Nowhere is the need for a discussion of the therapeutic process itself more essential than when dealing with a client's repeated requests that the therapist talk about herself.

**Self-Definition**   *I am me. I can think for myself. My feelings are my own.* The need for self-definition is the need to know and express one's own uniqueness and to receive acknowledgment and acceptance of that uniqueness from others. Many clients come to therapy hungry for validation of their uniqueness. They have been discounted, treated as unimportant or second-best, not allowed to argue or to say "No." They are not so much interested in other people's similar experiences as in having their own experiences attended to. At moments when this need for self-definition arises, therapist self-disclosure is not only irrelevant; it is evidence that the therapist does not understand the client's needs or is not fully invested in the therapeutic relationship. Failure to support the need for self-definition can be a further reinforcement of the client's script belief that he is unimportant and that nobody really cares about him.

As was pointed out in chapter 3, the need for self-definition is the complement of the need for mutuality. A client experiencing the need for mutuality may want to know about the therapist in order to gain a sense of closeness and similarity; when the need is for self-definition, the client needs the focus to be on himself. If the client appears impatient when the therapist shares her own thoughts or feelings, or if he seems to withdraw, the therapist may have misjudged his state of relational need. At such a moment, it is a good idea to shift back, ask him what it's like for him when she talks about herself, and use the exchange as an opportunity to validate his need to be who he is. Encouraging his disagreements with or challenges of the therapist will encourage him to define himself as different and valuable in his own right.

**Making an Impact**   Clients can do a great deal of self-exploration by keeping a journal or by talking into a tape recorder. One problem with this strategy is that the journal or the tape recorder does not answer back—is not impacted by the client's input. Relationships in which one does not experience having an impact on the other person are one-sided if not actually abusive; just as with a thwarted need for self-definition, they foster the belief that one is unimportant and that others don't care. The therapeutic relationship is no exception: just as the therapist, in order to feel valued and competent, needs to feel that her behaviors have an effect on the client, so the client needs to feel that he can make an impact on the therapist—can attract her attention and can influence the way she thinks and/or feels about things that are important to him.

Unlike the "blank screen" therapist model espoused by traditional psychoanalytic theory, relationship-focused integrative psychotherapy insists that the therapist be present as a person, caring about the client, willing to be changed by what happens in the relationship. If she is moved to tears, she allows those tears to show; if she is angry on the client's behalf, the client knows about her anger; if the client corrects her, she is willing to be corrected and to think seriously about what change may be required. If the client demands a greater impact than the therapist is willing or able to allow, she acknowledges his desire and shares her honest response to that desire. Whether the need is actually met, or simply recognized, her acknowledgment is a validation of the legitimacy of the client's need and proof that he does, indeed, have an impact on her.

**Other-Initiation**  When the need for the other to initiate is foreground, the client needs the therapist to do just that: step in and make the first move. He wants her to offer a new idea, suggest a direction, reach out a hand. Sometimes clients will signal this need by closing down and becoming silent, and sometimes they will do the opposite: talk faster, jump from one topic to another, do whatever they think will please the therapist. Clients who are starved for other-initiation expect to be ignored, tolerated, or forced to prove themselves; and that expectation limits and distorts their relationships with others—including their therapist.

"The therapist's willingness to initiate interpersonal contact or to take responsiblity for a major share of the therapeutic work normalizes the client's relational need to have someone else put energy into reaching out to him or her" (Erskine, 1998a, pp. 240–241). There are many ways to accomplish this. In the therapy session, the therapist can break a silence (rather than always waiting for the client to speak), or choose a topic (rather than expecting the client to decide what to talk about), or respond to some nonverbal request (rather than insisting that the client express his needs directly). She can suggest a more frequent appointment schedule or ask her client if he would like a different length session. She can phone him to ask about an important life event that she knows has occurred—a hospitalization, a job change, a public performance. Overdoing this sort of initiation is, of course, countertherapeutic; it can be an invitation to dependency and may constitute a quite unwarranted intrusion into the client's private life. However, when the client's need for the therapist to initiate is genuine, taking that first step can provide a corrective emotional experience that effectively challenges his whole script pattern.

**Expressing Love**  Of all the relational needs that are dealt with in therapy, this is perhaps the most difficult—and how ironic! Expressing love and appreciation—and receiving that expression—should be a joyful experience. When the therapist has been close to the client, seen his confusion and his pain, accepted him and valued him, and helped him to grow and heal, it is only natural that the client should feel loving and appreciative; to stifle such feelings

would be to retreat into phoniness and fragmentation again. Yet, most therapists have been trained to be suspicious and distrustful of their clients' gestures
of affection, always looking for some underlying motivation, some toxic transferential remnant that must be rooted out and done away with.

It is usually not difficult to tell the difference between a manipulation and
a genuine expression of caring. When a client, out of such genuine feeling,
thanks his therapist or tells her how much she has meant to him, or brings her
a gift, she should accept it gracefully and let him see her pleasure. It *does* feel
good to be appreciated; being real in the relationship means enjoying the good
parts as well as being impacted by the bad.

## Attunement Errors

Relational needs shift from moment to moment, and being attuned to those
shifts requires close attention to the client's responses to the therapist's behavior. What begins as an attuned response to, say, the need for mutuality or other-
initiation can change into a failure to deal with the need for self-definition.
Because therapists are human—and imperfect—such misses are inevitable;
when they occur, we simply go back and talk about the miss.

"Go back and talk about it" is good advice for failures in every facet of
attunement. Missing an affective shift, not understanding a cognitive process,
misjudging the client's psychological level of development, moving too quickly
or too slowly—all are bound to occur sooner or later. The therapist who cas-
tigates herself internally for her error, or tries to gloss it over so the client
won't notice that it happened, takes herself away from the client and distorts
the contact between them. This sort of contact distortion, in turn, is likely to
create a repeat for the client of the very kinds of relational experience that support his script and have gotten him into the situation that brought him to therapy in the first place. In contrast, the therapist's acknowledgment of what has
happened and re-attuning (to herself and to the client) allow the therapeutic
process to move on.

## INQUIRY

Of all the things that therapists do, asking questions and listening to the
answers are probably the most common. Questions are asked at all stages of
therapy, from initial diagnosis to the final termination process; and question
asking cuts across all theoretical approaches (though it is a more central activity in some than in others). By "questions," we do not refer just to those sentences that end in a question mark; questions include any sort of intervention
that requests the client to search for information. Replying with an "Oh?" or
a "Hmmm," repeating what the client has just said, lifting an eyebrow or smil-
ing encouragingly, even waiting patiently for what may come next—all of
these are forms of inquiry. Indeed, insofar as the essence of therapy is to help
the client explore his internal world and re-establish contact with self and others, most of what we do as therapists can be seen as a kind of inquiry.

Asking questions is easy. Questions occur naturally in conversations between friends, in consultations with professionals, in the classroom, and in the workplace. Children learn to ask questions as soon as they learn to talk, as anyone who has faced the endless "why" of a preschooler can tell you. Asking questions therapeutically, on the other hand, can be more difficult. It requires, among other things, that we know—and remember—the purpose of our inquiry. Questions can be asked for a variety of reasons: to provide the questioner with some information ("Where do you keep the napkins?"), to continue an argument ("Why won't you let me have the car tonight?"), as an implied criticism ("Why are you watching TV when you have homework?"), or simply to demand attention ("What are you doing, Mommy?"). In relationship-focused integrative psychotherapy, inquiry has but one purpose: to assist clients in expanding awareness, increasing internal and external contact, and enhancing the sense of self-in-relationship.

If the purpose of inquiry is to expand the client's awareness, it follows that what the therapist may learn from the client's answer is secondary. While we certainly listen to the answers to our questions (verbal and nonverbal) and learn from those answers, what the client learns is much more important. Part of the skill involved in therapeutic inquiry is that of getting out of the client's way, postponing our need to understand fully in order not to interrupt his process of discovery. It also follows that the easily answered question, the question to which the client already knows the answer, is generally less valuable than the question that requires him to search for a response. Clients do not learn much from stating what they already know; they learn by being challenged to discover something new. Uncertainty and ambiguity stimulate people to learn more, to solve the problem, and to clarify what is happening. Questions that ask about what is not yet known tend to invite the client into his areas of uncertainty and ambiguity and challenge him to explore those areas. Well-executed inquiry is a spiral process, with each response leading to a new question, and each question opening the door to a previously out-of-awareness response.

## Characteristics of Effective Inquiry

The most basic characteristic of therapeutic inquiry is that of respect. The questions the therapist asks, and the way in which she asks them, must be respectful—respectful of the client's needs, of his problem-solving efforts, and of his internal wisdom. Her respect springs from what Rogers (1951) has termed "unconditional positive regard," a fundamental conviction that all clients are doing and have done the best they are capable of at any given moment. Without this kind of respect, inquiry is likely to turn into interrogation, the therapist becomes "she-who-knows-better," and the whole process can disintegrate into advice giving or sermonizing. Respecting the client's wisdom and intentions, in contrast, leads to genuine interest and healthy curiosity about how the client experiences his world. Interest and curiosity, in turn, are vital in helping the therapist to frame the sorts of questions that will further the client's explorations.

Inquiry should be open-ended. The therapist's questions and her questioning behaviors invite the client to search for answers; they do not restrict him or demand that the answers meet the therapist's expectations. Indeed, willingness to abandon expectations and let go of preconceived ideas is another hallmark of successful inquiry. Even though the therapist's theoretical training and clinical experience may lead her to expect a certain kind of answer (and may have suggested her question or comment in the first place), she is glad to be surprised. Getting a response that she did not expect whets her curiosity, pops her out of the rut of the conventional, and allows her as well as her client to discover something new.

Neimeier (1995) recommends "a willingness to use the client's personal knowledge system, to see the problem and the world through his or her eyes, though not necessarily to be encapsulated by it. To this is added . . . a curiosity or fascination with the client's perspective and its implications" (p. 114). The therapist's theoretical and clinical expectations provide a background for this fascination but must not blind her to what the client is really telling her. Open-ended questions help to keep the *therapist* open to learning something new from the client, something not predicted by her past experience.

What does a therapist do when the client tells her something that she finds difficult to believe? When he changes the subject; insists on telling long, rambling stories; or simply says "I don't know" and then waits? These sorts of behavior suggest that the client may be retreating into an old defensive system rather than being honest with himself. The first rule of good inquiry is: do not argue. The therapist should never try to persuade the client that his answer is wrong. How could it be "wrong" when it came from him? It is *his* response, and the therapist's job is to help him understand it. She may express curiosity, or confusion; she may ask him about what he means or what lies behind his response. "You surprised me; help me to understand how you came to that conclusion," "What happened inside, just before you said that?" "How is this story related to the problems you were talking about earlier?"

Inquiry grows out of a constant attention to contact. Its goal is contact enhancement; all of the therapist's questions are designed to help the client establish and maintain contact of some sort. The focus at one point may be on his internal contact ("What are you experiencing?") or at another on his external contact ("Tell me what you are noticing and attending to right now"); often, we deal with the contact between therapist and client ("What's it like for you to hear me say that?"). Contact leads to health and growth, and lack of contact leads to fragmentation, constriction, and shutting down. To the degree that our inquiry promotes the former and moves away from the latter, it will be therapeutic.

## Areas of Inquiry

Attending to contact and remembering that her purpose is to enhance it helps the therapist to construct and frame her inquiry. She must be careful, though, not to neglect one aspect of contact as she pursues another. Therapeutic inquiry is like a web, spun out of many strands; the therapist follow first this strand, then that; but, eventually, all must be woven into the pattern. Let us look, for a moment, at these strands.

One of the most obvious strands is that of affect: therapists are used to asking clients about their feelings, helping clients to explore and deepen their emotional responses. Many clients, though, are relatively closed to affect. They do not know what they are feeling; they have learned to disavow or close off their awareness of painful emotions and do not know how to open those doors. For such clients, inquiring about physical sensations and reactions can be useful. The therapist can invite her client to be aware of his body, and of what his body is doing. Is he breathing shallowly? What does that shallow breathing feel like? Is he aware of a swinging foot or a balled fist? Simply noticing and talking about physical experiences are a first step toward increased contact with self.

Cognition is another natural area of inquiry. What is the client thinking? What are those thoughts connected to, and how does he get from one thought to another? What is he remembering? What decisions is he making, and how is he making them? Thoughts, memories, and decisions (past and present) often weave back into affect, just as affect can take him into thinking and remembering.

Inquiry about fantasies provides another window into the client's phe-nomenological world. Fantasies involve thinking, feeling, and sensation. They are not only the client's daydreams and night dreams; they also include the client's hopes, fears, and expectations. They are his imaginings about what has happened in the past and about what is yet to come. Because they are built upon past experience, experience that has often been blocked from awareness, they can help him re-connect with himself, with long-buried thoughts and feel-ings. Fantasies and expectations determine the way in which he makes and maintains relationships with others, and they shape the therapeutic relation-ship as well. Clients use fantasy to transform painful internal experiencing into that which can be born; to provide substitute gratification of needs that can-not be met in reality; and to manage behaviors that they fear may run out of control. It is a rich vein of information, and mining it can lead to rich rewards.

Finally, and perhaps most important of all, is inquiry related to the thera-peutic relationship itself. As we said in chapter 5, the experience of being in a relationship that is qualitatively different from past, script-forming relation-ships is a key factor in dissolving that script. The impact of this relationship experience is heightened when inquiry is used to call attention to it. Questions like "What are you wanting from me right now?" or "How do you feel about what I just said?" or "What do you think my response would be if you told me the whole story?" invite the client to explore his reactions to what the ther-apist is offering. Is he defending against a level of contact that would be too threatening? He and the therapist can talk about the threat, as well as the means of defense. Does he disagree with, disbelieve, or discount what the ther-apist says? The therapist asks about his disagreement, disbelief, or discount-ing. She is open to the client's criticism, cares about his disbelief, and is interested in the ways in which he supports the discount. She is also interested in how the client experiences her support and concern. She needs the client's feedback in order to maintain and enhance her attunement to him. "Therapists need to continually engage in process diagnosis to determine when and how to communicate empathic understanding and at what level to focus their empathic responses from one moment to the next," advise Greenberg and colleagues (Greenberg et. al., 2001, p. 383). Process diagnosis includes asking about the ongoing relationship as the client experiences it. The therapist inquires about this, just as she inquires about everthing else.

As the therapist improves her inquiry skills, learns to gather up the various strands of experiencing and help the client to explore their interrelationships, she is guided by attunement. She notices the client's rhythms, his thinking and feeling, his developmental level, and his moment-to-moment relational needs. What she notices directs what she asks about and how she does the asking. But there is another element at work here. Therapists are not simply skilled machines, taking in information and forming interventions. The therapeutic process is a relationship, formed in the in-between of two living, thinking, and feeling human beings. The therapist, as well as the client, is involved in that process. Involvement, then, is the third aspect/extention/subdivision of empathy that characterizes relationship-focused integrative psychotherapy.

## INVOLVEMENT

*Involvement* is one of those words that most of us think we understand but that turns out to be very difficult to define. The *involved* therapist is there for her client, present in the relationship, real, honest. She cares what happens to this person, and she is willing to put energy and effort into helping him achieve his goals. She is genuinely interested in this client's intrapsychic and interpersonal worlds and communicates that interest through attentiveness, patience, and respectful inquiry. She risks being vulnerable: she does not insulate herself from contact but, instead, allows herself to be emotionally touched. She does not hide behind a mask of phony professionalism; she lets her caring show, talks about her feelings, and admits to her errors. "By embracing a technique of self-disclosure," says Billow (2000), "the patient may feel the analyst's emotion, without which emotion an authentic analysis is impossible" (p. 62). Involvement, then, involves emotion and authenticity—emotion and authenticity that arise out of commitment to and genuine caring about the client. Involvement is best understood in terms of the client's perception: his sense of his therapist as contactful and truly committed to his welfare.

### Acknowledgment

Four therapist activities are especially crucial in maintaining and demonstrating involvement. The first of these—and the one that tends to be called for earliest in therapy—is *acknowledgment*. The therapist acknowledges the client by means of her attunement to his thoughts, feelings, behaviors, and desires, and her sensitive inquiry about all of those facets of his experience. She hears what he is telling her, and she lets him know that she hears. She is willing to talk about what is important to him; she doesn't force him to deal with her agenda. While she is listening to him she is also listening to herself, in full contact with her own internal experience and willing to acknowledge that as well. Again, there is no pretending, no hiding behind some sort of clinical mask. "The analyst is not a blank screen, but a quite human other presence whose emotionality the patient both correctly perceives as well as misperceives" (Billow, 2000, p. 63).

Acknowledgment of the client's affect, relational needs, and physical sensations helps him to reclaim his own phenomenological experience. He is in the presence of a respectful other who recognizes and talks about his nonverbal responses, his muscular tensions, his feelings, and even his fantasies. Through this kind of sensitivity the therapist can guide the client toward awareness and expression of needs and feelings; she can help the client understand that emotions and physical sensations may be a form of memory—the only kind of memory that may be available to him right now. In essence, acknowledgment of the client's internal experience reverses the relational failures of the past, providing permission and protection for him to express that which was ignored or punished in previous relationships.

Perhaps most important of all, the therapist acknowledges her part in the creation of the therapeutic relationship. What happens during the therapy session is jointly created; therapist and client both are responsible for the successes and the failures, the stuck spots, and the leaps ahead. They both are responsible for the misunderstandings, the insights, and the feelings of care and closeness. Acknowledging our own contribution to relationship issues, as well as the client's contribution, breathes life into that relationship. Such acknowledgment requires, enhances, and demonstrates authentic involvement.

## Validation

*Validation* communicates to the client that his affect, defenses, physical sensations, or behavioral patterns are related to something significant. The involved therapist lets the client know that what he says or does is important and that his internal experience has meaning, even though she may not yet understand what that meaning is. One of the tenets of relationship-focused integrative psychotherapy is that every behavior—every act, thought, and feeling—has a function; people do not behave randomly. The therapist validates the function of the client's behaviors and of his reported internal experiences. The behavior itself may appear hurtful to self or others—telling oneself that life is hopeless, or feeling panic when crossing a bridge, or sending poison pen letters are not desirable behaviors—but there is an underlying purpose to even the most irrational-appearing response. Moreover, that purpose is positive; ultimately, the behavior was acquired and is maintained in order to protect the client from some danger or to achieve some important goal. It is this positive function that the therapist validates.

Sometimes simple acknowledgment serves as a validation. By attending to the client's story, believing that what he says is true as he understands it (or, if he is being untruthful, that the untruth too serves an important function), the therapist lets the client know that she values his communication. Greenberg and Paivio (1997) characterize this aspect of the therapeutic relationship as a new experience for most clients: ". . . feeling that a fragile sense of oneself is heard, received, validated, and accepted is a source of new transformative experience" (p. 83).

Going beyond simply acknowledging what the client is saying and doing, the therapist may explicitly validate some client behavior. This is a particularly useful intervention when the client himself discounts the behavior. "I don't know why I react that way," or "I keep doing the same dumb thing over and over," says the client; the therapist responds with "There's an important reason for that reaction/behavior. Part of our job is to discover what that reason is."

It is a truism that clients often experience the therapeutic relationship in the same way that they have experienced important relationships in the past. These past relationships have taught them how to be with people, how to communicate their needs and respond to the needs of others, and what to expect and what to avoid in human interactions. Inevitably, some of those learnings and expectations will generalize to the therapeutic relationship and the therapist will be understood in light of how other people have behaved in the client's past. It is especially important, then, to note and to validate the client's responses to the therapist—the way the client deals with the therapeutic relationship—since these responses may have more to do with old, script-determined functions than with actual here-and-now events. Uncovering script-determined functions is a first step in dissolving that script and re-establishing the spontaneity and creativity of full internal and external contact.

A final aspect of therapeutic validation is *confrontation*. Confrontation involves calling attention to a discrepancy—between words and behaviors, between what the client actually does and how he or she describes it, between thoughts and affect, between expectations and actual events. Like geological fault lines, discrepancies signal something important going on beneath the surface. The confrontation, implicitly or explicitly, calls attention to the underlying process. Again, we assert that a purpose is being served, that the discrepancy has a function. Far from being a punitive "gotcha!", confrontation that validates an underlying positive goal respectfully invites the client to look more closely at what he is thinking, feeling, doing, and saying and to value the purpose of that behavior even as he may strive to change the behavior itself.

## Normalization

The involved therapist *normalizes* her clients' responses. Clients need reassurance that their behavior is not crazy, not shameful or disgusting. They come for treatment because they are doing/thinking/feeling things that they do not want to do/think/feel and because they have not been able to change their responses; they are likely to believe that they are different from (and less than) other people, who obviously are much better able to take care of themselves. Normalizing interventions point out the similarities between clients and others: "Given the situation you were in, and the resources available to you, it makes sense that you would have acted (thought, felt) as you did. Anybody would."

The intent of normalization is to counter a client's categorization or definition of his internal experience or his behaviors from a pathological, "something's-wrong-with-me" perspective. Instead, the therapist presents a point of view that respects the client's attempts—archaic though they may be—to resolve conflicts and to protect himself. The client's confusion, panic, defensiveness, memory flashbacks, or bizarre fantasies all derive from coping strategies developed in difficult and painful situations. It is imperative that the therapist let the client know that his experience is a normal, self-protective reaction and that others experiencing similar life circumstances might well respond in similar ways. Normalization involves both acknowledgment and validation. The therapist acknowledges what the client is telling her, verbally or nonverbally. Validating the function of the behavior implies that the function is a reasonable and rational one; this paves the way for talking about how the client did the best he could do, under the circumstances, to maintain that function. His choices may not have been good ones, but they were the best that he—or anyone else in his situation—could have made. Now that the situation is changing, he is in a position to do something different.

## Presence

Acknowledgment, validation, and normalization are specific therapist behaviors that emerge naturally and inevitably from the conviction that every client is fundamentally a good person, doing the best he can given his history, belief system, and current resources. These therapist behaviors emerge because the therapist is *present* in the relationship, willing to be known as well as to know, in contact both with the client and with her own experience. *Presence* is the fourth ingredient of involvement, and it is fundamental to the process of relationship-focused integrative psychotherapy.

Presence is provided through the therapist's sustained attunement to the client's verbal and non-verbal communication and through her constant respect for and enhancement of the client's integrity. It is an expression of the therapist's full internal and external contactfulness, and it communicates her dependability and her willingness to take responsibillity for her part in whatever happens in this relationship. It includes receptivity to the client's affect: willingness to be impacted by the client's emotions, to be deeply moved while not becoming anxious, depressed, or angry.

There is a kind of duality to presence, a duality that we have touched on before: a simultaneous attending to other and to self. The therapist de-centers from her own needs, feelings, fantasies, or desires and makes the client's process her primary focus; but she does not lose touch with her own internal process and reactions. "The therapist's history, relational needs, sensitivities, theories, professional experience, own psychotherapy, and reading interests all shape unique reactions to the client. Each of these thoughts and feelings within the therapist are an essential part of therapeutic presence" (Erskine, Moursund, & Trautmann, 1999,

p. 242). It is not just that the therapist has a unique history—a unique set of past experiences, present interests, needs, and wants. She also uses her experience as a kind of reference library that sheds light upon the client, upon her responses to him, and upon their interactions with each other. Most importantly, the therapist is willing to be transparent in her uniqueness, willing to let the client see who she is and what she is experiencing, willing to be impacted by that which impacts the client, and willing for that impact, too, to be seen. The respectful interplay between self-awareness and de-centering opens the way for what Buber (1958) calls an "I-thou" relationship, a relationship between two connected, contactful, self-and-other-aware individuals. The "I-thou" relationship, in turn, is the primary source of the transformative potential of relationship-focused integrative psychotherapy.

One of the immediate consequences of therapeutic presence is that it serves as a model. The client, seeing that the therapist is willing to be open and vulnerable, is encouraged in his own openness and vulnerability. Presence also serves as a container for the therapeutic interaction (Schneider, 1998); it is a sort of psychological safety net, marking an interpersonal space that supports without constraining and protects without demeaning the client.

Attunement, inquiry, and involvement are the basic elements of a relationship-focused integrative psychotherapy. They are based on a set of beliefs—a set of attitudes—about people in general and clients in particular. They grow out of a commitment to the premise that each client strives to be the best he can be, and that his problems and pains have developed out of a set of beliefs and decisions, acquired over time, that constrict and distort his way of being in the world. Yet, these basic elements are more than attitudes, more than just a general way of thinking and feeling about clients: they involve skills, skills that can be acquired, skills that are applied through all the stages and phases of the therapeutic endeavor. It is time now to turn to those stages and phases, to consider the various tasks and challenges that arise as therapist and client journey together toward growth and change.

## SUMMARY

Attunement, inquiry, and involvement are extensions of empathy. They allow the therapist to use herself, her own personhood, to develop and maintain an effective therapeutic relationship.

The attuned therapist resonates to the client's process. She not only attends to what the client presents, but reciprocates, meeting the client's thoughts and feelings with her own affective and cognitive response. When the client is joined by an attuned therapist, he feels respected and safe and is encouraged to expand his awareness of self and of others. The therapist attunes to the client's affect, cognition, psychological developmental level, ryhthm, and relational needs.

Inquiry includes not only questions but also every intervention that invites the client to deepen his awareness of his own internal process. In this sense, every therapeutic intervention can be a form of inquiry. Effective inquiry is crafted so as to enhance the client's self-discovery; what the therapist learns is secondary. Therapeutic inquiries are respectful and open-ended, and they encourage the client to correct the therapist's misunderstandings or misconceptions. The goal of inquiry is to expand the client's contact with self and others. Areas of inquiry include the client's affect, physical sensations, cognition, fantasies, and relationships.

Involvement has to do with the therapist's commitment to being an active, caring, vulnerable, and authentic participant in the therapeutic process. It is reflected in the therapist's acknowledgment, validation, and normalization of what the client presents, and by her being fully present, emotionally available, self-aware and willing to be known as well as to know.

# 7 CHAPTER | **Beginning the Work**

The first session with a new client is an interesting time. For an inexperienced therapist, it can also be an anxious time. The therapist is about to meet someone with whom she hopes to develop a very close and intimate relationship. She will come to know him very well—better, perhaps, than anyone else in his life. And he will come to know the therapist, too. Each will be making a decision as to whether to work together: each is feeling the other out, drawing conclusions. *What sort of person is this? What will he or she expect of me? How will we work together?* Beginning therapy is a step into the unknown of contact-in-relationship. It is only reasonable that the therapist should feel both excited and uneasy about it.

The therapist's uneasiness is minor, though, compared to what the client is likely to be feeling. After all, the therapist is the professional here. She isn't the one who is hurting, who is admitting that he cannot handle things on his own. She has been here before (or, at least, the client thinks she has), while he can only imagine what this therapy business will be like.

## FIRST-SESSION TASKS

Several tasks need to be attended to in an initial session, and the first of these has to do with the feelings that the therapist and the client are experiencing. The client needs to be given some sense of what therapy will be like, what the procedures and the expectations are, and what kind of person the therapist is. He needs to begin to experience contact with the therapist as safe and supportive and, at the same time, as a relationship where something is going to be accomplished. As the therapist goes about responding to these needs, both she and the client will begin to feel more comfortable. Anxiety lessens when something can be done about what is causing the anxiety, and here something is being done about it. Therapist and client are beginning to build a working relationship. Horvath (2001) reports that meta-analysis of more than two decades of psychotherapy research indicates that "developing the [therapeutic] alliance takes precedence over technical interventions in the beginning of therapy" (p. 369). The working relationship is the single most important ingredient in successful therapy, and beginning to build it is the single most important task of the initial session.

The primary activity through which the working relationship begins to develop is the therapist's gathering of information. She needs to learn about this client in order to respond to his needs and to help him clarify his goals in therapy. She needs to learn what he wants, why he has come to her, what he expects, how he has attempted to solve his problems in the past, and how those attempts have succeeded or failed. She does not question or find fault with what he tells her; she suspends any disbelief that may arise in her (time for that later, perhaps); he is introducing her to his world, and she is respectfully aware that he knows much more about that world than she does. Here, the client is the expert, and the therapist is the student. Her attitude is "more inquisitive than disputational, more approving than disapproving, and more exploratory than demonstrative" (Neimeier, 1995, p. 115).

The therapist is not the only person who needs to gather information during this first encounter. Another task of the first session is to give the client a sense of what therapy—and, specifically, therapy with this therapist—will be like. He will decide, sometime during this first session, whether he wants to work with this therapist; and, to make that decision, he needs to have a sense of who she is, how she works, what it feels like to be with her. He also needs some specific facts: he needs to weigh the costs (monetary, time, emotional) against the probable benefits, and he needs to know what will be expected of him (we talk more about this issue later on). Exchanging information is the most obvious task of an initial session; it is also the vehicle by means of which the therapeutic relationship will begin to grow.

The final (but by no means least important) task for this first session is to provide the client with a sense of hope. Hope is what will bring him back for further sessions; hope is what makes it worthwhile for him to invest in and bear the inevitable discomforts of therapy. Hope is born of the kind of contact that happens between therapist and client, the kind of relationship that is begun. Before the client leaves, the therapist needs to establish herself as someone who is present, respectful, and willing to be involved; as someone who understands what this client wants and has an idea of how to accomplish it; and as someone who knows how to build and maintain an effective therapeutic relationship.

# ESTABLISHING A SAFE WORKING ENVIRONMENT

Security is born out of a sense of trust. When people can trust their environment and, especially, the other people in that environment, they feel safe. According to Erikson (1968), the most fundamental attitude toward the world, as well as toward oneself, is a sense of basic trust. Basic trust begins to be established during the first year of life, emerging out of the mutual regulation of needs by both the infant and the mother (Stern, 1985). The interactions through which this earliest of relationships is shaped are similar, in many ways, to what happens at the outset of a relationship-focused therapy. The therapist, by her attunement and involvement, by the skill with which she inquires and gives information, establishes her trustworthiness. Simultaneously, the client's responses help the therapist to know how she is being received, whether she is respected, and what kind of expectations this client has about therapy. Like mother and infant, therapist and client calibrate themselves to each other; and, in that calibration, mutual trust can grow.

Watson and Greenberg (1994) have provided a description of some of the elements that go into providing a safe and trustworthy therapeutic environment. According to them, therapists need to "first, perceive the clients' verbal and nonverbal communications accurately; second, communicate and seek confirmation of their understanding; third, negotiate a shared understanding or otherwise readjust their understanding in line with their clients' phenomenological perspective; and fourth, refrain from expressing critical, intrusive, or hostile thoughts during the session" (p. 165). These are the basics, the foundation upon which a sense of safety is built. Understanding the client, and making sure he knows that you understand; being willing to see the world from his point of view; and maintaining an attitude that is supportive rather than hostile or critical—all of these encourage the client to say more, explore further. They are the concrete, experiencable evidence that the therapist can be trusted, that this is indeed a safe place. They pave the way for building the kind of relationship within which healing and growth are possible.

## Joining

How can we describe the sense of being joined by another? It feels supportive, understanding, and caring; but none of those words really captures the essence of therapeutic joining. Joining involves the creation of an in-between, a therapeutic space that is more than the sum of what each person contributes. For the client who truly feels joined, the therapist is more than a technician, more than a friend—she is the co-creator of a unique relationship, a partner in exploring the most private and personal aspects of the client's life. She is, says Mitchell (1988), "not simply a vehicle for managing internal pressures and states; interactive exchanges with and ties to the other become the fundamental psychological reality itself" (p. 25).

Joining a client in this way requires careful attention to attunement, willingness to put one's own style and preferences on hold in the service of attending to the client's needs. Yet, the therapist must not move so completely into the client's frame of reference that she loses her own individuality. She too must be present, real, knowable. "It is important for clients to see their therapists as their 'own person.' That is, they need to see their therapists as persons who are able and willing to state their true positions on things, to agree or disagree, to cooperate or confront, and to set self-respecting limits on what they will and will not do in relation to the client" (Bergner, 1999, p. 205). Contact is possible only when there is something to be contacted; joining is possible only when there is some-one with whom to join. The therapist treads a delicate line between being too swept into the client's world (which does not allow the client an authentic other with whom to interact) and being too wedded to her own perspective (and thus relatively closed and noncontactful). In the region where these two extremes come together, therapeutic joining is possible.

## Maintaining a Healing Presence

In his first contact with a therapist, the client forms a sense of what this help-ing person will be like and what kind of relationship will be possible with her. First impressions, while not indelible, have a strong influence on the course of therapy; it is important that this first impression be one that will invite the client to invest himself in the process that they are beginning together. The client needs to experience the therapist as a healing presence: someone who is both competent and caring, with whom the client can join without losing him-self. Says Breggin (1997), "The creation of a healing presence focuses on our-selves rather than on the person we are trying to heal or to help. In creating healing presence, we don't change the other person as much as we transform ourselves in response to the other person. We find within ourselves the inner resources that speak directly to the other person's psychological and spiritual needs" (p. 5). Embedded in Breggin's description is, again, the notion of inter-nal and external contact. Finding inner resources within oneself requires that one be aware of one's history, one's wants, one's thoughts and feelings; of what one has learned from previous work and study; and of the ways in which friends and mentors have touched one in the past. The therapist uses that awareness not to present herself to the client as an expert, an authority, but rather to organize her resources, to "transform herself" in response to him, to his needs, his fears, his hopes.

It is tempting, particularly if we are inexperienced therapists, to attempt to present ourselves to clients as wiser or more experienced than we really are. After all, clients have come for help; they might not want to work with us if they think we don't have answers for them or don't fully understand what they tell us. So we try to fake it, try to appear calm, composed, and sure of our-selves. Unfortunately, faking simply does not work. Not only is the client (who is highly invested in finding out what sort of person we are) likely to see through the false veneer, but also the dissimulation interrupts and distorts the very sort of contact that therapist and client need to establish. "We should not try to carry ourselves as if we're adequate to anything and everything," says

Breggin (1997). "Faking undermines healing presence. An acceptance of our limits contributes positively to a healing aura, making us more comfortable with ourselves and allowing others to face their vulnerabilities without shame" (p. 27). The client needs a competent therapist, but he does not need an infallible one; he needs a therapist who can make mistakes and admit to them, can get it wrong and then go back and repair the damage (Guistolese, 1997). The therapist's willingness to be human, with all the warts and blemishes that humans have, allows her to create a truly healing presence.

## Attending to Feelings, Thoughts, and Behaviors

Clients vary enormously in the degree of emotion they display. They will use the therapist's response to their emotion (or lack of it) in the initial session to figure out how they are supposed to behave in therapy: should they put feelings aside and try to be logical problem solvers? Does the therapist expect them to dissolve into tears during every session? Is she more interested in their feelings or in what they are thinking and doing? Many of the client's conclusions will be wrong; if the therapist is doing her job properly, she does not have a pre-set agenda for what her clients ought to be discovering. What she would like them to decide is that whatever emerges for them is what they need to attend to and that she will support their exploration and help them to use it constructively.

Clients need to be able both to think and to feel to fully benefit from therapy. They need to think about their emotions, and they need to be aware of their emotional responses to their thoughts. To the degree that they have fragmented themselves, closed off parts of themselves in order to protect themselves from pain, they may not have full access to all of these awarenesses. The therapist's job is to help them to regain their contact with themselves and to use that internal contact in their interactions with others.

Most people—therapists included—have little trouble with sharing information, talking about things, and relating stories of who did what. That is what folks do, for the most part, when they are with others: they talk about what is happening in their lives, they attempt to solve problems or make plans, and they "pass the time of day." Sometimes they tell others some of what they feel, either in words or nonverbally; but the deepest feelings are seldom shared; in fact, people often go to a great deal of trouble to hide those feelings. In many subcultures, it is not socially acceptable to be "too emotional." Children (especially boys) are trained to hide their vulnerabilities, to be brave, to make the best of things. Society tends to reward those who do not cause a fuss or make others uncomfortable. For all of these reasons, clients are likely to hide or tone down their emotionality when they first meet with a therapist. If they are unable to do so—if the feelings break through—the client may be ashamed or even apologize.

One of the therapist's tasks is to teach clients that dealing with feelings is a central part of the therapeutic process. Far from being shameful, experiencing and expressing affect is simply part of being a whole person. When a client cries, the therapist does not try to get him to stop; if he appears frightened or angry, the therapist accepts his fear or anger as an important facet of who he is at that moment. If he tells his story with no emotion, the therapist may ask about his feelings; and, when the therapist is emotionally impacted, she does not hide her feelings from the client.

Of course, some clients are very emotionally labile and their emotionality interferes with thinking clearly and effectively. They have learned not to use their cognitive abilities; have learned, rather, to use only feelings to communicate with the world. They, too, need to find a better balance. With such a client, the therapist asks for information, for history, for ideas and beliefs. She does not criticize, directly or by impliction, his display of emotion; rather, she asks him to think about his feelings—when they arise, how long they have been around, what they are connected to, and what effect their expression has on others. She is not interested in helping the client to "get rid of" some distressing emotion; she is interested in discovering the function served by that emotion and in developing alternative ways of accomplishing the same thing. To do that, both therapist and client need to be able to think as well as to feel.

Frequently, clients attribute unwanted behaviors to their feelings. "I did it because I was angry." "I felt so bad, I just couldn't help myself." "When I'm real scared, I just have to have a drink." Miller and DeShazer (2000) point out that while emotions may be *reasons* for behaviors, they are not *causes* of behaviors. Thinking of actions as caused by feelings takes away the ability to make choices about what to do; people who think this way experience themselves as uncontrollably driven by their affect. Again, this way of being in the world is out of balance. Learning to feel and to express emotion without having one's behavior controlled by it is another integrative task, another step on the road to becoming whole. Effective therapists ask questions that invite clear thinking, support the client's emotions without making them all-powerful, and deal with behaviors as being related to but not caused by feelings. They also model that sort of balance in their own behavior, from the outset, in building relationships with their clients.

## Exploring Expectations

The work of the first session sets the stage for the work to come. Just as the therapist is learning about the client and forming hypotheses about what sort of approach will be most helpful, so the client is learning about the therapist. These learnings will be colored by what he already believes about therapy, and these beliefs are often formed from fairly dubious sources: television programs, novels, and even jokes on the Internet. Even if a client's ideas about therapy in general are reasonably accurate, they still may not fit with this particular therapist's style. Say Callaghan, Naugle, and Folette (1996), "The information the client brings with him/her to the therapy may not accurately correspond to the way the clinician conducts treatment and can hinder the development of the therapeutic relationship" (p. 385). The client may, for example, expect the therapist to behave like a physician, asking questions and gathering information and then prescribing some sort of treatment; he will be confused and bewildered if the therapist simply waits patiently for him to talk about whatever is foreground for him. The therapist, in turn, may wonder why this client is so reticent, so unwilling to take the lead in bringing up the issues that are important for him; she experiences his confusion as resistant or even hostile—not the best start for a therapeutic partnership!

One way to avoid this sort of mismatch is to talk about expectations. It can be useful to find out what the client thinks psychotherapy will be like, and to let him know how these expectations are similar to and different from the therapist's own. This is especially important if the client has been in therapy with someone else; people who have learned how to be a client with one therapist naturally expect other therapists to behave the same way. If the therapist's own style appears to be different from what the client expects, she can talk about those differences and explain why she works as she does. Giving clients a rationale, rather than simply telling them that things will be different here and expecting them to conform, is reasonable and respectful.

The goal of all of this discussion is, of course, to find a way for therapist and client to develop an effective therapeutic relationship. When both share the same expectations, misunderstandings will be minimized. The client will have a sense of why the therapist acts as she does and will be more inclined to give her the benefit of the doubt when she does or says something unexpected. She is not mysteriously pursuing some goal that the clients cannot or should not know about; she has a sensible reason for her questions and her silences.

Shared expectations allow people to experience their similarities: we both want the same thing, and we are both pleased when we make progress. Perceived similarities, in turn, allow each of us to identify with the other, and this identification helps the joining process. Particularly at the beginning of treatment, partial identifications (of client with therapist, and of therapist with client) "act as pathways to a deeper resonance between the unconscious worlds of the patient and the therapist" (Kainer, 1999, p. 10). Here, again, it is all about contact, about what will enhance the client's ability to make contact with the therapist and, through that relationship, regain contact with himself.

Above all, the client needs to believe that therapy can work for him and that this therapist is someone who will be able to be helpful. No one knows how much of the success in any given psychotherapeutic treatment is due to a *placebo effect*—the client achieving his goals simply because he expects to—but there is little doubt that the expectation of a favorable outcome is extremely important. Conversely, without such an expectation, the likelihood of success is significantly lessened. One of our tasks is that of mobilizing the client's belief in therapy and in our ability to conduct therapy, for without that belief there will be little motivation to do the hard work that successful therapy requires. Weinberger and Eig (1999) paraphrase Jerome Frank's summary of what is needed to maximize the client's sense of hope: "(a) an emotionally charged healing relationship; (b) a healing setting; (c) a rationale or myth that plausibly explains the patient's difficulties and offers a sensible solution; and (d) a believable treatment or ritual for restoring health" (p. 368). When all of these are present, the client can believe in the possibility of change, and therapy has begun.

# THE DECISION TO WORK TOGETHER

Before plunging into the work, though, both therapist and client need to be clear about whether they are in fact going to continue. Showing up for a first session does not guarantee that the client will want to come back; seeing a client once does not mean that the therapist is required to continue with him. Another major goal of the initial session is that both parties make a clear decision about working together. If possible, it should be a *mutual* decision, one that both therapist and client agree upon.

## An Informed Choice

Sensible people do not agree to buy something until they know what that something is, how much it will cost, and what it will do for them. "Buying" therapy works the same way: clients need to know what therapy is, how much it will cost them, and how it is likely to be helpful. It is the therapist's responsibility to provide them with this information. In a sense, though, therapists can never tell clients exactly what their therapy will be like: therapy is a journey into the unknown. Exploring that unknown is not a precursor to therapy—it *is* therapy. Nevertheless, therapists are obligated—legally and ethically—to give clients the best description possible: how they work, what may happen, how long it is likely to take, what the cost (in money, time, and energy) will be.

Many therapists, in fact, go farther than simply telling the client about what therapy will be like. They have a written description that the client is expected to read and to sign so that the therapist has evidence that the client has been given the information. This is the *informed consent form,* and it is a wise precaution in the litigious climate in which therapists now find themselves; it protects the therapist from accusations of misleading the client about costs, expectations, or other aspects of therapy. The problem with informed consent materials is that, in order to include all the things that the client may want to know about therapy, the forms can be quite long and quite complicated. Research indicates that the more readable and the more personalized the informed consent document is, the more comfortable the client is about working with that therapist (Wagner, Davis, & Handelsman, 1998). Informed consent, then, must be a compromise between telling everything that the client may find relevant, on the one hand, and being brief and readable, on the other.

Telling a client how the therapist works is important, but showing him is even more so. From the moment he walks into the therapist's office (and perhaps earlier, if she has spoken with him on the telephone to set up the appointment), he is responding to a host of verbal and nonverbal cues—many out of his conscious awareness—that tell him what the therapy experience will be like; these cues will influence his decision even more than the facts the therapist provides. He is deciding if he likes this therapist and if she is going to like him; if she knows what she is doing; and if her style of working will meet his needs. What he experiences in her should be a reasonably accurate sample of what things will be like if the therapy continues.

As an example of the sort of thing that clients may use to form their idea of what therapy will be like, consider the way in which the therapist chooses to begin the session. Less-experienced therapists often begin an initial session with some sort of "small talk"—comments about the weather, the traffic, or some upcoming public event. Asked why they do this, they are likely to say that they are trying to put the client at ease. In fact, this sort of conversational beginning is probably more for the benefit of the therapist (who may be feeling somewhat awkward, and anxious for the client's approval) than for the client. Starting the session with small talk suggests that this is how therapy is done; it sets up a mistaken expectation about the work. "Counseling is not a social conversation," comments Patterson (1985), "and for the counselor to begin it as such is misleading in terms of structuring and reinforces such an approach by the client" (p. 108). What the therapist does, and invites the client to do, during the first session does structure what is to come; and this structure is a large part of what the client will use to make his decision about continuing.

## To Refer or Not to Refer

What about the therapist's decision whether or not to work with this client? Generally, this question boils down to one of when *not* to take on a particular client; most therapists (certainly when their practices are beginning) hope to continue with the clients who come to them unless there is some specific reason for not doing so. The most important of these reasons, the one therapists are ethically and legally bound to observe, has to do with the limits of their competence. A therapist does not agree to work with a client when she does not have the expertise needed to help him. Some therapists may, for example, not be trained to work with seriously thought-disordered (psychotic) individuals, or with children, or with the elderly. Working with certain kinds of problems requires special training: training regarding sexual dysfunction, for example, or eating disorders, or substance abuse. If a client presents with a problem that one is not trained to handle, it is an ethical obligation to refer him elsewhere.

A second reason for referring a prospective client is a mismatch in values. We have mentioned this before, but it bears repeating: if there is something about this client that prevents the therapist from honestly joining with him in an authentic and supportive relationship, from honestly believing that he is doing the best he can given his circumstances, then she should not work with him. If the therapist finds herself feeling critical of this client–of *him*, not of his behavior—she will not be able to offer him the respect and valuing that he needs. Rogers (1951) posited "unconditional positive regard" as a necessary condition for therapeutic growth; if that unconditional positive regard is not available for a particular individual, then that individual deserves a different therapist.

Fortunately, finding oneself unable to feel positive regard for a client is a rare event for most therapists. If the therapist (or her secretary, or someone at her agency) does a good job of screening prospective clients over the phone, being confronted with someone she is not qualified to work with will be equally rare. When it does happen, the therapist should simply be honest about it. "I don't think I'm the best person for you to work with." "You need to see someone who has been trained to deal with xxx, and I don't have that specialized training." She makes the referral (preferably giving the client two or three names rather than just one), thanks him for his interest in seeing her, gives him an opportunity to respond, and ends the session. The experience may not feel good, for either client or therapist. But, minimally, the client will be given a better chance to meet his needs, and the therapist will know that she has done what is best for him.

Ideally, the decision to work together is a clear one on both sides. The client agrees to commit to at least some number of sessions or for some length of time, or until his goals have been met, or until a decision is made that the therapy is no longer helpful; the therapist makes the same commitment. When that sort of agreement cannot be reached, agreeing on a trial period still may be possible—one or more sessions during which both client and therapist will have an opportunity to get to know the other better and have more information upon which to base a longer-term commitment. This sort of tentative agreement should be clearly spelled out and, if possible, included in the informed consent document. When the trial period has expired, it is the therapist's responsibility to bring up the topic and ask the client whether he wants to continue.

## THE THERAPEUTIC CONTRACT

Once therapist and client have decided (at least tentatively) to work together, the next order of business is to develop a therapeutic contract: a joint agreement about the nature of the problem to be solved and what will be done to solve it. The notion of therapeutic contracting was a key element in Berne's (1966) early writings and in the work of other transactional analysts (Steiner, 1974). Behavioral and cognitive behavioral therapists, too, have emphasized the importance of developing a contract that outlines the specific goals of therapy, along with how client and therapist will recognize when those goals have been accomplished.

Therapeutic contracts are useful for at least four reasons. First, without such a contract, therapy tends to jump from one topic to another and neither therapist nor client has a clear sense of direction. For the therapist, the contract is a tool for keeping on course, a sort of internal beeper that signals when things are wandering away from the psychological glide path. Second, the contract-making process firms up the client's sense that something is going to be accomplished here, that this is not simply a conversation that may or may not be helpful. Setting a goal creates an expectancy that the goal can be accomplished; and, as Weinberger and Eig (1999) point out, "it seems clear that expectancies are a force in human functioning generally and in psychotherapy in particular" (p. 367).

Developing a contract does more than simply create an expectancy of productive work, though: it is another step toward forging a therapeutic relationship. Says Bordin (1994), "Reaching an understood and mutually agreed-on change goal is the key process in building an initial, viable alliance" (p. 21). The best way to learn is by doing; one of the best ways to learn to be in relationship together in therapy is to do the work of contract building.

Finally, in these days of managed care, clear contracting may be a requirement for third-party reimbursement. Health-maintenance organizations (HMOs) usually demand regular reports on each client, including a list of specific treatment goals and progress made on each. Of course, many of the benefits of therapy cannot be laid out in objective, measurable terms. Some of the most important therapeutic events may not even be predictable before they actually occur. Still, concrete goals and objectives provide a useful framework for therapy; they tie the work together, make it comprehensible, and give it a structure that the client can understand and commit to—and they provide a responsible form of communication with third-party payers.

## Gathering Information

To build a useful contract, one must have information. The therapist is starting from zero; she needs to find out what is going on for this client. The client may not (consciously) be much better off; he has a great deal of information, but much of it is disorganized or out of awareness.

The information needed for good contracting—and for good therapy, as well—consists of the answers to four questions: (a) How are you? (b) How do you want to be different? (c) How did you get to be the way you are? (d) How will we know when you have accomplished your goals? It would be nice if the answers to these questions could be as short and simple as the questions themselves (or maybe not; if they were, we therapists might have to look for another profession!), but just the opposite is usually true. In fact, neither client nor therapist will probably ever have a complete set of answers to any of them; discovering more and more of the answers is a large part of the therapeutic process. However, some part of the answers—the part that the client can, at the outset, call to conscious awareness—will form the basis of the therapeutic contract.

It is not just the client who begins to answer these questions; just as therapist and client are co-creators of the therapeutic relationship, so they are co-creators of the contract. The therapist helps the client to discover his answers by suggesting where to look and by talking with the client about what he finds when he looks there. The therapist's language is a powerful influence in this process: the way she expresses her understanding of what the client is telling her will shape what the client thinks, feels, and believes about himself and his world (Hanna, 1996). It is essential that the therapist not import her own biases into the information-gathering process, and that she remember to regard her inferences as hypotheses rather than as facts. Grove (1991) talks about the importance of using "clean language" in therapy, of making sure that we approach any topic from the client's point of view rather than our own. Listening in this way requires constant self-monitoring and constant "course correction" when we veer off into an unfounded assumption.

"How are you?" has to do with what the client's life is like right now: his thoughts, his feelings, and his beliefs. What goes through his mind as he wakes to begin another day? What are the significant relationships in his life? What does he care about? Hope for? Fear? When does he feel good, and when does he hurt? There are a thousand answers to "How are you?," and each can lead to dozens more. Discovering all of the shifting and changing internal experiences that answer this question is the very stuff of therapy, and that discovery continues long beyond the point at which an initial contract has been developed.

Unlike the answers to "How are you?," the answer to "How do you want to be different?" may—initially, at least—be short and specific. "I want to stop being depressed." "I want to be able to be with people and not feel anxious." "I want to have an intimate relationship." These short and simple answers form the basis for setting therapeutic goals. The wise therapist, though, does not expect such initial goals to remain unchanged through the entire course of treatment. An initial goal is often just the tip of the iceberg; what the client knows (but is afraid to say) that he wants, and what he wants but cannot yet express, lie below the surface. As the work unfolds, the therapist must be prepared to revise and expand her understanding of what the client wants and needs.

The next question—"How did you get that way?"—begins the process of unraveling the tangle of life experiences that have led to the client's present distress. It has at least as many answers as "How are you?," for it asks about the "How are you?" of all of the years and months and days of the client's past. The client may not—usually does not—know which of his past experiences have been most important in forming the schemas and script that order his life today. Much of that past experience, or at least its significance, is no longer consciously available to him. Script is, by definition, out of awareness; people do not know why they think and feel as they do any more than they know why they believe that grass is green or why they cry when they are sad. "How did you learn to rage at people when you get upset?" or "How did you come to feel so down on yourself?" may seem unanswerable questions to a client, but it is often in finding the answers that change begins. "Sorting out the different strands of interpersonal history that form the standards used for negative self-evaluation allows a person to gain a perspective on the power of such standards" (Jack, 1999, p. 241). Not only negative self-evaluation but also every other relational response grows out of "strands of interpersonal history." These are the strands we trace as we explore "How did you get that way?"

Finally, "How will we know when you have accomplished your goals?" looks forward to the end of therapy. As is discussed in chapter 11, the question of ending treatment is (or should be) dealt with from the outset. Therapy is not an endless process; it is not a way of life. It is an enterprise with a purpose; and, when that purpose has been accomplished, the client should be encouraged to go ahead on his own. There are many reasons, however, that terminating therapy can be difficult; spelling out, at the beginning, the criteria for termination can help both client and therapist to know when it is time to say good-bye.

## Beyond the Facts

People who seek therapy (and many who don't!) live in a world artifically constricted by old, outworn beliefs and rules. The "facts" they present may be accurate, but "facts" will almost certainly provide an incomplete picture of their experience. The therapist's job is to help the client go beyond the facts into the realm of internal experience, of supposition, of memory, and of fantasy. Some clients need little encouragement to enter this world; their stories come gushing out, words tumbling over words, so fast that it is hard to keep up. Others may have trouble finding words or may be too angry, anxious, or embarrassed to talk freely, and the therapist will need to provide more help, more direction. She will do so in the context of the developing relationship; her questions and comments are respectful, interested, and attuned to the client's communication style and rhythm. Whatever that style, everything the client says is important, significant, and meaningful; it is his story, his way of describing who he is. The therapist listens to it all, alert to any hint of the needs, hopes, relational conflicts, and protective strategies that lie at the core of the client's present way of being.

Often, parts of the client's story will become confused. He will reveal himself as believing things, feeling emotions, and behaving in ways that seem strange—self-destructive, hurtful to others, simply nonsensical. When such things happen, they should signal the therapist that this material deserves special attention. Responses and reactions that don't match up, that seem at odds with what has gone before or with how the world works, are often the first clues about script, those internal and out-of-awareness structures that govern people's perceptions, feelings, and relationships. At the same time, the therapist needs to direct her attention inward, toward her own reactions to the client's confusing story. One of the most serious misconceptions that can trap a therapist is that of believing that a client's behavior makes no sense or is silly or even evil. Bergner (1999) reminds us that each client is "an individual whose every emotion, judgment, and action has a logic which is in principle reconstructable, and whose every perception is an understandable way of looking at things. The client is regarded as eligible to be mistaken in his or her perceptions and judgments at times, but not eligible to make no sense" (p. 206). To respond to him otherwise puts client and therapist on opposite sides of the fence, either as adversaries or as judge versus person to be judged. A story that sounds weird or destructive deserves the therapist's full and respectful attention, not her internal criticism or condemnation.

With all of this attending to do, switching to a "sending mode" and making an appropriate response is sometimes difficult. What does the therapist say when her client tells her that he has been abducted by aliens, or that he gets drunk and then goes joy-riding in his car, or that he would like to kill his infant son? Whatever words you find, make sure to avoid two things: phonyness and judgment. "Most patients," says Strupp (1996), "particularly more seriously disturbed ones, are exquisitely sensitive to even minimal slights and criticisms. To cope with these exigencies, a therapist must be correspondingly sensitive" (p. 137). Clients are also on the alert for any cue that the therapist may be insincere, faking a supportive or understanding response that she does not really feel. Rather than offer insincere support, the wise therapist asks for more information and/or responds to the quality of the client's experience: "Can you tell me more about it?" "How do you feel about doing that?" "It sounds like you've been in a lot of pain."

Even silence may be taken as a negative response by a client who has just shared some important bit of information. Imagine that you are the client and that you have told your therapist something about yourself, something that you do not usually share with others, or something that others have reacted to negatively. How the therapist answers will be a sign of her trustworthiness, of her ability to understand you. But she's not saying anything! Doesn't she get it? Or does she think you're really stupid? Or bad? "When clients pause in their talk, they usually (though not always) expect and desire a response from the therapist. Not to receive a response may be perceived by clients as rejection. Or, it may be seen as an indication that they were not talking about what they should be talking about" (Patterson, 1985, p. 111). Much better, then, that the therapist tell the client what her silence is all about: "I didn't expect to hear you say that; let me think about it for a moment" or "What you are saying seems very important. I need a few seconds to fit it in with the other things you've been telling me." Later, when the client knows the therapist better, he will understand her pauses and her silences; for now, she must make sure he does not misinterpret them.

In sum, then, what a client says is never "wrong"—mistaken, perhaps; at odds with the facts. The behavior that he reports may be hurtful and ill-advised. His pain-producing responses may be unfortunate and deserving of change. His goals may be unattainable, and what he wants from the therapist may not be possible. Safran and Muran (2000) deal with this latter point, what the client wants from the therapist: "It is important for the therapist to be empathic and understanding while acknowledging the limitations of the therapeutic relationship. It is important for therapists to see patients' nonfulfillable wishes for union or nurturance as a normal part of the human experience, rather than to view them pejoratively as infantile wishes" (p. 242). By treating the client's wishes as normal human experiences, his responses as intended to serve a positive function, the therapist encourages him to explore further; and as he does so, the therapist can travel with him into his unknown, his once-known, and his yet-to-be.

## Diagnosis

The word *diagnosis* most often refers to determining what "disease" someone is suffering from. Some doctors diagnose strep throat or hypertension or cancer; doctors of psychiatry diagnose major depression or dementia or dissociative identity disorder. Other mental health workers may also need to make these sorts of psychiatric diagnoses, since most insurance companies and HMOs require them. However, unlike the diagnoses of physical disorders,

*DSM-IV-TR* (2000)[1] diagnoses seldom take into account either the origin of a given disorder or the most effective treatment for it. The *DSM-IV-TR* is a category system, in which each diagnosis is based on a description of a set of symptoms that form a commonly occurring pattern.

While *DSM-IV-TR* diagnoses can help us know what sorts of things to look for and can also help professionals communicate with each other about their clients, other sorts of diagnosis may be more useful in developing a therapeutic contract and building a treatment plan. In this sense, "diagnosis" means any organized system of describing whatever a client presents in therapy. Often, the therapist will share this sort of diagnosis with the client; even though the client may not understand all the implications of the therapist's description, its overall content will allow him to hear (and perhaps correct) the therapist's assessment of the situation. Breggin (1997), who refers to therapist and client as "partners" in the work of therapy, comments, "The understanding that the therapist shares with a partner may contain nuances that, while compatible with their shared understanding, go far beyond it. As the partner with greater knowledge and experience, these differences, when there, are to be expected. Instead of a hidden agenda, which can be damaging to an alliance, they represent an asset of knowledge of the terrain over which a journey will pass" (p. 22).

One common ingredient of these less formal, non-*DSM-IV-TR* diagnoses is a description of the client's strengths and resources. *DSM-IV-TR*, based on a medical model, focuses on pathology—on what is wrong. Psychotherapists are equally interested in what is right: in what areas the client is doing well, under what conditions he feels good, what sorts of supportive and health-giving relationships he has. Not only do these things provide a more well-rounded picture of the client, but they also yield information that can be utilized in actually working with him. "Clients seem to listen better if the therapist has not only understood their view of themselves and their situation, but also finds something positive in what they have been doing" (Chevalier, 1995, p. 43). Building on strengths is generally more effective than building on weaknesses.

We have said over and over again in these pages that relationship is essential to health and that contact is essential to relationship. Part of the diagnosis in relationship-focused integrative psychotherapy involves an assessment of where the client is open to contact and where he is closed to it. Openness to contact is a strength and can be used as a doorway into those areas that are less available. Ultimately, a goal of therapy is that all aspects of the client's functioning be available: that the client have full internal and external contact, be fully aware of his own experiencing and of the world around him. A fixated life script causes distortion of contact, and contact distortion is required in order to maintain such script. As the client expands the areas in which he has contact, he also begins to break up the patterns that have been restricting his thinking, feeling, behavior, and relationships.

---

[1]The *DSM-IV-TR* (2000) is the *Diagnostic and Statistical Manual of Mental Disorders* (4th edition, text revision), published by the American Psychiatric Association. It is the standardly accepted source for psychiatric diagnosis in the United States.

This leads us to one last area of diagnosis: life script. Formulating hypotheses about the nature of the client's script beliefs and patterns is useful. The more we know about the client's life script, the better equipped we are to provide and/or prescribe experiences that can counter it. The client who has a basic script belief that "people can't be trusted," for instance, can experience the therapist's trustworthiness through her consistent attention to the client, her willingness to take responsibility for errors, and her sensitivity to the client's relational needs; the client can also be invited to notice situations in which other people have behaved in a trustworthy fashion. Clients may be helped to make script changes through suggesting experiments with new behaviors (that do not fit the script system), by rewriting script-supporting fantasies and ruminations, by planned regressions in which the client re-visits the site and time of the original decision and challenges it at that level (Erskine & Moursund, 1988/1998; Erskine, 1974/1997a; Goulding & Goulding, 1979). All of these strategies are most effective when the therapist understands the various parts of the client's script and how they fit together. Mismatches and incongruencies in the client's presentation often signal the operation of script, as do distortions and disruptions of contact. Much valuable script information can be found in the client's history, his account of the important events of his life and the meanings he has assigned to those events.

As much as possible, the client should be a partner in the diagnostic process. Talking with them about *DSM-IV* diagnosis may not be useful, but his input and his corrections are vital to the other, more dynamic kinds of diagnosis. This is especially true because contracts evolve out of diagnosis, and the contract must be a joint product of client and therapist. The therapist does not figure out what is wrong and what the client needs to do, and then tell him to do it (even though many clients would be delighted if it were that easy). Rather, therapist and client together develop both the diagnosis (what is wrong here) and the contract (what we will do about it).

Many clients have histories in which they were not allowed to negotiate to get their needs met; as a result, they anticipate either being overwhelmed or having to use strong methods of manipulation and control with their therapists (as was true with their caretakers). Joint contracting allows these individuals to negotiate, giving them a new experience and obviating the need for the old patterns (Erskine, 1993/1997c, p. 38). Even for people who have learned to negotiate, to engage in the give and take that is essential in healthy relationships, the contract-building process is therapeutic in and of itself. It fosters a sense of purpose and of possibility, a belief that change can happen, and a commitment to achieving personal goals.

## Kinds of Contracts

Contracts may involve both long- and short-term goals, and short-term contracts are most likely to shift and change over the course of therapy. As a result of completing one short-term contract, the client may realize that there is more work to be done. "I want to learn more constructive uses for my anger," for example, is an achievable contract; the client who achieves that goal may then become aware that one function of his anger has been to cover a deeper sense of sadness and loss, and will want to build a new contract to explore and deal with those feelings. "Local goals," say Stern and colleagues (1998), "perform almost constant course corrections that act to redirect, repair, test, probe, or verify the direction of the interactive flow towards the intermediate goal" (p. 910). Intermediate, longer-term contracts and goals tend to be more general and are less likely to shift and change: "I want to regain a sense of competence and self-esteem" and "I want to overcome my depression" are examples of such goals. Whether goals are long- or short-term, articulation of those goals (as well as reaching them) will be facilitated by a caring, involved therapeutic presence.

A short-term contract not yet discussed is the session contract. Many therapists open each session with the question "What would you like to accomplish in our work today?" The answer to this question is, or can lead to, a contract for the session. Again, such contracts tend to be springboards into the work rather than being rigidly held to. They are valuable partly because they give shape to the early part of the session. They help both client and therapist to avoid the "what shall we talk about today" that can lead into a confusion of nonproblems, eating up time and distracting from what is really wanted and needed. A session contract invites the client to take the work seriously from the outset—to consider what is achievable and what he would like to achieve. It invites him to become aware of his internal processes, his wants, and his needs. Not infrequently, developing a session contract *is* the work of the session; exploring the "what would you like to accomplish" can be, for someone closed to internal contact, a difficult and lengthy process. Alternatively, the work initiated by the session contract can shift, leading into areas unanticipated by either client or therapist. By the end of the hour, work may have been done that seems far, indeed, from the initial session contract. It is illuminating, though, at the end of such a session, to ask the client about the relationship between what he is dealing with now (at the end of the hour) and what he initially wanted to do. Invariably, we have found, the client knows and can describe how the two are related—even when the therapist cannot.

"Homework" can be a useful part of therapy; it adds to the credibility of the therapist, and it keeps the client working between sessions and, thus, extends the therapeutic influence beyond that which occurs in the therapist's office. A homework assignment is also a kind of contract, one in which the client accepts responsibility for carrying out some task before he and the therapist meet again. Homework usually involves either trying out some new or unfamiliar behavior or observing (and often writing about) current behavior patterns. It can be designed to explore patterns of thinking ("Notice every time you discount yourself, and figure out what you would rather be believing about yourself"), of feeling ("As soon as you become aware of those angry feelings coming up, stop and write down what you have just been doing, thinking, and believing"), or behavior ("Will you agree to spend at least one hour each day this week doing something that you enjoy?"). Sometimes homework is paradoxical, inviting the client in one way or another to do the very thing that he has been trying to avoid (for instance, the client who fears being criticized may be asked to deliberately request criticism from his boss); this can provide insight into the function of his unwanted behavior, as well as breaking up the logjam of futile struggling that has immobilized him. Whatever the nature of the homework, it must—like any other contract—be agreed upon by both client and therapist. When it is completed, the results can be used in building the next session's contract. When it is not, discussing the noncompletion often leads to new and useful insights, which in turn provide a foundation for the next homework contract.

As any salesman can tell you, "closing" a contract is one of the most important parts of the contracting process. Closing a therapeutic contract involves making sure that the client fully intends to carry it out and that any reservations he has about it have been aired and dealt with. Therapeutically useful contracts nearly always involve some sort of cost (either real or fantasized); if there were no cost, the client would have long ago achieved the contracted-for goal on his own. Discovering the costs—working through the fears and prohibitions—does not precede therapy; it *is* therapy. Indeed, developing and closing a contract may require much more than a single session. The contracting process begun in the initial session shapes what is to come; in future work, the client will face, appreciate, and work through the obstacles to his chosen contract. With that completed, the rest of therapy may turn out to be just coasting home.

One last word about therapeutic contracting is that part of contract negotiating is *re*negotiating. An initial contract is really a jumping-off point, the first in a series of emerging therapeutic goals. A good therapeutic contract is an ongoing process rather than a finished product; it shifts and changes as the work opens up new vistas, new possibilities, and new areas to be explored.

## SAYING GOOD-BYE

The final task of the first session with a new client is that of saying good-bye. The getting-acquainted process is well under way, some initial diagnoses have been made, client and therapist have decided—for now, at least—that they will work together, an initial therapeutic contract has been (or is being) developed, and a relationship has begun to come into being. Much has been done, and it is time for this session to end.

The single most important criterion for a good session ending of an initial session is that the client wants to return. No matter how difficult, painful, or confrontive some of the earlier moments may have been (and it is hoped that, in an initial session, this kind of negative experience is at a minimum), the end of the session is a time for support and appreciation. To feel good about coming back, the client needs to feel that he has gotten something; that he has been understood, respected, and valued; and that something worthwhile can come of this experience.

Beginning therapists need to beware, though, of the temptation to end a session with some stroke of therapeutic genius that will demonstrate how wise and far-seeing they are. Such interpretations are likely to do more harm than good: they may simply echo what the client already knows, leaving him wondering why the therapist would think he needs to be told; they may go further than the client is ready to look, raising his defenses and lowering his trust level; or they may miss the mark entirely and leave the client confused and the therapist looking foolish. Moreover, such endings tend to disempower the client, implying that the therapist (not the client) is responsible for figuring things out. It is much better for the client to be impressed with his own wisdom than with that of the therapist; asking him what has stood out for him in the work that has been done or how he expects to use the work in the days to come is generally more useful than telling him something about himself. (And the answer to the latter question, about using the work in his out-of-therapy life, is a fine lead-in to a homework suggestion.)

The client should leave the therapist's office feeling like a partner in the work rather than like a patient being worked on. He is the boss, the CEO, and the therapist is his assistant. He is the expert on himself, the only one with access to what is to be explored. Respecting him as the primary change-maker will keep him active and involved in the therapeutic process, and his activity and involvement will increase the likelihood of a successful outcome (Hanna, 1996, p. 231).

How the first session is ended sets the tone of endings for the duration of the work. The client should be given some warning that the time is almost up ("I see we have about ten minutes left; is there anything more that you want to be sure to tell me about today?") and then, when it *is* up, the session ends. Ordinarily, it is not useful to allow the client to drag out the session, either with small talk ("Looks like a nice weekend coming up; hope you've got something good planned . . .") or with last-minute requests ("Oh, I forgot, there's just one thing I really wanted to ask you . . ."). The session is over. The therapist may have enjoyed meeting this person; she may be glad to be working with him, or she may have trepidations about the work. In either case, she knows that she and the client stand at the beginning of a journey together. She smiles, she ushers him out, perhaps they shake hands. The door closes. The next time it opens for this client, the work will truly have begun.

## SUMMARY

Major tasks for the first session with a new client include beginning to build a therapeutic environment, gathering and giving information, and establishing a sense of hope. To do this, the therapist must join the client, attending to his thoughts, feelings, behaviors, and expectations. All of this helps to create and maintain a healing presence.

Both client and therapist must make a decision as to whether they want to work together. For the client, this requires that he be informed about what therapy will be like and what the relative costs and benefits may be. The therapist should refer the client elsewhere if she is not trained to work with this sort of person and/or these sorts of problems or if there is a mismatch of attitudes or values that will prevent her from joining the client in an authentic and caring therapeutic relationship.

Goals of therapy are defined by the therapeutic contract. Contracts are built around the answers to four questions: (a) How are you? (b) How would you like things to be different? (c) How did things get to be the way they are? (d) How will we know when you have accomplished your goals? In finding answers to these questions, a formal diagnosis may be helpful; it can also be helpful to evaluate the client's resources and to begin to develop a sense of his life script. Contracts may be long- or short-term or may even be set up for a single session's work; they frequently need to be renegotiated.

The final task of the initial session is saying good-bye. This should be done in such a way that the client leaves feeling respected and supported, a partner in the therapeutic task.

# 8 CHAPTER | Moving In

In Shakespeare's *Julius Caesar,* Cassius says to Brutus:

> And since you cannot see yourself,
> So well as by reflection,
> I, your glass,
> Will modestly discover to yourself that of
> Yourself which you
> Yet know not of.

Although psychotherapy was unknown in Cassius' day (or in Shakespeare's, for that matter), Cassius' remark was an eloquent description of the task of the psychotherapist. The therapist serves as a mirror that helps her clients discover that of themselves that they do not yet know. More often than not, what must be discovered is something that the client has hidden from himself, and has good reason to keep hidden—were this not so, he would have no need of our help in rediscovering it.

So the client comes to therapy both wanting to know and wanting not to know. He has worked hard to keep parts of himself—memories, thoughts, feelings—out of awareness, yet he needs to rediscover those parts if he is to make the changes he wants. To help him in the discovery process, we must also help him to move past his don't-want-to-know. That is what this chapter is about—getting past the barriers to knowing and accessing the thoughts, feelings, memories, and physical sensations that the client has hidden from himself.

Strupp (1969) has asserted that "for therapeutic learning to occur, the most important precondition is the patient's *openness* to the therapist's influence" (p. 210). If therapist and client, working together, can create a relationship in which the client feels safe to be open—as far as he is able, at any given moment—the therapist can then guide him into the kinds of exploration and experimentation that lead to more and more full contact with himself. This will involve helping him to move away from the safe but fruitless questions that he has been asking himself, away from the behavior patterns that are keeping him stuck, into new and different ways of knowing himself. The new ways are often uncomfortable and may at first seem unrelated to his primary goal, and their discomfort and strangeness often invite him to resist and to fall back into the old and familiar. Yet, if the therapeutic relationship is solid and ongoing, and the therapist well attuned to the client's needs and fears, discomfort and strangeness can become signs of progress rather than barriers.

A major task in the early stages of psychotherapy is teaching the client how to be a client—how to look inside and begin to reconnect with himself and to welcome the reconnections when they occur. Most new clients expect therapy to give them "answers." They ask "why" questions: Why do these things happen to me? Why do people act that way? Why do I get myself into such a mess? They have forgotten how to simply observe themselves—what they are feeling, thinking, and wanting—without trying to explain. The explanations that they create generally push them back into their old defenses and away from contact with their ongoing experiencing. Words like "because" and "probably" and "should" take the client into the realm of explanation and self-criticism and distract him from full contact with himself and with the therapist. As we go about helping the client access himself, we continually bring him back to phenomenology, to what he is aware of at the moment (Guidano, 1991, p. 158). Attending to one's ongoing phenomenology leads to contact; contact leads to awareness; awareness opens the door to change and growth.

## AFFECT AND AWARENESS

One of the paradoxes of psychotherapy is that clients, who have usually sought treatment because they want to stop feeling bad in some way or another, generally do not know in detail just what they are feeling or when they are feeling it. A client may describe his depression but have no awareness of the anger and resentment that underlie it; or he may talk about his frequent angry outbursts but not mention (or even notice) that he is afraid of losing his job, his wife, or his friends as a result of those outbursts. Affects and emotions are complicated things: they slide into each other; they overlap; they have layers and underlayers; they can change in an instant or stay with us for hours. They make our lives worthwhile (who would want to live with no feelings at all?); they make our lives miserable. Strict behaviorists may assert that affect is simply a matter of chemical events in the body; yet, the experience of affect is deeply and personally connected to our sense of being-in-the-world.

## Feelings and Beliefs

Infants appear to be on much better terms with their affect than are most adults. They neither hide their feelings nor hang on to them; they live what is going on for them in the moment. Internal awareness of affect leads immediately and naturally into outward expression of emotion. There are no "bad" or "good" feelings, no shame or should-ness about them; what is, is. Over time, though, children learn that some feelings are bad or wrong and should not be expressed—maybe should not even be experienced; after all, nice/normal/strong/worthwhile people do not react to things that way. They may learn that some kinds of feelings are uncomfortable or painful and are best not attended to; or they may come to believe that feelings can make them do things that cause them trouble: can make them hit people, or steal, or abuse themselves.

What people believe about their feelings either magnifies or attenuates those feelings (Lee, 1998, p. 145). By the time an adult client appears in a therapist's office, his ability to observe his own affect is so papered over with beliefs about that affect that the feelings themselves may be quite unaccessible to his awareness: he is "feeling thoughts" (Therapist: "What are you feeling?" Client: "I feel that I shouldn't have done it.") or "thinking about feelings" (Therapist: "What are you feeling?" Client: "I think I'm all mixed up.") and has lost touch with his raw experience. His affective experience, as well as his emotional expression of that experience, is confused with his beliefs, hopes, and memories. He says—and believes—that he wants to change the way he feels; but, in fact, he does not know what he is feeling. The worst feelings—the most painful fears, angers, and sadnesses—are hidden away, too unpleasant to allow into awareness. Keeping those feelings out of awareness has required that he distort and disrupt contact with himself and with others; and, without contact, the pain and the problems can only grow.

Relationship-focused psychotherapy is designed to help the client reverse the process: to restore contact, to bring the hidden thoughts, feelings, and memories back into awareness, so that the mistaken learnings and beliefs that surround them—the life script—can be dissolved. This means doing precisely what the client has worked so hard to avoid: going into the affective experiences that he has blocked from awareness. Say Greenberg and Paivio (1997), "The primary maladaptive feelings of badness, weakness, or insecurity and the fears of annihilation, disintegration, and abandonment have to be accessed in order to allow for change. It is only through experience of the emotion that emotional distress can be cured" (p. 123).

## Working with Feelings

Accessing painful feelings is not, for many clients, simply a matter of enduring something unpleasant. Early trauma, either acute or cumulative, can bring about reactions that seem to threaten one's very self, one's very existence. Keeping those feelings out of awareness is, to such a client, a survival issue. Yet—and here is the paradox, again—true survival, as a whole person, requires that feelings be experienced and assimilated. The poison must be drained from the memories—the intensity of the affect reduced—to free the client to be spontaneously himself in the here and now.

Not just single emotional responses but whole patterns of emotion as well can become a part of the don't-want-to-go-there phenomenon. Greenberg and Paivio (1997) describe some of these patterns: rage following shame (and blotting out the pain of feeling ashamed), for instance, or fear following intimacy (inhibiting further contact). Again, these patterns must be activated and brought into awareness in order to be reorganized. By experiencing them, facing them, and working them through, the client frees himself from their constrictions.

*Working through* is a vague sort of concept—necessarily so, since the working-through process is different for each person and can even be different for different aspects of script within the same person. Yet one part of working through tends to be constant: working through requires talking about what one is discovering. "Experience is not simply 'in' us, fully formed," say Greenberg and Pascual-Leone (1991). "Rather, we need to put words to our feelings to bring them to full awareness" (p. 171). Not only the *putting into words* is important here but also the *sharing* of those words with a supportive and protective other. The healing process involves a shuttling between internal and external contact, between focusing on what one is discovering inside and daring to share those discoveries with another person. The therapist's job is to create a psychological space in which that shuttling can occur, to co-inhabit that space with the client, to both lead (suggesting, inquiring, directing) and follow (attuned to the client's needs and rhythms, respecting the client's wisdom and autonomy) as the client learns to know himself.

## Supporting Emotional Accessibility

In the early days of psychotherapy, as we have mentioned before, the therapist (analyst) was advised to be a "blank screen," to let as little as possible of herself be visible to the client. It was thought that keeping the therapist distant and impersonal would facilitate the client's using her as a kind of psychological stand-in for other important people in the client's life, people with whom the client needed to work through old relationship issues. A major problem with this strategy, though, is that it deprives the client of the opportunity to form a real relationship with the therapist. One cannot be distant and impersonal and at the same time enter into a contactful relationship. Moreover, in the social climate of the 2000s, maintaining this kind of psychological distance is likely to be perceived by the client as disapproving or even hostile; and, as Henry and Strupp (1994) point out, "interventions designed to enhance the immediacy and depth of emotional experiencing are likely to fail if the underlying process is one of hostile separation or interpersonal distance between patient and therapist" (p. 72). We cannot effectively support the client in accessing and expressing his feelings unless we are willing to be active participants in the relationship, letting ourselves be known and impacted by the client's emotional experience.

For some clients, accessing and expressing emotions is a slow, cumulative process. At first tentative, often ashamed of what they are experiencing, they are alert to any sign that the therapist regards their feelings as odd, wrong, or out of place. Not infrequently, they will apologize: "I'm sorry for getting so upset," or "Excuse me for breaking down this way." If they sense respect and receptivity in the therapist, they are encouraged to go more and more deeply into their affective experience. Other clients tend to stop and start: they share some deep feeling, then pull back and "get control," then dip again into their emotions. When the therapist is contactful, yet willing to be governed by the client's self-pacing, each of these new excursions into feeling can be a bit deeper than the one before.

Expressing feelings that have been hidden away for months or years can be a frightening experience, an emotional roller coaster that threatens to go out of control, overwhelming the client or pushing him into impulsive and perhaps hurtful behaviors. In addition to supporting the client in his affective exploration, the therapist must also help him to contain the feelings, taking over some of the responsibility for control, so that the client does not have to try to hold back and forge ahead at the same time. In order to feel safe, the client needs to know that the therapist will not be swept up in the storm of emotional expression; will not be overwhelmed by the client's sadness, intimidated by his anger, or immobilized by his fear. Glickauf-Hughes, Wells, and Chance (1996) recommend that the therapist speak slowly and calmly, so that the client can sense her confidence that the problem can be managed (p. 434)

Therapists as well as clients can be reassured by their own tone and pace. Slowing down allows us to listen rather than simply react; it lets us bring our focus back to the client's experience rather than our own response, helps us to stay with the client's perspective instead of leaping into problem solving. It reminds us of why we are here: to support and empower the client in his own journey of discovery. It may be that the process of discovery will be all that is needed, for "the very acts of approaching, attending to, and accepting or positively evaluating feelings leads to their transformation" (Greenberg & Paivio, 1997, p. 98). Even when further work is necessary, that work will go more smoothly when the therapist acts—and feels—calm and competent.

"Calm and competent," though, can be overdone if they create artificiality in the therapist's manner. The therapist's external calmness must not be used as a cover-up for her true reaction; the client will sense that something is wrong, and the therapist's dissimulation will be more alarming than if she shared her feelings. "As you tell me that, I find myself getting angry too," or "when you talk about what happened to that little boy, I feel sad" are responses that can be given calmly and still reflect the therapist's honest reaction. An effective therapist continually monitors her own expressions of affect, attuning those expressions to the needs of the client, yet remaining an authentic participant in the therapeutic relationship. She does not so much hide her feelings as select among them, choosing to express that aspect of herself that will best facilitate the client's exploration of his own affective experience.

## FEAR AND ANXIETY

A certain amount of fear and anxiety is almost a given in psychotherapy. Clients arrive fearful: afraid of their own feelings and/or behaviors, which they can no longer control; afraid of the future and what it will bring if they cannot change; afraid of therapy itself. They know or suspect that they will have to look at things that they would rather avoid, and they fear what they may see. Sometimes it seems that their very selves will be shattered if they allow themselves to truly face what they have been denying—and, in a sense, that fear is justified; making life script changes, major changes in the way one organizes one's world, does involve changing oneself in ways that cannot be anticipated.

Unpleasant as it is to experience, though, anxiety is not always a hinderance to psychotherapy. Without a certain amount of anxiety, people would probably not be motivated to do the hard work required in order to change and grow. Within a certain range of intensity, anxiety also seems to heighten one's sensitivity and one's ability to retain and integrate new information. Says Lee (1998), "There is a curvilinear relationship between fear and learning. . . . As fear increases, learning does until the apex is reached, after which as fear further increases, learning declines . . . excessive anxiety can inhibit development but, if brought down to a satisfactory level, it is a spur to growth" (p. 133). One consequence of this relationship between anxiety and learning is that the therapist may, on occasion, have to not only tolerate but even stimulate a certain amount of anxiety in her client. This requires, of course, that the therapeutic relationship be solid and positive: few clients would accept a therapist's anxiety-creating behaviors unless they were quite certain that the therapist was acting in their best interest. "A willingness to create discomfort *in a situation where both members can recognize and identify a history of rapport and caring* is a necessary part of therapy" (Callaghan, Naugle, & Folette, 1996, p. 385; italics ours). Without a history of rapport and caring, the therapist who creates discomfort will be seen as insensitive or cruel, and therapy is likely to go nowhere. Even with such a history, it is important that the client understand the rationale underlying the therapist's behavior, and that the therapist eventually move back into a more supportive and receptive stance.

Although some anxiety, some discomfort, may be useful in therapy, too much anxiety can immobilize a client or lead him to barricade himself from his feelings rather than explore them. Many clients come to therapy in order to deal with anxiety that threatens to overwhelm them. These clients are looking for a way to reduce and/or control anxiety; the last thing they want is to intensify it. Yet, it is essential that they talk about their problems and work through their memories of pain and trauma. It is often helpful to suggest to such clients that they can work on just one issue or incident at a time, putting all the others temporarily on hold; this allows them to keep their anxiety at a bearable level (Erskine, 1993/1997c). Similarly, clients can be assisted to move into anxiety-generating content gradually, getting the "feel" of the anxiety and learning that they need not be devastated by it. Hanna (1996) suggests using "Gestalt approaches such as 'stay with it' [to] help a client to be able to tolerate anxiety to the point of simply seeing it as a kind of sensation, without the gloomy or intimidating aspects normally associated with it" (pp. 252–253). A significant part of the experience of anxiety has to do with one's efforts to avoid it or turn it off; anxious feelings that one chooses to move into, describing them fully to a supportive therapist, are a quite different experience than anxious feelings that one tries (usually without success) to escape.

Notice, in that last sentence, that the anxious feelings are not only invited, entered into willingly, but are also put into words. The therapist's presence as a caring and involved other changes the quality of any strong emotion, including anxiety. An anxious child instinctively seeks help and protection from an older, stronger, wiser person. The experience of trauma, rejection, or betrayal may stifle that natural response, and many anxious adults have taught themselves to suffer alone. One of the functions of the therapeutic relationship is to allow the client to regain the ability to seek help and comfort in relationship. The therapist becomes the caring adult who was not available at the time of the original trauma—the adult who should have been there to listen, sympathize, and protect the child. As the client regains the ability to use the therapeutic relationship to mitigate his discomfort, that discomfort (along with his learned ways of relating to others) begins to be transformed.

## RESISTANCE AND REPRESSION

Nobody likes to hurt. Even a so-called masochist chooses to endure one kind of pain in order to avoid something even more painful. It is a given that clients, throughout therapy, will sometimes resist the therapist's invitation to explore their situation because they believe (consciously or unconsciously) that doing so will be difficult and uncomfortable. It is much easier to talk about trivialities or to complain about other people than to open up long-hidden parts of oneself; often, the very thing that most needs to be looked at and talked about is the thing one most desperately wants to avoid.

Most of us had the experience, as children, of falling and skinning a knee. It hurt! And the sight of that hurt knee, with all its dirt and blood, was frightening, too. I (JM) remember crying and running into the house, wailing that I had hurt myself. My mother was there, and I ran to her, wanting her to comfort me and make the pain go away. But, instead, she wanted to look at the raw knee—wash it off—put disinfectant on it. *NO, MOM! Don't touch it! Don't even get near it!*

Clients can be expected to resist the pain of self-exploration just as a child resists the pain of cleaning up a hurt knee. A major theme of the early stages of therapy is moving through that resistance, getting to the place where the work needs to be done.

## Resistance

Resistance, says Freyd (1996), has many names. "Whatever we call it—repression, dissociation, psychological defense, denial, amnesia, unawareness, or betrayal blindness—the failure to know some significant and negative aspect of reality is an aspect of human experience that remains at once elusive and of central importance" (p. 16). Resistance is not an abnormal reaction, not something to criticize the client about, not something that should surprise or dismay a therapist. It is what people do. It is what therapists are paid to help clients work through. Helping them do so is one of the most important parts of our job.

Why is resistance such a universal phenomenon? Why should it be so difficult to look into oneself? To answer this question, we go back to the notion of life script: the patterns of thoughts, feelings, and behaviors that one has established throughout life in order to manage and make sense of the world. Changing those script patterns threatens one's sense of who one is and how one gets along in life. "Resistance," Janoff-Bulman (1993) notes, "actually reflects our powerful tendency to maintain rather than change the fundamental beliefs that have enabled us to make sense of ourselves and our world" (p. 40). Changing the interior decorations of one's psychological home—putting on some new paint, getting a few different pieces of furniture—is one thing; shaking its very foundations is something else again! Fundamental changes threaten our stability, our ability to predict and prepare ourselves for what may come next. Things may be miserable right now; we may be acutely uncomfortable; but at least the misery and the discomfort are familiar—we know them, we know what to expect.

In chapter 2, we discussed the benefits of maintaining a life script, and we introduced the PICS acronym. *PICS* applies to resistance as well (resistance is a means whereby script is maintained): resistance helps us to maintain *predictability,* of ourselves and of others. It helps us to maintain our *identity,* our sense of who we are. It provides us with *continuity* from one moment to the next, protecting us from the disruptions of change. It gives us the illusion of *stability* in a kaleidoscope of feelings and needs. Predictability, identity, continuity, stability—without them, where would we be? *Who* would we be? So, we twist ourselves around, pushing away any internal or external awareness that might threaten to disrupt our fragile equilibrium. "The trade-off of a distorted awareness for a sense of security is, I believe, an organizing principle operating over many levels and realms of human life" (Goleman, 1985, p. 21). People—all people—tend to disrupt or deny any contact with themselves and others that would threaten the script patterns they guard with such vigilance. That disruption or denial is the essence of resistance.

## Repression

Resistance involves not allowing oneself to know what one knows, to feel what one feels, or to recognize what one sees; it is a close relative of repression, a concept we introduced in chapter 2. Denial of thoughts, disavowal of feelings, and desensitization of our bodies are the mechanisms by means of which repression is accomplished; they are also the mechanisms by means of which people resist change. Resistance protects repression; it is an out-of-awareness attempt to keep the repressive processes intact. At the same time, resistance is protected by repression: clients must keep their resistant maneuvers out of awareness if those maneuvers are to be successful. Each maintains the other; if one fails, the other is weakened. To understand how a relationship-focused integrative psychotherapy helps clients to overcome their resistance, then, we shall need to revisit the idea of repression, how it works, and what its consequences may be.

Freud (1915/1963), who originated the notion of repression, said that "the essence of repression lies simply in the function of rejecting and keeping something out of consciousness" (p. 105). Repression is more than simply forgetting something: it is an active and ongoing process, even though it takes place outside of conscious awareness. Freud's descriptions of repression make it sound like a sort of psychic wrestling match, with repressed elements struggling to make their way into consciousness and the ego's defenses struggling with equal vigor to keep them out. Since the whole process is, by definition, out of awareness, we shall probably never know how accurate Freud's picture is. What practitioners now agree upon is that, in repression, there is a failure to access something that we once knew. Moreover, that something is significant: it relates in some important way to our present situation. Our inability to access it is not a random error, a coincidence; it is motivated by our need to protect ourselves from the consequences of bringing it to consciousness.

"Repression," say Atwood and Stolorow (1984), "is understood as a process whereby particular configurations of self and object are prevented from crystallizing in awareness . . . because of their association with emotional conflict and subjective danger" (p. 35). Notice that phrase, "configurations of self and object": repression is about child and parent, husband and wife, client and therapist, me and you. Repression is *relational*; it involves patterns of self-other, of internal-external. The elements of the pattern—who is involved, and how—are just outside the client's awareness, ready to form, but he prevents that formation by keeping them separate, unrelated, and—by virtue of their unrelatedness—without meaning and without threat.

**Memory As an Active Process**    Repression is a motivated failure to remember something of significance. To understand just how this works, we need to remind ourselves that remembering is not simply the conjuring up of some sort of mental picture album. We do not register images like a camera and store them away to be reviewed at a later time. Rather, both our first awareness of something and our later recall of it are active, creative processes. We notice things that have meaning for us—that is, things that relate to our previous store of experiences in some way. What we notice, as well as what we believe and remember about it, is strongly influenced by those previous experiences. Imagine, for instance, that you are walking in the woods when you hear a cracking noise behind you. What could it be? Your answer will depend largely upon your previous experiences. If you have just seen a movie or a television program about people shooting at each other, you may hear the noise as a shot. The next day, you may tell a friend that you heard shooting in the woods; a year later, you may remember the day someone shot at you while you were out walking. Now, stop here and ask yourself what mental image you have constructed as you read about this incident. What kind of trees are you imagining in the woods? What was the time of day? If we now say that the trees are fir trees, that their branches are covered with snow, and that the cracking noise is one of the branches breaking under the weight of the load, do you have to adjust your picture? Even the way we read a written description is selective and creative: we fill in the blanks with our own story. Every time we recall something—whether it happened a few seconds ago or many years ago—we continue to fill in the blanks. We are involved in "the continual re-membering of our memories of our memories" (Clocksin, 1998, p. 114). Repression is not only the failure to bring up some stored image; it is also the active mistaken perceiving or re-membering of what happened. We can repress one memory, one awareness, by papering it over with a memory or a perception of something that never happened—or at least never happened in the way we now believe it did.

It would be impossible to remember everything. Even people with eidetic memories do not remember every impression, every sight or sound or idea that has passed through their conscious awareness. There is simply too much; trying to remember it all would jam our circuits. We remember the things that are relevant, that may be useful in the future, that help us to find things we want and avoid things that could be dangerous. Usually, this information is encoded as traces, key ideas that we use as frameworks upon which to reconstruct the memory—much as a good comedian remembers only the punch lines of jokes, rebuilding the rest as needed. We do not forget something entirely when we repress it; we merely suppress the reconstruction process. But the framework is still there, ready to be built up again whenever repression fails.

**Knowing and Not Knowing**    It is all out of awareness, of course, all the complex ways in which memory operates. We are unaware, for the most part, of the shortcuts and strategies we use as we encode a memory trace and of the reconstruction activity we use to bring it back into consciousness. We are equally—and necessarily—unaware of the ways in which we distort, delete, and add to what we originally experienced.

The net result of all of this resembles an elaborate filing system, files within files—some relatively complete and some with instructions about which other files must be opened in order to gather all the wanted information. Many of these files are easily accessible; others must be tracked down through the network; still others are locked tight, their information hidden from conscious awareness. Goleman (1985) describes the locked-up information this way: "The memories are grouped in 'themes,' a particularly rich set of schemas, like a file of documents. Each theme is arranged like layers of an onion around the core of forbidden information. The nearer to that core one probes, the stronger is the resistance. The deepest schemas encode the most painful memories, and are the hardest to activate" (p. 113).

All of this complexity is at odds with what most of us would like to believe about knowing and remembering. Things would be much simpler if we either knew or did not know, remembered or did not remember. But it does not work that way. Says Freyd (1996), "We know things we cannot articulate, and we know things we do not even know we know. *To know* is not unitary" (p. 80). One of the most familiar examples of the know-but-don't-know experience is the "tip-of-the-tongue" phenomenon: that word you cannot quite think of but can *almost* remember.

## How Repression Is Accomplished

It is all very well to talk about the complexities of memory and to assert that one can know something without being consciously aware of it; but how, precisely, do people manage to block specific ideas and memories from awareness? Knowing how we do something can help us develop ways of undoing it; knowing how memories are repressed may assist us in re-accessing them.

Memories are most easily accessed when they are well assimilated, well integrated into one's total store of knowledge. The more thoroughly we integrate some bit of information, the more pathways there are to access it; when one pathway is blocked, we can use another. It follows that one way to keep a memory out of awareness is to prevent its being assimilated, to freeze it somehow so that it cannot interact with all of the other things one knows and can remember. According to Goleman (1985), this is precisely what we are able to do when we experience something that is traumatic or dangerous: "Whenever we are faced with an overwhelming experience that we sense as potentially disintegrating, we have the ability to suspend it and 'freeze' it in an unassimilated, inchoate form and maintain it in that state indefinitely, or for as long as necessary" (p. 27).

Even unassimilated, inchoate, and frozen memories, however, are not completely lost. They still have the power to disturb us, to knock at the door of awareness. They stir up affect; we feel sad, or frightened, or angry but do not know why. They threaten to break out when we experience something closely associated with the original experience: a particular smell, a tone of voice, or a bit of music.

**State-Dependent Memories**   One's internal and external surround, one's moment-to-moment phenomenology, can link strongly to a repressed memory. Incidents experienced in a particular place are best recalled when one is in that same place; memories laid down when one was in a particular emotional state may be triggered by a return to that state. Many students discover that they do better on a test if they can study in the same room where the test will later be given: the smells and sounds of the exam room trigger memories of things learned earlier in that same room. Internal states, too, can trigger memories of previous experiences: anxious persons may remember things that happened the last time they were anxious, for instance. This is the *state-dependent* phenomenon. "Memories acquired in one state are accessible mainly in that state but are 'dissociated' or not available for recall in an alternative state. It is as though the two states constitute different libraries into which a person places memory records, and a given memory record can be retrieved only by returning to that library, or physiological state, in which the event was first stored" (Bower, 1981, p. 130).

Rossi (1990) believes that the state-dependent nature of memories has to do with actual substances that affect the brain's information-coding process. "Under the impact of stress (any form of emotional or novel experience), many information substances are released throughout the body. Many of these substances can reach the neural networks of the brain to encode our life experiences in a state-dependent manner; that is, what we remember, learn, and experience is dependent on the different psychological states encoded in the brain by informational substances." (p. 357).

Whether or not future research will validate Rossi's theory, it is nevertheless clear that one's psychological state, as well as one's physical surroundings, is a critical factor in one's ability to access stored information. Other things being equal, the more similar one's present state is to the state in which a memory was acquired, the more easily that memory can be retrieved. This is especially important when dealing with life script information, patterns of beliefs and behaviors that were often acquired and coded early in life and/or at times of great stress. A neglected or abused child, for instance, lays down memories of neglect or abuse and makes life-determining decisions about himself, others, and the quality of life in a state of extreme stress; moreover, it is the stress state of a young child (Erskine & Moursund, 1988/1998). It is a small wonder that, as an adult, this person might have difficulty accessing either the child's experiences or the decisions and beliefs those experiences led to; yet, in the presence of a respectful and contactful therapist, the same person may re-enter his earlier psychological state and remember fully both the painful events and his responses to them.

**Selective Experiencing**    Entering into a given state helps one to access memories laid down in a past similar state. Some of those memories have the capacity to make us uncomfortable. It makes sense, then, that our self-protective mechanisms should also lead us to avoid those memory-triggering states—especially when they are painful in and of themselves. Resistance serves to protect repression. We are drawn to experiences that fit comfortably with what we know and want to know; we avoid experiences that do not fit and remind us of a world we would rather not believe in. "Persons use 'selective noticing' of experiences," says Atwood (1999), "scanning the environment and taking in only those aspects that are in agreement with their socially constructed realities" (p. 16).

How can a person know in advance that some experience should be not noticed? How do we evaluate a perception for its potential dangerousness without letting ourselves know what it is? Browne (1990) suggests that it is the affective component of an experience that warns us; the first hint of an emotional reaction sets off a train of events in the central nervous system that ultimately results in a kind of selective perception and allows us to notice only that which is "safe." As for the rest—the door slams shut, experience is walled off, and even the affect that initiated the process may be banished from awareness.

## Consequences of Repression

Repression—and all of the mechanisms that make repression possible—allows one to know without knowing, to remember without being aware of one's memories. Moreover, the repressive process does not stop with the single, original experience that is being restrained. Repression spreads into other cognitive activities and eventually impacts perception, recognition, learning, judgment, and behavior (Cloitre, 1997). The result: psychiatric symptoms, the emotional, cognitive, and often even physical distress that brings clients to a therapist's office.

Even though repressive processes tend to ripple out and affect broader and broader areas of one's life, they usually prove to be imperfect barriers to memory. Repressed information leaks through, entering our conscious awareness by means of dreams, fantasies, or flashbacks. "Because the original traumatic event has been actually perceived, and a trace has been laid down (in some form of unstable, short-term storage) but not worked through in reflection to long-term memory, it remains 'active,' and, again, in spite of denial, it leaks, breaks through, and causes 'flashbacks' on the screen of perception" (Browne, 1990, p. 28). Flashbacks are at best uncomfortable; more often they are terrifying. An individual suffering from flashbacks feels out of control of his own thoughts. Disjointed fragments of memory leap into awareness, vivid and compelling. He is trapped by these fragments, forced to re-experience and helpless to change them. His very attempt (out of awareness) to protect himself has resulted in a solution more painful than the problem itself.

Even when actual flashbacks do not occur, repression is likely to cause other sorts of perceptual distortions. Repression requires that one block off information about current reality (lest the current reality trigger the memory that must be repressed). Blocked information cannot be fully integrated; some parts of the self are literally not allowed to know what other parts are doing, thinking, or feeling. This can lead to a sense of *depersonalization*—feeling detached from one's own body—or dissociation (Freyd, 1996). In the most extreme cases, multiple personalities can develop.

Whether it results in obvious pathology such as dissociation or flashbacks, or in less dramatic alterations of affective and cognitive functioning, the net result of repression is that it interferes with the natural cycle of need arousal and satisfaction. Individuals who must keep themselves from knowing and remembering can no longer be spontaneous and flexible in problem solving or in maintaining a healthy lifestyle. Their social relationships are constrained; because they cannot allow themselves full internal awareness, they cannot be contactful with others.

Therapists are among those "others" with whom the repression-bound person cannot be contactful. Therapists are dangerous to repression; they threaten the walls behind which painful memories are hidden. This brings us back to the notion of resistance—the attempt to hold off the therapist, and her interventions, lest they break through one's repression and allow all that forbidden material into awareness.

## ACCESSING

The benefits of accessing and sharing previously repressed material are (at least) threefold: First, as the defensive walls come down, the individual is no longer divided within himself. He can use all of his cognitive skills, all of his affect, all of his perceptions and memories as he moves through his daily life. Second, because he no longer must restrict internal contact, he can also relate to others more openly, and can use those others as a resource. Finally, as he shares his new awarenesses with others, old feelings and memories change. Sharing what was private requires that it be recoded, languaged; the recoding process is in itself detoxifying. What was an amorphous, forbidding, unknowable mass becomes a set of discrete thoughts, feelings, and behaviors, each of which can now be integrated into the whole of his sense of self.

All of these benefits notwithstanding, though, the therapist must tread very carefully in dealing with a client's resistant behaviors. One of the problems with words like "resistance" and "repression" is that they can be misunderstood as some sort of conscious and deliberate process. Comments such as "he's resistant" or "she's repressing old memories" have a pejorative air about them, as if the client is somehow trying to thwart the therapist's efforts. Nothing could be farther from the truth: resistance, like repression, takes place outside of awareness, insulated from one's will or intentions. They are products of the organism's innate tendency to protect itself from pain or danger. Often, the more strongly one consciously tries to overcome them, the more stubbornly they persist. Our task as therapists is not to blame or criticize the client for resisting, or to try to crash through his resistance, but to help him accept resistance as a natural and normal self-protective skill. We respect his resistance, and we invite him to do so as well: this respect is part of the safety provided within the therapeutic relationship. Says Schneider (1998), ". . . it is crucial to respect resistances. Resistances are lifelines to clients and as miserable as clients' patterns may be, they are the scaffoldings of their existence, both known and familiar" ( p. 115).

### The Internal Landscape

Respecting resistance is easy to talk about; it is more difficult to actually accomplish. Again, the therapist walks a narrow line: valuing the client's resistance, on the one hand, and understanding the need to go beyond it, on the other. Helping clients to find their own way past resistances, as well as to access their hidden information, is one of the therapist's primary challenges. For clients who want more than a small change in external behavior, or whose ability to make even a small change is blocked by the repressive processes we have described, little long-term growth will occur until the log-jam of repression is broken and internal contact is restored. But how can this accessing be accomplished? As Goleman (1985) reminds us, "the contents of awareness come to us picked over, sorted through, and pre-packaged. The whole process takes a fraction of a second" (p. 65). If the client is to make changes in his basic ways of experiencing and organizing the world, he will have to go beyond this picked-over terrain into a richer internal landscape.

In that internal landscape, deeper than that which the client knows that he knows, there exists a complex pattern of concepts, meanings, and decisions. Theorists have used a variety of terms to describe these patterns: "personal construct systems" (Kelly, 1955); "personal meaning organizations" (Guidano, 1991); "core ordering processes" (Mahoney, 1991). Whatever we call them, they are the ways in which the client has come to understand himself and the world around him. They are the rules that make sense of things; they tell him who and when and where he is. In a very real sense, his pattern *is* the client; without it, he would not be who he knows himself to be. It is central to his functioning out in the world and within himself.

Embedded in this structure, though, like a cancer spreading its cells through healthy tissue, are the mistaken notions, early childhood conclusions, and survival reactions that constitute the client's life script. As we have seen, script beliefs have to do with the self, with others, and with the quality of life. They tend to be rigid (many were formed during a developmental period in which cognition was concrete, things were either black or white, with no shades of gray) and harsh. They often define the client as less than he should be, yet helpless to change, and the world as punitive and inhospitable. Frequently based on early traumatic experiences, script beliefs are no more directly knowable than any other core cognitive processes—perhaps even less so, since they are so often connected to painful memories that must be kept out of awareness.

Script beliefs are self-perpetuating: under their influence, the client filters and distorts new information so as not to challenge the familiar structure of the world as he knows it. One of the therapist's responsibilities, then, is to interfere with this unaware censorship so that new perceptions and experiences can move in to upset the old, dysfunctional patterns. By interrupting the familiar cognitive sequences—the rules and beliefs that squeeze every new experience into the same old pattern—we help the client to construct new ways of understanding himself and his world (Greenberg & Pascual-Leone, 1991, p. 181).

Changing well-established patterns is not easy. No one enjoys having familiar ways of thinking and understanding disrupted. "Radical reconstruction of current meanings, particularly those central to the self, is customarily and understandably resisted," says Neimeier (1995, p. 116). Again, the therapist's task is twofold: respect the resistance, while helping the client to move through it.

## Communication Patterns

**Implicit Relational Knowing**  The earlier in life a cognitive structure has been laid down, the more difficult it is to access or to change. This is true partly because the earlier structures are overlaid by more recent ones, so that accessing may require a kind of progression through stratum after stratum of beliefs and decisions. Moreover, the earliest structures are not verbal; they were acquired before the individual had language and are thus virtually impervious to languaged, logical challenge. Stern and his colleagues (1998) describe the "ongoing process of negotiation" that occurs between infants and their caregivers. The give and take of these early relationships determines how the infant will organize his way of interacting with the world, and that organization (which Stern and colleagues call "implicit relational knowing") provides the foundation for all later schema. What is internalized at this very early age is not so much information about the caretakers or their treatment of the infant but, rather, the whole process of mutual regulation—the back-and-forth-ing, the way in which each responds and adapts to the other, the whole nonverbal texture of being a human in a world full of other humans.

When the infant-caretaker relationship is healthy, when the infant's needs are generally acknowledged and dealt with, the developing pattern of implicit relational knowing becomes a solid foundation upon which later learnings about relationship can be built. In contrast, many clients' earliest relationships did not acknowledge needs, did not have a consistency of give and take. Their implicit relational knowing has incorporated this dysfunction, and later relationships have been built upon the same patterns—and more than just built upon: what one expects in relationships is what one actually creates. An individual's communication style demands responses that will confirm his expectations; and, when those responses do not occur, he is uncomfortable and tends to leave that relationship and find someone who does fit what he is used to. He can be expected to play out the same drama with his therapist: selective perception of therapist's communications, so as to confirm his script beliefs, and rejection and withdrawal (real or threatened) when the selective perception fails to significantly disguise the reality of what the therapist is offering.

**Ostensible and Underlying Messages**  Every communication contains two levels of message. The most obvious level is the *ostensible* content of the communication: "Breakfast is on the table." "You stepped on my foot." "I love you." Less obvious, and less generally consciously attended to, is an underlying message that describes or defines the relationship between the two individuals. "You stepped on my foot" may be an almost apologetic message from a one-down to a one-up, a warning to a rambunctious child, or a surprised and outraged response to a presumptuous underling. The underlying message is nonverbal, conveyed through voice tone, facial expression, and body language; like all nonverbal communications, it nearly always carries more meaning and force than the words it accompanies.

The communications of psychotherapy have the same two levels, ostensible and underlying. As in any other relationship, when the underlying messages fit the receiver's relational expectations, those messages remain largely unnoticed. When they do not fit—when they violate the client's or the therapist's beliefs about the nature of the relationship—they create discomfort. When an elderly, motherly client says to her young therapist, "You look nice today, dear," the therapist's discomfort probably has to do with the underlying messages about role and relationship expectations conveyed by that message. Similarly, the therapist's understanding and genuine interest may create discomfort in a client whose unconscious relational expectation is that he will be disliked and eventually rejected.

## Relationship and Accessing

Therapists learn to attend to the underlying, relationship-describing part of a communication at least as carefully as to the ostensible content of the message—in both therapist-to-client and client-to-therapist transactions. Say VanKessel and Lietaer (1998), "The therapist will . . . try to reverse the importance of these two levels and not primarily pay attention to the communication content but rather to the signals defining the relationship between the client and him-/herself" (p. 160). It is the underlying, nonverbal part of the client's message that helps the therapist to understand the relational expectations governing the client's world of relationships, the expectations that must be guarded and defended at almost any cost.

In her own underlying communication messages, the therapist refuses to fall into an expected negative relational pattern. She listens, she acknowledges the client's needs, she does not punish or humiliate. She attends to the nonverbal messages sent by the client, but does not allow her responses to be determined by them. She invites the client to stay in relationship with her and to notice the ways in which this relationship is different from others he has known. She invites him to *feel* as well as to think about what is happening between them. By refusing to be shaped by the client's underlying relational messages, the therapist creates a dissonance that shakes that client's basic relational structure. Sometimes with awareness—more often without—he must gradually shift his relational style and expectations in order to be with the therapist in this new way. As he does so, new awareness emerges and access to old structures grows.

Overcoming resistance, melting defenses, accessing underlying script patterns—all of these outcomes are facilitated by a skillful attention to communication patterns. Gently, imperceptibly, the therapist's responses wear away at the client's old expectations, making resistance less and less necessary. Gradually, like rocks emerging as a hill erodes, script beliefs (and memories of the experiences from which they grew) become accessible.

The melting of resistance, as well as the penetration of repressive barriers, marks the middle phase of therapy. There is no clear boundary here, no this-side-or-that marker; the transition, like the wearing away of resistance, is gradual. Progress is uneven and relapses into not knowing are frequent. Through it all, the therapeutic relationship provides the safety that the client needs in order to do his work. Watson and Greenberg (1994) comment that "while the empathic relationship is curative in and of itself, it also provides an optimal environment for completing specific therapeutic tasks" (p. 155). The nature of those specific tasks and the interventions that facilitate their accomplishment vary from one theoretical orientation to another. In chapter 9, we look at some of the tasks and interventions that are most typical of a relationship-focused integrative psychotherapy; in chapter 10, we return to a consideration of the relationship itself as a therapeutic intervention.

## SUMMARY

One of the most important factors in successful therapy is the client's openness, his willingness and ability to look within and begin to reconnect with himself. A central task for the therapist is to enhance client openness and accessibility. Many clients are unaware of their feelings and beliefs; the therapist, through her own emotional and cognitive availability, helps them bring those thoughts and feelings back into awareness. Resistance is a normal and universal process, emerging from our need to maintain what we know and have learned to deal with; repressing disquieting ideas and feelings can provide predictability, identity, continuity, and stability. Repression is a way of maintaining resistance, and resistance protects the process of repression. Memory is an active process; memories are created rather than simply stored. By means of repression, people screen and/or distort the memories to which they have access. Some memories may not be consciously available because, originally laid down while the individual was in a particular psychological state, they can only be retrieved when he re-enters that state. Repressed and state-dependent material can never be kept completely isolated; repressed thoughts and feelings leak into awareness, causing discomfort and distress.

Repression requires that some parts of the self be kept separated from the aware ego and, thus, restricts one's ability to function spontaneously and to be fully available in relationships. Accessing previously repressed material reduces internal division and conflict, enhances relational ability, and invites script change. Accessing and dissolving script can be difficult to accomplish, especially if the script patterns were laid down early in life and have been strongly repressed. The underlying, nonverbal messages embedded in a supportive and authentic therapeutic relationship can bypass resistance, challenge repressed patterns of thinking and feeling, and initiate the process of script change.

# 9 CHAPTER | **Therapeutic Interventions**

"Many therapies fail or are terminated," say Stern and colleagues (1998), "not because of incorrect or unaccepted interpretations, but because of missed opportunities for a meaningful connection between two people" (p. 904). The same could be said of any other sort of intervention, either made in the session or given as homework. The connection between therapist and client is the most important tool that a therapist has, and interventions are, first of all, made in such a way as to preserve and enhance that connection. Henry and Strupp (1994) criticize those who describe therapeutic work simply in terms of its technicalities or its theoretical orientation, saying that such descriptions are "artificially truncated" because they do not deal with the complexities of the human relationship that forms the basis of therapy.

As we discuss some of the kinds of interventions that may prove useful in helping a client access and work with his hidden-from-self beliefs and feelings, then, we must keep in mind that these interventions are useful only in the context of the therapeutic relationship within which they occur. Relationship gives an intervention its impact, makes it believable, encourages the client to use it as a way of experimenting with new ways of thinking and feeling about himself and his world.

## INTERVENTION GUIDELINES

In addition to maintaining the therapeutic relationship, there are some other general concerns to which the therapist needs to attend. The first of these has to do with contact: interventions should be designed so as to enhance the client's contact with himself, with the therapist, and, ultimately with the other people in his world. Whatever the client's specific presenting problem, and whatever specific techniques the therapist may use to help him deal with that problem, healing ultimately comes about through the client's increasing ability to establish and maintain contact with himself and with others and through the emotional experiences that both signal and deepen that contact. The therapeutic relationship itself, when well managed, invites contact; it also provides a safe environment within which other contact-enhancing activities can occur (Gold, 1996).

A second general guideline grows out of the concept of life script, the set of beliefs and decisions that, out of awareness, limit spontaneity and creativity and keep people stuck in old, pain-producing patterns. As contact and awareness increase, the therapist helps the client to challenge his script beliefs, change his script behaviors, and create new experiences that are inconsistent with script. Whether or not they use "script language," most therapeutic approaches are aimed at this sort of change: ". . . different orientations can all be considered attempts to get the client to question and change old assumptions and construals of reality" (Janoff-Bulman, 1993, p. 39). Tending the therapeutic relationship, fostering contact, and dissolving script are interrelated activities; each promotes the others.

A third general intervention principle is that, whenever possible, the client should be allowed to make decisions and discoveries for himself. Making one's own decisions also means choosing one's own goals. People generally work harder and succeed more often when they are pursuing their own goals rather than following someone else's plan, just as they best remember the things they have discovered for themselves. Once a goal (or set of goals) has been agreed upon, the most effective therapists continually invite the client to choose a starting point for his explorations and to follow the avenue that seems most promising to him. If the exploration takes him down a blind alley or off on what seems to be a tangent, the therapist may invite the client to describe the connection between what he is now talking about and what he wants to accomplish. Usually there is such a connection, even if neither client nor therapist recognized it until the question was asked.

Letting the client choose his own path and make his own discoveries helps him to gain confidence in himself and spurs him to further exploration. Conversely, suggesting answers and telling him about himself (even though it may make the therapist feel wise) can undermine the client's self-confidence and increase his passive dependence on the therapist. By telling him what she has figured out, the therapist is tacitly informing the client that she knows better than he does; she is teaching him to wait for the next therapeutic pronouncement.

## Client As Expert

The truth is, of course, that the therapist cannot know the client in the same way that he knows himself. She may hypothesize on the basis of her training and experience, and her hypotheses may turn out to be correct—but there are many other things that the client knows about himself, of which the therapist is quite ignorant. She cannot possibly experience the world exactly as he does, any more than she can share the life history that has shaped his experiencing. Fortunately, the therapist does not need to understand everything about the client; her job is to help *him* to know himself more fully. If she has tended the relationship successfully, the client will trust her enough to share with her what he is learning. If she pretends to know more than she really does, or if she leaps in to share her ideas before the client has a chance to discover his own, she will erode his trust.

The client may choose not to talk about some discoveries or will only talk about them much later in the course of treatment. That is his choice, and the therapist must respect it. If she senses that the client is holding back in a way that interferes with their work together, she may comment on that sense, but the comment will have to do with her concern rather than being a criticism of his behavior. "When we're dealing with a human psyche, we must approach it, if at all, in the same way we would approach a skittish bird during mating season: with enormous respect for its privacy. And if we're going to learn about the bird, we must set aside our own assumptions about what's going on and pay enough attention to find out what's really happening" (Breggin, 1997, p. 13).

Whatever else we may do, then, whatever strategies we may use to enhance contact and assist in dissolving script, we must also promote the client's self-respect: his confidence in his ultimate ability to discover himself, and his valuing of the strength and courage that have allowed him to survive in a difficult world. No matter how hurtful or odd his behavior may seem, this behavior must be understood as an essentially good and competent person's response to a confusing and threatening world. Too often, warns Wile (1984), "clients are seen as gratifying infantile impulses, being defensive, having developmental defects, and resisting the therapy. . . . Therapists who conceptualize people in these ways may have a hard time making interpretations that do not communicate at least some element of this pejorative view" (p. 353).

But wait, you may be saying—the client doesn't know how to discover himself; that's why he has come to therapy. If he could do it on his own, he wouldn't be here. Clients *do* sometimes get into trouble by "gratifying infantile impulses," and their therapy *can* bog down when they are "defensive" and "resistant." How can we help a client get past all this, if we are not supposed to lead or direct him? And you would be right; a part of the therapist's job is indeed to get the client into and through and beyond his defenses, reclaiming those parts of himself that he resists knowing about. Whenever possible, though, we accomplish this not by directing but by inviting, not by answering but by asking. Rather than trying to tell a client what he doesn't know, the therapist encourages him to attend to what he does know. Internal experience is not an either-or sort of thing, with a clear demarcation between what is known and what is kept from awareness. Instead, there is a broad band of almost-known, of could-know-but-never-noticed, between what is available to awareness and what is not. "By helping clients to actively attend to and represent their inner experience," say Watson and Greenberg (1994), "therapists support clients in realizing more hidden or latent parts of themselves" (p. 154). Successful interventions bring to a client's attention that which he is capable of knowing at this moment. By attending to what he can know, he gradually expands the borders of his awareness. The therapist points and invites, and the client looks. The *client* decides how far to go; *he* is in charge.

All this being said, all cautions given, though, there are some strategies and techniques that a therapist can use to make the treatment more efficient. Particularly in these days of managed care and time-limited therapy, most clients can no longer afford a leisurely, take-lots-of-detours sort of treatment— even though they might well benefit from having more time and taking more excursions. Therapists are expected to help clients make as much progress as possible in as short a time as possible; and, to do so, they often must become active in suggesting, inviting, and sharing ideas.

## INTERPRETATION

Interpretation is probably the most common of all active therapeutic strategies. In an interpretation, the therapist shares with the client her own perspective about the client's dynamics. She tells him, in one way or another, what she thinks is going on and/or what might be useful in dealing with it. She may comment, for instance, on the similarity between the client's feelings toward his wife and his feelings toward his mother; or she may talk about an early decision and how it seems to be affecting his current behavior, or describe a recurring pattern that she has seen in the way the client relates to her. Whenever the therapist goes beyond what the client currently knows, talking instead about what *she* believes to be true about him, she is making an interpretation.

Used well (that is, accurately and sparingly), interpretation can be helpful in a number of ways. Obviously, one of these ways is simply providing information. Interpretations help the client to understand himself—his feelings, his behaviors, his relationships. They help him to make sense of what has been frustrating and confusing. When the information is provided in the context of a caring and respectful relationship, there is also an affective component: the client feels understood and in contact with the therapist. Moreover, say Buirski and Haglund (1999), "new cognitive understanding [i.e., accurate interpretation by the therapist] not only satisfies the longing to be understood, but the function of making sense of the totality of one's life experience also promotes self-understanding, self-delineation, self-continuity, and self-cohesion. Furthermore, new self-understanding contributes to the construction of new organizations of experience" (p. 33).

While most interpretations are primarily aimed at understanding—that is, they are cognitively oriented—the best interpretations invite other responses as well. They must "resonate emotionally" (Buirski & Haglund, 1999): the client has a sense of recognition, an affective "jolt." Effective interpretations take the client beyond what he knows into the not-yet-known, and excursions into hidden areas nearly always have an emotional charge. Excitement, apprehension, and anger are common, as is the release of some affect connected to a memory long held out of awareness.

Interpretations should not be made lightly or casually; they have major significance for the client and can affect both the therapeutic relationship and the course of therapy. They are often taken by the client as pronouncements of "truth," to be believed whether or not they fit his own internal experience. Made too frequently, interpretations begin to train the client to wait for the therapist's opinion rather than form his own. If interpretations come from a distant, noncontactful position, they may never connect with the client's experience, remaining superficial or even creating new resistance to awareness. "A sterile interpretation may have been correct or well formulated but it will most likely not have landed or taken root" (Stern et al., 1998, p. 914). Whether or not an interpretation is accurate in reflecting some aspect of the client's dynamics is much less important than how the client experiences it. If it has enhanced and encouraged his internal awareness, as well as his experience of contact within the therapeutic relationship, and has not undermined his sense of competence and self-worth, it has served its purpose well.

## Kinds of Interpretation

While direct statements of the therapist's observations or opinions are the most common kind of intervention, they are by no means the only kind. Indeed, it could be argued that there is some degree of interpretation in every therapist intervention, since everything the therapist says or does is partly the product of her own understanding of the client. We might even hypothesize an interpretation continuum, with "pure" reflections of client statements at one end and "pure" statements of the therapist's opinions at the other; most of what the therapist does—statements, questions, body language—would fall somewhere between these two extremes.

**Confrontation**   One of the more frequently maligned varieties of therapist comment is the *confrontation*. The word itself has a negative connotation: we tend to think of a confrontation as forcing us to look at or deal with something we would rather avoid, something that makes us feel uncomfortable. A therapeutic confrontation, however, does not necessarily cause discomfort in the client: it is simply a comment about a discrepancy, a mismatch, in what the client is presenting (Berne, 1966). The client's facial expression may not match his voice tone, for instance, and neither of them may fit with the content of what he is saying. He may believe that he is pursuing a particular goal but be acting in such a way as to make that goal unreachable; or his behavior during the therapy session may be quite different from the behavior that he reports outside of therapy. Calling attention to any of these discrepancies is a therapeutic confrontation (Patterson, 1985, p. 76).

Like any other interpretation, confrontation seeks to broaden and deepen the client's awareness. It calls to his attention something that—on the surface, at least—does not seem to fit, and invites him to look at it more closely. It is not intended as a criticism, and the therapist must be careful to phrase it so that the client will not feel criticized or humiliated. If the client experiences a confrontation as something intended to help him, to expand his awareness and enhance his well-being, and if he experiences the therapist as respectful and competent, then the confrontation can become a confirmation as well: a confirmation of his own commitment to growth and of the therapist's concern and involvement.

**Metaphor**    *Metaphor,* too, may be used in making an interpretation. Buirski and Haglund (1999) point out that "an interpretation framed as a metaphor may link modalities of touch, hearing, and sight; it can bridge past and present experiences simultaneously; it might connect affect with a narration of experience, and it could allow for associations among different developmental levels of cognitive processing (such as preverbal sensorimotor experiences and, later, more advanced levels of symbolic representation)" (p. 35). Metaphors may be quite short and succinct ("you remind me of a flower that always turns toward the sun") or may involve a long and intricate story or even a joke. They may be explicitly linked to the client's situation, or the connection may be left rather vague: instead of commenting directly on a client's self-defeating behaviors, for example, the therapist may tell a story about an obese man who avoided shopping for clothes because he was embarassed by his weight and who always fortified himself for the shopping ordeal by consuming several pieces of cake and a big glass of whole milk. Milton Erikson was a master at delivering this latter sort of metaphor (Haley, 1986), and his work clearly demonstrates that a metaphoric interpretation need not even be consciously understood in order to be effective; the client can take in and use the information at a level quite out of awareness.

Interpretations can be delivered in the form of *questions* (have you ever thought about a possible relationship between your problems at work and what happened to you when you were a kid at school?) or of *directives* (I'd like you to stop and think about what you just said and how it fits with what you told me about your son). In each case, the therapist's intervention goes beyond what the client is currently aware of, adding (to a greater or lesser degree) information or conjecture from the therapist's point of view.

## Cautions

Like any other powerful form of intervention, interpretations can, when badly used, do harm rather than good. We have already mentioned the need for an interpretation to be made within the context of a caring and supportive therapeutic relationship. When the client experiences the therapist as authentically involved in the relationship, committed to the client's well-being, he benefits not only from the cognitive awareness provided by an interpretation but also emotionally: he is being thought about, helped with his problems, no longer alone in his struggle. This can be a corrective emotional experience, a way of being-in-relationship that challenges the rigid life script beliefs that have been keeping him stuck. In contrast, if the interpretation is delivered from an intellectualized, distant, or one-up position, the old script beliefs are likely to be strengthened and the client's automatic defensive reaction will prevent the therapist's comments from "getting in" to the tender and vulnerable place where new growth occurs.

Another caution with regard to interpretation has to do with its accuracy. It is not necessary that every interpretation be a correct representation of the client's process (although getting it wrong too often can erode the client's sense of confidence in the therapist), but it *is* necessary that the therapist be willing to be corrected—willing to change or even abandon an interpretation—if the client disagrees (Guistolese, 1997). Interpretations are not some sort of truth, handed down from a higher authority; they are hypotheses to be tested in the laboratory of the therapeutic environment. They should be framed tentatively, often with a "perhaps" or "have you looked at it this way?" or "it seems to me," and always followed with an invitation to the client to correct or clarify what was said or to reject it entirely.

In a number of therapeutic approaches—notably, Gestalt therapy and person-centered therapy—direct interpretations are not used. Fritz Perls (1969a) warned that inexperienced therapists are likely to make an interpretation at a time when the client is open and vulnerable to suggestions, and at such times he is likely to accept the interpretation without pausing to discover what fits and what does not. This kind of swallowing whole is known as *introjection,* and it is perhaps the most serious danger inherent in the use of interpretation. In introjection, the client uncritically takes in the therapist's ideas, swallowing them whole, encapsulating them within his internal system. Kainer (1999) describes introjections as "characterized by a loss of freedom and choice" (p. 3). The swallowed-whole material is as rigid as the life script— indeed, it becomes a part of the life script. It sits within, often out of awareness, impervious to the integrative processes that are ordinarily used on newly acquired information, yet casting its shadow over a growing constellation of thoughts and feelings and behaviors.

To prevent introjection, the therapist must make certain that the therapeutic relationship has developed to the point where the client feels safe to say "no" to the interpretation—he must feel free to disagree, to reject part or all of what the therapist is saying (Perls, Hefferline, & Goodman, 1951). Rather than introjecting, the client is encouraged to assimilate: to chew up the therapist's ideas, spit out what doesn't feel right, and only accept what is useful. Assimilation not only prevents introjection but is also a means of attacking and dissolving previously introjected material. "Because of the introject's theoretically central role in maintaining problematic affective/interpersonal cycles, it would stand to reason that any successful therapy would likely alter a patient's introject state by some means" (Henry & Strupp, 1994, p. 70). "Problematic affective/interpersonal cycles" are parts of the life script, as is the "introject state," and a successful interpretation may relax or dissolve such cycles and states.

The three most important ingredients for effective interpretation, then, are (in order of importance) a supportive therapeutic relationship; the therapist's willingness to be corrected; and a general level of accuracy. If the therapist's interpretations are consistently inaccurate, the client will eventually stop listening or will begin to doubt his own self-knowledge. Therapeutic support without accuracy and a willingness to be corrected is an impossibility, and accuracy without support and caring is likely to go nowhere. When all three are present, interpretation becomes a collaborative process: client and therapist work together to understand how things are, and the process itself is as healing as the content of the interpretation.

## ENACTMENT AND EXPERIMENT

No learning exists without novelty. If all we see is what we are already aware of, we learn nothing new. In fact, one of the most common ways in which a client may exhibit resistance in therapy is by talking only about what he already knows, staying with that which is safe and will not propel him into unpredictability. A part of the therapeutic invitation may be to suggest experiments that will help the client to "move sideways" into unknown areas, going around the resistance rather than trying to smash through it. One of the first therapists to write extensively about such experiments was Fritz Perls (1973), the founder of Gestalt therapy, who suggested that therapist and client together can create "safe emergencies" in which the client is pushed into new ways of experiencing and responding to the world around him. Probably the most familiar of such situations is "two-chair work," in which clients are encouraged to talk with other (fantasied) people or to create dialogs between split-off parts of themselves.

### Benefits of the Therapeutic Experiment

When a client moves into a new experience or enters an old one in a new way, he becomes his own laboratory. He no longer has to speculate about what things were like, or how he might have responded, or what he hoped or feared would happen next—he is there; he can go to his immediate experience and awareness. Experiments like two-chair work or guided imagery allow clients to "get data on their own reactions to new behaviors, how they go about it, what is experienced in the new behavior, what resistances come up, what unfinished business from earlier periods of life emerge from the background as a result of the new activity, and so forth" (Yontef, 1998, p. 101).

Another useful aspect of therapeutic experiments is that they allow client and therapist to escape, temporarily, the constraints of reality. "Although the act of experiencing takes place contemporaneously, the reference of the experience can be past, present, or future—in the room or anywhere in the universe" (Yontef, 1998, p. 84). The client can re-create experiences from childhood, or project himself into situations that have never occurred at all. He can take the roles of old antagonists or allies or give voice to fantasized persecutors and protectors. He can, in the safety of the therapeutic relationship, turn and face his demons; he can journey in imagination to places that would be far too risky to visit on his own. These adventures, fantastic and unreal in a literal sense, have a psychological reality that can speak far more compellingly than reasonable, rational conversation.

The nature of the therapeutic interchange itself can also be changed by a well-selected therapeutic experiment. Giving voice to an internal dialogue, or allowing his body and his feelings to enter into the story he is telling, not only gives the client a chance to escape from the painful familiarity of everyday interactions: the therapist's support and participation in the experiment, too, is different from what the client has come to expect from others. VanKessel and Lietaer (1998) observe that "the client's typical style of communication calls for a response from the other which will allow this typical form of communication to continue. . . . By adopting a noncommittal stance in the therapeutic dialogue [and, we would add, in the therapeutic experiment as well], the therapist creates room for him-/herself to steer clear of the role that the client is trying to force on him/her. . . . in which the client almost 'trains' her/his conversation partners" (p. 161). And sometimes more than "noncommittal"—the therapist may actually enter into the fantasy, lending her own emotional intensity to that of the client, guiding him into new ways of being in relationship.

## Strategies for Creating a Therapeutic Experiment

Bohart & Tallman (1998) suggest several general strategies that will encourage clients' experiential involvement in therapy—strategies that will help clients to actively experience their hidden feelings and the script beliefs that accompany those feelings, and then explore the quality of that experience. To accomplish this, they recommend "(1) vividly reevoking experience; (2) engaging in exercises that allow experiential exploration, such as two-chair or empty-chair work; (3) responding in an empathic, experiential manner; (4) turning clients inward to their own experiencing; or (5) using guided imagery" (p. 195). Each of these is a way to move clients away from simply talking about (which is relatively safe and involves little that is novel) and into *being* their experience.

The client's body language is also a rich source for therapeutic experiments. Body language stands at the border between awareness and out-of-awareness; often one is only partially aware of the signals that one's body is sending. Therapists can attend to such signals and invite their clients to repeat or exaggerate or put words to them. "Swing your foot even harder, now—what is that foot trying to say?" "Let that hand keep moving; let it go wherever it wants . . . and give it a voice, so it can ask for what it wants. . . ."

Alternatively, a client can be invited to change some part of what his body is doing and to attend to that experience: to slow down and deepen his breathing, for instance, or to relax a muscle group that has tightened. He can be invited to change his body's position so as to match his voice tone ("Your voice sounds scared—will you let your body be scared too?") or the content of his words ("You are saying that you were really angry at your brother. Will you tell me again and this time let your voice and your body show that anger?").

Notice that none of these interventions attempts to explain or define what the client is experiencing or to suggest what he "should" be experiencing. Each simply suggests an experiment, something to try out and see what happens. If it leads to something useful, it may move the therapeutic process forward; if it does not, it has still provided some additional awareness, something new that may serve as background for further self-discovery. Experiments like these involve relatively small changes and do not push clients to do something that would violate their values or their sense of what behaviors are acceptable. "The effective therapist contributes a knowledge of how to proceed in sequential steps that do not exceed the patient's external or self-support and that take into account the structure of the patient's personality as well as personal and cultural values. This means helping the patient identify both with what *is* and with what is *emerging*, so that the patient can grow without disclaiming or artificially pushing him-/herself" (Yontef, 1998, p. 90).

Putting language and voice to one's internal conflicts can be an awareness-enhancing experiment. Clients who frequently use the word "but" in describing their experience ("I don't want to yell at them, *but* . . ." "I feel scared sometimes, *but* other times I just get mad . . .") are signaling a tension within themselves, two or more desires pulling them in different directions. Similarly, negative self-talk ("I get so disgusted with myself . . ." "I always do stupid things like that . . .") can be an indication of a dialogue between an internal "top dog" and "under dog"—a controlling and critical part versus a submissive and apologetic part of the self (Perls, 1969a). Inner dialogues like this tend to be carried on at the edges of awareness; they have been a part of the client's internal experience so long that they are like familiar background noises that are no longer consciously attended to; yet they mask and distort one's ability to hear clearly what else is happening. Inviting the client to act out the conflict, to play the part of first one side and then the other (perhaps designating different seats for each voice—thus the term *two-chair work*) allows him to attend to what he is saying to himself and to begin to experience the connections between this ongoing struggle and the underlying life script that supports it.

Greenberg and Paivio (1997) suggest that increasing the overall intensity of a client's descriptions and/or dialogues also enhances awareness and helps him to feel as well as to think about what he is saying. "In addition to empathic attunement, appropriate degrees of stimulation or intensification are used at appropriate times to increase arousal and to prime the schemes for activation, allowing clients easier access to their experience" (p. 6). Asking the client to "say it louder" or "repeat that, and this time let your body say it too" invites him to let go of the control that he usually uses to protect himself from awareness, allowing his emotions, too, to be experienced and expressed. Again, the goal is to dissolve the barriers that have kept him split, divided within himself, opening the doors to archaic memories, beliefs, and decisions so that they can be re-worked and integrated with his current abilities, resources, and goals.

In a real sense, the whole of therapy is a kind of experiment, an excursion into an arena set apart from everyday reality, an interaction with someone who refuses to behave in the old, predictable ways. The therapist attends to and comments on things that other people (including the client himself) seldom notice; she encourages him to do and say things that he would never do and say anywhere else; she does not discount him and will not allow him to discount himself or her. She is not frightened or disgusted by what he says but consistently treats him as a competent and respect-worthy partner in the therapeutic enterprise. She invites him to value these new kinds of interactions, to attend to his internal experience as he participates in them, and to describe that internal experience in detail.

The net result of all this, when it is working well, is that the client becomes more and more aware of his own internal process. He begins to notice connections, contrasts, and contradictions. Feelings begin to emerge, and memories— and more connections and contrasts and contradictions. He becomes increasingly open to himself, and with that openness to self comes increasing openness to the therapist: increasing trust, increasing willingness to share even that which is tentative and not yet fully known. Openness leads to contact, and contact encourages yet more openness. Optimal therapeutic responses, say Broucek and Ricci (1998), may well be defined as those that "simultaneously diminish the patient's estrangement from himself or herself and bring about greater communicative contact with the analyst" (p. 429) Therapeutic experiments and enactments, as well as the relationship out of which they emerge, are designed to do exactly that. They enhance internal and external contact, so that the client can finally come to grips with the life script that has for so long constricted and distorted his ability to be fully himself.

## REGRESSION

One of the most common phenomena in relationship-focused integrative psychotherapy is *regression*: as a client begins to drop his defenses, allowing himself to express more fully the totality of his experiencing, he finds himself feeling, acting, and thinking in ways that have been blocked from awareness and are now re-emerging. These patterns of thinking, feeling, and acting are often repetitions of patterns that were common for him during previous developmental stages: he re-creates ways of being that belong to earlier times of his life. It is as if, psychologically, he has gone back in time, back to the incidents and experiences during which he formed the beliefs and made the decisions upon which his life script is based.

When a client is regressed, he has an opportunity to re-visit his decision-making process. Areas of feeling and knowing that are closed off to his normal conscious state are open and available now; he can work through old traumas, reconsider old decisions, update old beliefs. "To regress is to go back," says Ohlsson (1998). "To do regressive therapy is to go back and work directly with how the client's past influences present life" (p. 83).

There has been a great deal of controversy in recent years about the accuracy of regressive memories. Can people "go back" and recall actual occurrences in the past, occurrences that they cannot remember in their ordinary states of awareness? Chamberlain (1990), among others, seems to think so: "Memory is limited and perhaps inaccurate, but, *in altered states*, it is sometimes remarkably reliable and clearly beyond previously accepted limits" (p. 11). Others (Socor, 1989; Hirt, Lynn, Payne, Krackow, & McCrea, 1999) point out that all memory is an active construction, strongly affected by subsequent experience and expectations. Our life script itself, based upon early experiences, shapes what we remember about those experiences and what we think and feel and do when we regress into them. Socor concludes that it is "an unwarranted and unverifiable assumption to view regression as an actual 'retrogression along a time dimension.' . . . [T]here appears no tangible way in which to grasp the elusive, objective truth" (p. 113).

Fortunately, it is not necessary to resolve this question; the historical accuracy of regressive experiences appears to be relatively unimportant in terms of their therapeutic usefulness. What the client is experiencing at any given moment is the world he knows—and this holds for regressive experiences as well. The memories that are tapped into during a therapeutic regression may well be distortions of what actually happened, but they are *his* distortions; they are what he has constructed and encoded, and they have shaped his way of being over the years. If we believe that this room is on fire and the doors are all locked, our thoughts and feelings and actions will all be based on that belief—it does not matter whether or not the belief is true. In the same way, the constructed reality into which a client regresses is his internal reality, and its correspondence with historical reality is quite beside the point.

## Therapeutic Usefulness of Regression

Why regress? Why should a client have to go back into painful experiences, reliving that which might best be forgotten? Isn't one trauma enough—does the therapist have to encourage him to do it again? To answer these questions, we should first point out that many therapeutic regressions occur quite spontaneously. The therapist does not "make" them happen or even invite them: the client simply goes there. James and Goulding (1998) assert that regression of some sort, spontaneous or planned, occurs in *all* therapies; it simply comes with the territory. As the client opens up bits of unfinished business, he naturally moves into a psychological space related to that unfinished business.

In contrast to these spontaneous regressions are the times when things do not open up; the unfinished business remains walled off and unfinished. The client has reached a dead end, and the therapy seems to be going nowhere. Sometimes a memory, as well as its associated decisions and beliefs, is simply unavailable. Consider our discussion (chapter 8) of state-dependent learning: a memory laid down in one context may not be retrievable in a different context. For such situations, regression provides a kind of context matching: regression re-creates the psychological surround of the original experience. In a planned regression, the client might be encouraged to think about the home he lived in as a child, the furnishings, the lighting, the smells and sounds and colors that were so familiar to him back then; he can be invited to imagine himself in that environment, and to recreate as vividly as possible all of those stimuli, and then to talk about what his experience is like. Not infrequently, this sort of imaginary rebuilding of an old context moves the client into regression and allows previously hidden memories to emerge.

**Contact, Script, and Regression**    When affect is experienced spontaneously and naturally, one moves through a series of stages. First, the feeling begins to build and emerges into awareness. It is accepted and owned, and one acts so as to express it. This action transforms the feeling from an internally experienced affect into a socially communicated emotion. When the expressive action is met with need satisfaction, one moves into completion: the feeling recedes, and one is free to move on to whatever next claims one's attention. "It is when this process is chronically interfered with—when, for example, emergence or identification is prevented, or experience is not symbolized in awareness, or expression is constantly interrupted and action and completion are repeatedly blocked—that people become stuck in a chronic bad feeling and become dysfunctional and chronically distressed" (Greenberg & Paivio, 1997, p. 27). This sort of distress is a direct consequence of disruption of internal contact, so that the client is unable to flow through a natural sequence. He has learned, through experiences repeated again and again, that his feelings do not lead to a sense of completion but, rather, to frustration and discomfort. The solution is to not feel them in the first place. Going back, psychologically, to the scenes of the original frustration, gives him the opportunity to do it differently: to re-create the natural sequence without interference and learn to welcome, rather than wall off, his awareness of needs, wants, and interests.

Disruption of internal contact is, of course, out of awareness. Similarly, people are largely unaware of the behaviors that they use to maintain the disruption. Script-generated behavior (and thoughts and feelings) does not feel like something one chooses to do; it is more likely to feel like the only possible response to a given situation. The client has no recollection of ever acting or feeling differently. Even when other possibilities are suggested (he sees other people reacting in other ways, or the therapist invites him to try something different for himself), such a change seems alien and frightening. The sense of danger is usually not realistic in the context of his current situation; it is an emotional response connected to an earlier trauma. Back then, it might well have been dangerous to behave differently, to speak up or leave the situation or even be aware of the feelings and needs that could prompt such action; so he learned how to act, think, and feel (or not act, not think, not feel) so as to make the best of things, to survive with the least amount of pain. He learned his lessons so well that he even forgot ever learning them. Regression experiences can help recapture that learning process, help the client remember what it was he decided to do or not do, and give him an opportunity to change that decision—to change his script.

**Change and Growth**   Script learnings and decisions are self-protective, and they often work—for a while. They were developed to keep us safe; when they are disrupted, the sense of danger is immediate and visceral. One of the major benefits of regressive therapy is that it provides a safe space in which to experiment with new ways of being and feeling that contradict script but would be far too threatening to try out in the real, outside-of-therapy world. Neimeier (1995) says that because such regressions take one to "a hypothetical place, a make-believe world, the client can feel free to experiment with changes without necessarily jeopardizing or assaulting existing meaning structures. New perspectives can be tried on without shedding present constructions, thereby circumventing much of the threat and anxiety associated with significant personal change" (p. 115).

There is no way, of course, that a client can actually undo his past or satisfy the unmet needs that he experienced decades ago. The pain of those events happened and cannot be changed. But the decisions he made in response to that pain, the beliefs he developed, and the fragmentation that grew out of them are things that therapy can address. In this sense, the traumas of the past are amended and healed in the present. Previously blocked memories can be brought into awareness and put into perspective, so that they can be remembered without having to repeat, over and over again, the emotions associated with them (Rhinehart, 1998, p. 21).

A regressed client can experience previously toxic relationships in new, nurturing, growth-producing ways. Instead of being a helpless child subject to the unpredictable behaviors of an indifferent, neglectful, or abusive caregiver, he is now working with a caring and protective therapist, an adult who has his best interests at heart and is competent to help him learn how to be fully himself. Blackstone (1995) describes a client who had been abused as a child and who, "working in the present but feeling the feelings she had in the past, [experienced] a positive environmental response. Since the client's self-affirmation was supported, not negated, her organismic reaction was overwhelmingly positive. Intense positive affect took the place of rage and terror. So now there is no need for self-negation or adaptation by the client to 'make the best of it.' She does not have to deny or exaggerate parts of the self, but is able to retain contact with core self and with the other at the same time" (p. 346).

The therapist does not need to know ahead of time what the blocked memories are or to what events the client needs to return. Because they have been central in the client's process of learning how he fits into the world, blocked experiences exert a kind of dynamic pull: when the client feels safe enough to drop his defenses, he will spontaneously go back to the times and places and relationships where script beliefs were formed. Says Freyd (1996), "The client spontaneously creates an episodic interpretation and integration of previously disjointed sensory and affective memories" (p. 170). Such reprocessing and restructuring allows the traumas of the past to remain in the past, while the dissociated parts of the personality identified with the traumas are reintegrated into the whole personality here and now (Sigmund, 1998).

Ultimately, the goal of regressive therapy is to dissolve script and to enhance internal and external contact. Returning to the scene of early script decisions, in the presence of a concerned and competent therapist and with the added awareness of an observing adult ego, allows a new dimension of experience within that scene. It is a kind of double vision, in which the regressed client feels as he did back then but can also be aware of new options, new resources, and new strengths. He is no longer alone in a world where the only possibility is to close down, mask his feelings from himself, and make the best of what cannot be altered. With the encouragement of the therapist, in a fantasy world where he is in charge, things can be different. Says Ohlsson (1998), "The aim of regressive therapy is to facilitate for the client an experience that allows him or her to realize that limiting early script decisions may be changed and/or given up and that redecisions affirming present life possibilities may take their place" (p. 83). The client cannot only *realize* that such changes can be made; he can actually make them! Within the context of regression, script can be changed, early decisions can be re-decided, and parts of self that were banished can be welcomed back.

## Inviting Regression

An observer, watching a regressive experience in therapy, might well criticize the therapist as cruel or unfeeling. The client is being led back into extremely uncomfortable situations and may be helped to accept a frame of reference in which he is relatively helpless to do much about it. He feels frustration, fear, anger, pain—all the emotions that one would ordinarily prefer to avoid. He does not just talk about how bad things were: he experiences them, he is there. "At times," say Greenberg and Paivio (1997), "we need to evoke traumatic emotional memories in order to reprocess and restructure them" (p. 5). One of the first things a therapist must do to facilitate this sort of work is to remind herself that the client's discomfort is serving an important purpose. She must not leap in to rescue him from his distress but must help him to work through it in a different way, making different decisions and regaining full internal contact. It is also well to remember Greenberg and Paivio's warning that working through feelings is a stage process; it does not happen all at once. Acknowledging and even expressing feeling is a first step, but moving through to a new resolution may require more than one trip back into the trauma of the past.

Mahrer (1998) suggests that three stages are involved in bringing about therapeutic change when working with long-buried feelings and beliefs. The first is to identify the scene in which the strong feelings occurred and to access and open up the feelings. This is the regressive experience, the shift in one's state of consciousness that allows one to re-experience past events as if they were occurring here and now. Second, we encourage the client to welcome and appreciate the deeper potential for experiencing and resolving the situation that he now brings to the problem. Finally, with the juxtaposition of new resources and awarenesses onto the old situation, the client "undergoes a radical shift into being the qualitatively new person in the context of past scenes and situations" (pp. 206–207).

When a client moves into a spontaneous regression, the therapist's first task is to recognize it. Berne (1961) has suggested four kinds of information that can be used to know when and to what degree a client has regressed. One of these is the client's personal history. If the therapist knows something of the client's developmental milestones and the relationships in place during each developmental phase, she can often match these to the content of the client's story and the manner in which he tells it. Another source of information is the therapist's general knowledge of child development. At what age can children be expected to speak with this sort of sentence construction? Using this tone of voice? Exhibiting these mannerisms? Third, the therapist uses her own social response system: how does she feel toward this person? How does she feel herself wanting to respond to him? If she temporarily blocks her awareness of an adult body sitting across from her, what age child does she see when she looks at him? All three of these sources provide clues that the client has indeed moved into a state of consciousness different from his ordinary adult way of being; these clues prompt the therapist to access the fourth and most accurate source of information about regression: the client's own report: "How old do you feel right now?" is a question that regressed clients can usually answer with little hesitation. "About 4 years old." "Like I did in the third grade." "Like a teenager, all awkward and confused." With this confirmation of her hypothesis, the therapist can encourage the client to continue and even heighten the regression, so that the work of reprocessing and restructuring can move forward.

Even when a spontaneous regression does not occur, client or therapist or both may recognize that a particular incident or relationship has been critical in forming the client's life script and that it would be helpful to reconstruct and revisit that incident or relationship. In such cases, the client may benefit from the therapist's help in making a shift of consciousness. For example, the therapist may invite the client to close his eyes and to visualize himself in a place familiar to him as a child, to see the other people who are there, or to choose to whom he wants or needs to talk. Some clients follow these directions easily and need little more encouragement than a simple "Close your eyes and tell Mama what it's like when she . . ." Others, more self-conscious or well defended, may need more extensive prompting; some require several attempts before learning to re-create an old memory or may need to return to the critical scene a number of times before resolving it. "When something happens to us, we do not experience all of it at once," says Browne (1990). "Experiencing is a process that takes place over time" (p. 21). Just as the original experience and its associated feelings and beliefs and decisions took time, so re-doing the feelings, beliefs, and decisions may take time, too.

Some clients are unwilling or unable to accept the invitation into a therapeutic regression. It feels wrong to them, they do not want to try it, or it just seems silly. "Why go back?" they ask. "All that is over now; it was bad back then but it's done; it's past history." Clients who voice these sorts of objections have a right to know the therapist's thinking, to know why the therapist believes a regression experience might be helpful. If, after having this explained, the client is still reluctant, the wise therapist does not push him. When he is ready, he will let her know.

The most essential requirement for a successful regression experience is safety. Regression is often a frightening experience. The client is going back to a place where resources and defenses were much more primitive than they are now, often to an incident involving severe trauma. Reexperiencing those early events means giving up all that he has learned to do to protect himself, and may feel like losing control altogether. The therapist must serve as an "auxiliary ego" (Glickauf-Hughes, Wells, & Chance, 1996), providing the protections that the client gives up during a regression. "I'll bring you back when you're ready," she tells him (sometimes in words, more often nonverbally), "and I won't let you die or stay crazy or hurt anyone while you're there." These protections allow the client to move fully into his experience, secure in the knowledge that he will be taken care of and will be able to return to his normal mode of functioning when the piece of work ends. He is giving up control temporarily and purposefully, not losing control (Nichols, 1986); and he will get it back again.

Sometimes, though, even the safety of a supportive therapeutic relationship is not enough to outweigh a client's visceral need to avoid the pain of old trauma. It is too much; going back to that experience would be as difficult as deliberately swallowing something horrid or walking off a cliff. The client finds himself at the doorway to an awareness that is too frightening, too painful, too dangerous to move into. He wants to turn and retreat, but that would take him back into the mess he came to therapy to get out of. He's stuck: he can't go back—can't un-know what he has learned thus far—and he resists going foward. Schneider (1998) suggests that bringing the resistance itself into awareness can be helpful at such a point. Instead of fighting against his resistance, the client is invited to respect it, to be curious, to learn as much as he can about it. Vivifying resistance in this way can act like a kind of psychic judo: with nothing to push against, the resistance loses its power. As the client explores how he blocks and sidetracks himself, he becomes more interested in how that process works than in how to defeat it; and, in learning how it works, he again expands the boundaries of awareness, often into the very regression experience that was originally being guarded against.

## Moving Out of Regression

Endings of regression work pieces are as varied as the regressions themselves. Many clients move out of the regression spontaneously. Sometimes, indeed, they move out sooner than the therapist wants them to, just when it seems they are on the brink of breaking through to new awareness. When this happens, the therapist may talk with the client about the feelings that precipitated the interruption and may suggest that the client go back, either now or during some future session. Ultimately, of course, the client's choice to return or not to return will be supported. Going into the regression took courage, and the client needs to be respected for that courage and for his own knowledge of when he has done enough. In fact, acknowledging the work that the client has done is an important ingredient in ending any regressive piece; this acknowledgment, as much as anything else, is what invites the client to continue his work.

When a client does not emerge from a regression spontaneously, bringing him back is generally a matter of simple invitation: "Come on back to this room and this time, and let's talk about what you discovered." Occasionally, a client may need help in grounding himself again in the present; suggesting that he make eye contact with the therapist or feel the physical sensations of his hands on the chair arms, his feet on the floor, or the pressure of his body against chair or couch can provide such help. Some clients need a few moments of silence, as they sort through and organize what they have experienced; others want to talk right away; still others want the therapist to talk to them while they "grow up."

One of the most useful ways in which to end a piece of regression therapy involves a technique developed by Erskine (1974/1997a), known as "disconnecting the rubber band." The client is interacting with someone or something from the past and has reached a point at which a script decision was made or reinforced. The therapist invites him to voice his needs, to demand what he wants, and to experience the rejection of that demand. With the therapist's encouragement, he intensifies the demand. Then the therapist prompts: "And tell xxx (Mother, Father, your teacher, Uncle George) what you're going to do if they won't do what you ask." Almost invariably, the response to this prompt is a script conclusion or decision, perhaps given actual voice for the first time. The therapist underscores this voicing, often asking the client to repeat the phrase and notice the decision that is being made. She then invites the client to tell the other person in the drama what his life will be like in the future, having made such a decision. The final move in the scenario is to remind the client that he need not stay with this decision, and that he may, if he wishes, tell the other person what new decision he is choosing to make. From this simple process often emerges significant script change; and, with resolution of the dilemma, the client spontaneously returns to his normal state of consciousness.

## Regression As a Continuum

Regression is not an either-or phenomenon, something that clients either do or do not do. Rather, it is a continuum, extending from simply talking about some past experience, with no associated affect, to fully experiencing the past event and all of the feelings that accompanied it. Most of the therapeutic work that involves old memories takes place somewhere between these two extremes; it is rare that a client will think that something in the past is significant enough to bring up in therapy and yet have no feelings about it. Additionally, full regression work is frequently both introduced and followed by a good deal of cognitive, affective, and phenomenological exploration.

Formal regression work is not necessary for everyone. Many clients move spontaneously into partial regression and gain significant insight and resolution from work at that level. Others seek therapy to resolve relatively straightforward, here-and-now dilemmas and neither need nor want to deal directly with life script issues. In contrast, clients whose ability to solve present problems is blocked by script decisions, whose spontaneity and creativity are constricted by lack of contact with self and others, may find formal regression work extremely helpful. Regressions should not be invited, however, until the therapeutic relationship has matured to the point where the therapist can offer effective protection and support. It is also useful to have a clear contract that specifies the issue to be dealt with and a plan for how the client is to return safely to his daily life at the end of each session involving regression (Sigmund, 1998).

## BEHAVIORAL INTERVENTIONS

The great fourplex of therapeutic interventions includes thoughts, feelings, physiology, and behavior. A successful intervention in any of these areas affects functioning in all the others: changing one's thinking stimulates changes in emotion, behavior, and physiology; changing how one feels affects how one thinks, how one acts, and how one's body functions; and, as pharmacologically based interventions clearly demonstrate, changing one's physiology can lead to significant shifts in thinking, feeling, and behavior. Up until now, we have been focusing on interventions aimed primarily at thinking (changing script beliefs and decisions), feeling (working with previously blocked affect), and physiology (increasing awareness of physical sensations and movements). It is time now to turn to behaviorally focused interventions.

There is no way that we can, in this volume, do justice to the myriad varieties of behavioral intervention that have been shown to be therapeutically useful. Behavioral therapists, basing their intervention strategies on both classical and operant conditioning, have developed scores of techniques that can be tailored to specific presenting problems, and many books are available that detail these techniques (Lazarus, 1989; Beck, 1991; Wolpe, 1969; Spiegler & Guevremont, 1993). We shall concentrate here on behavioral interventions designed specifically to enhance contact and impact life script.

A behavioral intervention involves an invitation to do something different: to change an old behavior or to try out a new one. What makes such changes effective is not the new behavior itself as much as the feedback, from self or others, that the new behavior stimulates. Frank (1991) says that everything we do, think, and feel is an element in an interactive system; we never operate in a vacuum but are always in the (real or fantasized) presence of others. Changes in our behavior result in changes in the whole system; everything shifts in order to reach a new equilibrium, and part of that shift includes feedback that serves to maintain, intensify, or diminish the behavior that started the whole process. This is as true for private behavioral changes as for public ones. Haley (1986) reports that Milton Erikson, one of the great psychotherapeutic wizards, asked a client which foot he stood on when he put on his trousers and then invited him to do it the opposite way. The internal feedback resulting from this relatively small behavioral change was enough to set off a chain of feedback interactions that eventually led to significant resolution of the client's problem.

"Meaning is made through action, through participation, and through concrete and representational manipulations of the world," says Neimeier (1995). "These manipulations yield novel experience, that is, perceived invalidations of present systems of knowing that require active efforts of meaning making to render them sensible within a coherent meaning structure" (p. 117). When a client experiments with some new behavior and receives the feedback resulting from that behavior, he is forced to adjust his understanding of self, others, and the world around him in order to accommodate the new experience. If the new experience conflicts with his life script, something has to give: either the script must change or the new experience must be discounted in some way. Either sort of shift is grist for the therapeutic mill, providing information and/or inviting further awareness.

In planning a behavioral intervention, it is important to select a behavioral change that will tend to challenge and disrupt script beliefs rather than reinforce them. Just any old change will not do (unless the client is dealing with a script belief that "nothing can ever be different"). Inviting a client who believes that "life is hard" or that "I will never succeed" to try a new and difficult task risks his failing at the task and confirming that life is indeed hard and that he cannot succeed. Behavioral assignments should build on strengths—strengths in the client and supports in his environment. Whenever possible, the assignments should be structured so that no matter what the client does with them, he will succeed. For instance, in a paradoxical intervention, an anxious client might be invited to figure out something that will make him even more anxious, right here and right now, and do it. If he succeeds, he can be helped to explore the nature of his experience of anxiety (an experience that he usually avoids, and, in avoiding it, makes it even more fearful and disruptive). If he does not become anxious, he has succeeded in doing a feared thing without fear and must adjust his belief system accordingly. If he cannot think of an anxiety-making behavior or refuses to experiment with one, he has succeeded in uncovering something important about himself and can be invited to explore the relationship between this inability/refusal and his stated goal in entering therapy.

The purpose of a behavioral intervention, then, is to set up a situation that will result in a success experience that challenges the client's script pattern. The behavior may be one that is contrary to his usual script-bound behaviors, or it may lead to feedback that will stimulate feelings or thoughts inconsistent with script-dictated feelings and/or script beliefs. This is true of in-session behavioral interventions as well as behavioral "homework," assignment of tasks to be completed outside of therapy and reported on at the next session.

In assigning tasks to be completed outside of the session, it is particularly important to be sure that the homework cannot be twisted or distorted so that it supports, rather than challenges, the client's script. People frequently create the very situations that they expect (Janoff-Bulman, 1993); and self-fulfilling prophecies are an important factor in maintaining script. The client who believes that "nobody cares about me" is likely to behave in ways that will make others reject him; the client whose script labels him as stupid and a failure sets himself up over and over again to fail and to look stupid. When a behavioral assignment is sabotaged during the session, the sabotage can be discussed then and there, and the whole situation may lead to positive change. When the sabotage occurs outside of therapy, though, the client has days or even weeks during which to use the sabotage to bolster his script.

No client deliberately tries to sabotage his work; people do not consciously set out to use behavioral homework to make themselves more miserable. Sabotage, like other defensive maneuvers, occurs out of awareness. To the therapist, it may appear that the client has deliberately set himself up to fail; to the client, his own behavior seems natural or even inevitable. A socially isolated client, for example, might be assigned the task of inviting a friend over to watch a sporting event on television. The client complies but is awkward to the point of rudeness. The visit is a social disaster; the homework assignment has confirmed his belief that he is unlovable and doomed to a life of loneliness. To avoid this sort of outcome, homework assignments should be crafted to build on client strengths rather than weaknesses and should involve small (and doable) changes rather than major shifts in behavior. Further, the homework should always be debriefed in the next session so that any unanticipated and unwanted outcomes can be dealt with.

## SUMMARY

A variety of psychotherapeutic interventions are available for use in treatment; all of them should be designed to enhance the client's internal and external contact, dissolve script, and support his sense of efficacy and self-worth.

The most common intervention, *interpretation*, involves sharing the therapist's hypothesis about the client's dynamics. Interpretations may take the form of simple statements, questions, directives, confrontations, or metaphor.

All should be given within the context of an authentic and supportive relationship, and the therapist must be willing to be corrected by the client if the client believes the interpretation to be off target. Interpretation should be used carefully and sparingly, lest the client introject the therapist rather than discover himself.

Enactment and experiments allow the client a new experience designed to clash with his script beliefs, enhancing his awareness of his internal processes within the safety of a protective therapeutic relationship. Regression involves moving into a pattern of thoughts, feelings, and behaviors common to an earlier developmental stage. It is not an either/or phenomenon; many clients regress partially or shift in and out of a regressive experience. Regression can help the client access walled-off or state-dependent memories, beliefs, and decisions; revisit old and toxic relationships with the support of a nurturing and protective therapist; recreate previously blocked sequences of behavior; and learn to express needs and wants. Clients can regress spontaneously or can be encouraged to regress by setting a scene that will be revisited in the regression. Similarly, the regressive experience can end spontaneously or by invitation from the therapist; the "disconnecting the rubber band" technique may be used to end a regression.

Behavioral interventions encourage changes in behavior that will, in turn, lead to changes in thoughts, feelings, and physiology. They usually involve trying out new behaviors in the therapy session or as homework assignments. The value of a behavioral intervention lies in the feedback the client receives, from self and others, as a result of the new behavior. Behavioral interventions should be chosen to build on the client's strengths while challenging his script pattern.

# 10 CHAPTER | **A Focus on Relationship**

Chapter 9 began with an assertion that any intervention, if it is to be effective, must be made in the context of a supportive therapeutic relationship. The chapter then discussed a number of intervention strategies, all of which are designed to dissolve script and enhance the client's ability to make internal and external contact. The therapeutic relationship itself, though, is perhaps the most potent "intervention" that can be made with a client: participating in a properly managed therapeutic relationship is in itself a script-dissolving and contact-enhancing experience.

Traditionally, the therapeutic relationship has been seen as a venue within which a client can work through the traumas that have shaped his life script, bringing to awareness old decisions and learned responses, so that he has the option of making changes in dysfunctional patterns of behavior. While relationship-focused integrative psychotherapy makes use of various sorts of interventions to facilitate this kind of working-through, it is most concerned with the ways in which the client manages his *present* relationships and, most particularly, his relationship with the therapist. Says Safran (1993), "From a technical perspective, the therapeutic focus appears to be shifting away from the exploration and working through of a major traumatic event with the therapist that is viewed as a re-enactment of a historical trauma, toward an ongoing exploration of what are often subtle fluctuations in the quality of client-therapist relatedness and the clarification of factors obstructing it" (p. 21). From this perspective, there is less need to return to past events in order to expose and dissolve script, because the client is acting out his script in the here and now.

The relationship between client and therapist is not simply an adjunct to the work of therapy; it is a living entity in which two involved individuals come together, both bringing their emotions, their thoughts, and their ways of reaching out and of pulling away from contact. The challenge to the therapist is to remain real and involved in this relationship, while at the same time attending to the dynamics of what is happening in the interaction. She invites the client to join her in what Plakun (1998) calls a "supraordinate context," a way of being together in which therapist and client act and react and, at the same time, observe their actions and reactions. From this supraordinate context, both participants can begin to notice the patterns that they are creating and recognize how those patterns are similar to and different from the patterns that the client establishes with the other people in his life.

## THREE RELATIONAL CONCERNS

In developing and maintaining an effective therapeutic space, the therapist must attend to three major concerns. The first of these is her own *authenticity*. She must not retreat into an artificial "professionalism," protecting herself from being impacted by the client. She must be aware of her own impulses to restrict contact (or, in contrast, to become over-involved). She must be fully herself, fully present, willing to know and to be known. At the same time, she must maintain her commitment to the well-being of the client—her *therapeutic intent*. She is responsible for creating a space in which the client is safe, supported, and nurtured. Here, she often becomes the parent-who-never-was, the caretaker whose absence meant that the client had to fend for himself. Self-protective patterns, growing out of inadequate resources and distorted perceptions, are the essence of script and most often develop in the absence of social support and nurturing. Such patterns can be disrupted when the client finds himself in an environment in which support and nurturing are consistently present. The therapist, in providing support and encouragement, helps the client to develop "adaptive emotion-regulation strategies" (Greenberg & Paivio, 1997): she allows the client to repeat interactional sequences similar to the ones of a healthy childhood. "Clients in therapy learn to self-regulate their emotions through the internalization of interactions with the therapist and developing self-empathy" (p. 5).

The third aspect of the therapist's relational task is technical and has to do with *attending* to that "superordinate context" that was mentioned earlier. The therapist notices, hypothesizes, and analyses. She attends to the dynamics of the session; she attempts to make sense of the myriad of transactions that flow through the therapeutic hour. She is like an observer in a window high above the crowd, watching the swirl of movement as individuals meet and part and meet again, trying to understand the underlying pattern of their movement. As she becomes aware of how she and the client are co-creating their interaction, she may shift her position so as to change the pattern. She may tell the client what she sees, and suggest that he experiment with something different, or she may simply use her process of being-in-relationship to invite him to change. "It is not necessary," say Safran and Muran (2000), "for the therapist and client to address explicitly the relationship issue that is being worked on through the therapeutic interaction. The message transmitted by the therapist's interpersonal stance is as important, if not more important, than any explicit messages" (p. 237). For her to be effective in creating such a change-inducing interpersonal stance, however, she must be able to see the overall pattern; thus it is necessary to be both in the relationship and standing outside of it at the same time.

## TRANSFERENCE AND COUNTERTRANSFERENCE REVISITED

Chapter 4 introduced the notions of transference and countertransference. Some of the ideas that follow repeat what was said in that short discussion; they bear reviewing because they are so fundamental to understanding the therapeutic relationship and how it can act as an intervention tool.

### Transference

The notions of transference and countertransference are among the many legacies that have come down from the theoretical insights of Sigmund Freud. Freud noticed that his patients often began to react to him in ways quite inconsistent with his position as their physician. Rather, they treated him as they had treated significant others in their lives years earlier; more important, they seemed to expect him to behave just as those significant others had behaved. Freud came to believe that his patients used him (or any other analyst) to re-enact past relationships, and he called this process *transference* because the patients seemed to transfer onto the therapist their feelings toward the person in the original relationship. Transference, Freud believed, offered an important means of understanding the patient's dynamics, and *analysis of the transference* became a staple of psychoanalysis.

Over the years, many therapists have come to believe that Freud's view of transference was too narrow. Since all of one's present relationships are shaped by the past, by the things one has learned about people and the ways one has learned to interact with others, it is sometimes difficult to distinguish clearly between a "transference" and a "non-transference" response. All of our here-and-now social interactions contain some historical elements, just as our interactions even when regressed are colored by our adult experience. Nevertheless, the idea of transference remains a highly useful one—particularly in the context of a therapy that focuses on the relationship between client and therapist.

Glassman and Anderson (1999) define transference in terms of the client's general patterns of organizing his world, of giving structure to the thousands of individual interactions and transactions in which he engages from day to day. "Transference," they say, "may be conceptualized as part of a basic meaning-making process for coming to understand the interpersonal world. . . . This meaning-making process reflects the interaction of stimuli in the social environment and previously acquired knowledge structures used to interpret ongoing experience. . . . Such knowledge structures may take the form of scripts, schemas, or prototypes encompassing the self, others, and social situations" (p. 105). Understanding a client's script can help make sense of the way in which he interacts with his therapist. Conversely (and of more practical importance), his ways of dealing with the therapist cast light on his life script: on his overall way of taking in, making sense of, and responding to the other people in his world.

In addition to meeting the universal psychological need to organize experience and create meaning, relationship-focused integrative psychotherapists see transference as a means whereby the client describes his past: the developmental needs that have not been met and the defenses that were created to compensate for those deficits. Transference expresses both an unaware enactment of childhood experiences and, simultaneously, a resistance to remembering the discomfort of those experiences. Because it involves both acting out an old experience and resistance to remembering the experience, there is always an element of internal conflict in a transference reaction. Finally, transference may represent a desire to satisfy relational needs that were unsatisfied in the past and to achieve closeness and trust in relationship (Erskine, 1993/1997c).

Transference, then, involves not only responses and reactions held over from the past but also current relational needs and expectations. Because the scripts that influence the client's current social interactions, as well as the old relationship experiences on which they are based, are not fully available to awareness, his transference behavior is a way of expressing something about himself that cannot be communicated in any other way. He may respond to the therapist as he might have responded to an abusive or neglectful or over-protective parent, but he is often unaware of the parallel between what he is doing and feeling now and what he did and felt back then. Reenacting the old pattern is literally the only way he can express what is going on for him.

Sands (1997) recommends that in dealing with transference we focus more on "how we are being used by patients as 'new,' longed-for objects . . . rather than on how we are being experienced (and are then invited to experience our-selves) as 'old,' pathogenic objects from the past" (p. 660). Focusing on the here-and-now relationship can help us to understand the blend of past and present that the transference represents and within which the client is immersed; it also helps sensitize us to the part that we ourselves are playing in creating and maintaining that relationship.

In transference behavior, the client enacts past patterns within the context of the present. Plakun (1998) says that "since enactments are inevitable and ubiquitous therapeutic phenomena, their detection, analysis, and interpretation offer an opportunity to understand something in a new way or to turn a corner in treatment" (p. 319). Analysis and interpretation, however, should be attempted only with caution: as was pointed out in chapter 9, providing them too quickly or in a way that the client may experience as nonsupportive or critical may intensify his defenses and leave him feeling misunderstood or criticized. It is best to begin with a gentle, respectful inquiry into the internal experience connected with the client's transference behavior. Such an inquiry may lead the client to discover for himself how his present reactions are connected to old experiences; self-discovery not only is less likely to stimulate defenses but also builds the client's sense of competence and autonomy.

## Countertransference

What about the therapist's feelings toward the client? It would be naïve to suppose that therapists can be neutral, without reactions of liking or disliking, approval or disapproval, being drawn toward or feeling repelled by their clients. Moreover, such a stance would be nontherapeutic: an emotionally neutral therapist would be unable to participate in an authentic therapeutic relationship, would be incapable of being impacted by her clients. For better or worse, therapists must be involved with their clients, experiencing real reactions toward them and dealing with real feelings about them. Countertransference, the sum of the therapist's reactions to the client, is as necessary and inevitable as are the client's transference reactions to the therapist.

When, as is most often the case, the therapist's initial reaction to a client is positive, she can proceed with the business of building a therapeutic relationship with relative ease. She likes the client, and her liking invites him to like and to trust her. When her first impression is negative, though, things may not run so smoothly. Strupp (1996) observes that therapists tend to develop a general attitude toward their clients within the first few minutes of their first meeting and that "this attitude has a profound influence on the . . . empathic quality of the therapist's hypothetical communications to the patient" (p. 135).

What should a therapist do, then, when she finds herself faced with a client toward whom, for whatever reasons, she finds it difficult to feel supportive? How does she deal with impulses to be judgmental, critical, or rejecting? First, she must recognize that her reaction has more to do with herself than with the client. An initial negative response is a signal about something going on inside the therapist, some internal pattern of thoughts and feelings that is being stimulated by this client. The therapist needs to look to herself, to bring to awareness the beliefs/needs/memories that are the source of her response. When she understands the basis of her feelings and owns her responsibility for them, she can begin to work through the problem without blaming the client or labeling him as wrong or bad or unlikable. If the negative feelings persist, consultation with a colleague may be the next step; she would also be well advised to seek therapy for herself in order to deal with the unfinished business that is intruding into her professional life. Without working through our own personal issues, our own script patterns, it is impossible to identify and deal with the ways in which those issues influence our therapeutic behaviors; ongoing personal therapy is one of the most important continuing educational experiences available to practicing therapists.

We may meet, rarely, a client whose values and beliefs are so directly and genuinely at odds with our own that an authentically respectful relationship is impossible to establish. When this happens, the client should be referred elsewhere. No matter how hard the therapist may try to be "therapeutic" in this sort of situation, the relationship will be basically flawed and her therapeutic involvement will be tainted. Again, it is essential that the therapist own her part in the mismatch: it is not that the client is wrong but, rather, that he and she differ in their views to such an extent that they would simply not work well together. Beware, though, if this sort of situation arises more than once in your early career; there may be more going on than you are aware of, and you would probably benefit from help in working it through.

Both client and therapist, then, may act out their unfinished business in the therapeutic relationship, using each other as screens on which to project their out-of-awareness feelings toward others in their past or present. It is quite usual for therapists to notice how a client's life script determines his way of being with and responding to others and how those script behaviors and responses are played out in the therapeutic hour. Less commonly recognized are the ways in which the therapist, equipped with her own life script, enters into that acting out. Plakun (1998) says that therapist and client together create a reciprocally supported pattern: the therapist "unwittingly participates by projecting back into the patient reciprocal unconscious conflicted countertransference material from the therapist's own life history. . . . Within such an enactment the therapist is as much an active participant as the patient" (p. 320). Because client and therapist are both unaware of their own contributions to the enactment, each may be puzzled by what happens in the interaction; frequent feelings of puzzlement or confusion are again a signal that the therapist may benefit from consultation and/or personal therapy.

Among the most notorious transference-countertransference situations arising in therapy are those involving sexual acting out. The very nature of the therapeutic relationship—its support and psychological intimacy—invites strong feelings. Clients may mistake the caring and attention they receive from their therapist as signs of romantic attachment; therapists may do the same. While it is normal and natural for a client to feel sexually attracted to his therapist, or vice versa, there are no circumstances under which it is appropriate to act on those feellings. This is one of the few therapeutic guidelines to which there are no exceptions: a therapist does not become sexually involved with a client. A client's sexual invitations must be respectfully declined and the client invited to discuss his response to that refusal. Say Callaghan, Naugle, and Folette (1996), "With clients who have difficulty relating to others without sexualizing the interaction, the therapist discusses openly the importance of the client being able to have a nonsexual relationship with the therapist, despite the fact that it may seem impossible to do this" (p. 387). A therapist who has difficulty respecting these guidelines, who is tempted to act on her sexual feelings toward a client or finds herself engaging in frequent sexual fantasies involving him, should certainly deal with this issue in her own personal therapy. Again, it is not the client who "causes" the feelings. The therapist is responding to unmet relational needs of the present or unfinished business from the past, either of which needs to be dealt with outside of her relationship with her clients.

## TOUCH

Perhaps because of the taboo surrounding therapist-client sexual contact, and because touching is such a potent and primitive way of conveying emotion, touch between therapist and client has been seen by some practitioners as dangerous if not actually improper. It has been regarded by others as an extremely useful, perhaps even necessary, part of the therapeutic experience (Rhinehart, 1998).

Touching is, as far as we know, the infant's earliest means of sensing the presence of another. Before birth, a mother's touch surrounds and protects her baby; her first instinct after the child is born is to hold and to cuddle. It is well known that many newborn mammals literally require the touch of the mother in order to survive: calves, for instance, must be "licked into shape" soon after birth, and anyone whose pet has had puppies or kittens can attest to how mother cats and dogs use their tongues to contact and caress their babies. Physical contact continues to be necessary long after birth, as Harlow (1958) so effectively demonstrated in his studies of primate babies. Humans are certainly not exempt from the need for touching; Spitz (1945) and others have noted infants' "failure to thrive" as the debilitating and sometimes fatal consequence of touch deprivation.

Touch, of course, can convey many different messages. It can be comforting, threatening, playful, or sexual. How the therapist's touch is experienced by a client will depend not only on how and where the therapist touches him, but also on the developmental level at which he is operating at the time he is touched: a touch that might express comfort or support to a child, for instance, could feel like a sexual invitation to an adult. One of the necessary elements involved in using touch therapeutically is the ability to diagnose such transitory developmental levels accurately and to calibrate one's touching to the client's current psychological age.

For an adult, touch can be a formal, almost ritualistic act (as in shaking hands with a stranger) or an essential component of deep intimacy. It can signal friendship, sympathy, or concern; or it can represent coercion, threat, or outright abuse. Depending on the circumstances, its absence can be a sign of respect or of coldness and distance. There is no formula, no clearly laid-out set of client behaviors, that will tell the therapist precisely when and how to touch and when to refrain from touching. One's empathic response to the client is probably the best indicator, along with constant sensitivity to how the client responds to one's first reaching out. It is wise to ask permission even if the therapist intends only to hold a frightened client's hand or put an arm around a grieving client's shoulder. "May I touch you?" is certainly appropriate for strong or protracted touching but would seem silly and artificial as a precursor to a light pat on the arm. Common sense, experience, and—again—sensitivity to feedback from the client are the best guides.

A regressed client experiences the world as a child does and may have the same sort of need to be touched and held. The therapist's support and caring can often be most clearly expressed through touching, and regressed clients may even ask directly to touch the therapist's hand or to be hugged or held. Rhinehart (1998) reports that, during regressive work, "I commonly place my hands on [the client's] knees or arms to provide a sense of grounding and physical contact with a safe person—especially important when frightening and "unsafe" memories are being accessed and released" (p. 59).

Needless to say, the therapist must never use any sort of physical contact to express sexual feelings. To do so with a regressed client would be tantamount to child abuse, as well as a violation of therapeutic ethics. If the physical contact appears to be becoming sexualized, the therapist can gently withdraw from touching and invite the client to talk about what he is experiencing; it may also be necessary to explain to the client that any romantic or sexual relationship would ultimately be detrimental to the client and will not, under any circumstances, be allowed to develop.

Sometimes a client regresses past childhood, into the world of infancy. A deeply regressed client, experiencing the world (temporarily) as a helpless infant, may be unable to communicate except through touch. Rhinehart (1998) observes that "our skin is not only our physical interface with the world but also the primary experiencer and mediator of life-giving or life-destroying messaging early in life" (p. 57). For a person who has survived severe trauma in infancy, nearly any touch may initially be threatening; yet such clients desperately need safe, supportive, and comforting touch experiences. The therapist must be enormously patient, offering touch yet allowing the client to decide when and how much of the touch to accept. Indeed, with any regressed client, it is important to remember that—in the client's perception, at least—there is a great power imbalance between the client and the therapist, and the therapist's offer of touch is likely to be experienced with significantly greater intensity than would be the case when the client is not in a regressed state. Touching should be gentle, gradual, and never insisted upon if the client seems to reject or be uncomfortable with it.

Like any other powerful tool, touch can do harm if used inappropriately. Touching a client against his will, using touch to establish a one-up position, or using touch to encourage the client's dependency past the point where it is productive are all countertherapeutic. Using touch to establish a sexual relationship with a client or to encourage the client's sexual feelings toward the therapist is one of the most damaging things that a therapist can do. Because of the potential for misuse (and, not incidentally, the potential for malpractice suits), a number of therapists choose never to touch their clients. While such practice provides safety for the therapist, it may deprive clients of the kind of contact that would be most healing for them. Yalom (1999), discussing a case in which he held hands with a grieving client, says, "I was sometimes uncomfortable about the hand-holding, though not because of all the legalistic proscriptions against ever touching a patient: to surrender one's clinical and creative judgment to such concerns is deeply corrupting" (p. 148).

In a truly contactful relationship, a relationship in which one's most private and painful experiences are to be explored, there will nearly always be a point at which physical touch will be helpful. When used appropriately, touch can invite the client into deeper awareness of his own internal process, as well as furthering the therapeutic relationship itself. Three basic guidelines can help the therapist to avoid inappropriate or damaging touch: (a) The client is in charge of when, how deeply, and for how long. Touch should be broken off if the client signals that he no longer wishes that sort of contact. (b) For anything more than light and short-duration touch, get prior permission. If there is a possibility that the client may need to be restrained during regressive anger therapy, a signal should be established beforehand that the client can use to indicate his need to move away from the therapist's touch, out of the regression, and back into an adult mode of functioning. (c) Under no circumstances should the therapist be sexual in her touching, or invite the client to respond sexually to her.

## THERAPIST ERROR

The therapeutic relationship is a potent tool for enhancing client accessibility, as well as a vehicle for the use of other tools and techniques. It is also a vulnerable relationship. Errors of omission or commission on the part of the therapist can seriously damage that relationship; even when errors are not made, the client may perceive the therapist's behavior differently than the therapist intended and begin to pull away from contact. Strupp (1996) notes ruefully that, while doing nothing wrong cannot guarantee success, making mistakes can easily lead to failure: "The presence of even relatively low frequencies of countertherapeutic interpersonal process does seem sufficient to prevent change. A little bit of bad process goes a long way" (p. 79).

"Bad process" is perhaps most clearly visible when the therapist persists in an interpretation or observation about the client that the client rejects. The therapist then labels the client as resistant, and the client feels misunderstood. In this sort of situation, the correctness of the therapist's intervention is almost irrelevant; the client believes that the therapist is wrong about him, and that belief defines the client's experience. The original therapist misunderstanding (from the client's perspective) is not the major problem here; much more disruptive to the process is the therapist's refusal to accept the client's correction. It is difficult to trust a therapist who misunderstands or makes false assumptions; it is nearly impossible to trust a therapist who will not back off from a mistaken assumption once that assumption has been challenged.

One of the most fertile grounds for misunderstanding involves interpretations about client-therapist interactions. As we have seen, the notion of transference suggests that what the client does vis-a-vis the therapist is likely to reflect, to some extent, interactions between that client and significant others in his life. The problem with this view is that it places responsibility for all such interactions solely with the client: if the client gets angry or suspicious or closes down and becomes distant, the therapist wonders who else he is angry at or suspicious about or distancing himself from. Yet the therapeutic relationship, and everything that happens within it, is co-created, a product of the interaction between client *and* therapist. The therapist with an angry or suspicious or distant client must share responsibility for her client's anger or suspicion or distance. To assume that the client's behavior in the therapy session is always and only a mirror of how he behaves with others is to ignore the therapist's contribution to that behavior, blaming (or praising) the client for something that is not wholly his creation. If the therapist persists in this one-sided perception, the client will inevitably feel misunderstood and is likely to withdraw from contact.

This does not imply that the therapist should avoid talking about the relationship between the client's in- and out-of-therapy behaviors—far from it! Exploring that relationship is a fundamental aspect of therapeutic work. It does suggest, though, that (as with any other interpretation) comments about in-therapy and out-of-therapy parallels are best made in the form of questions about the process itself, rather than just the client's behavior. The most effective process questions assume a shared responsibility for what happens between client and therapist; they also invite the client to express his own perceptions of the process. "By maintaining a stance that leaves the degree of parallel between the transference or the in-session cognitive-interpersonal cycle and other patterns in the client's life open, therapists are better able to approach clients in a nonblaming fashion that accepts responsibility for their own contributions to the interaction" (Safran & Muran, 2000, p. 239). In dealing with process issues, asking is generally more useful than telling, and asking about *us* is generally more useful than asking about *you*. "How are we creating this?" is a better question than "What are you doing?"; "Am I responding to you the way your wife/mother/son does?" engenders much less defensiveness than "Do you act this way with your wife/mother/son?"

It is inevitable that a client will, at some time or another, believe that his therapist has misunderstood him or made some other sort of mistake; it is equally inevitable that sometimes he will be correct in that assessment. Guistolese (1996) described therapeutic errors as "inevitable and necessary" in the course of therapy. Errors are inevitable because therapists, like everyone else, are fallible; they are necessary because, for many clients, working through and repairing the rift in the relationship caused by the error may be a fundamental part of the therapeutic process (Safran et. al., 2001).

"Misunderstanding is not the logical opposite to understanding," says Orange (1995). "Instead, misunderstanding is inherent in the process of understanding, and it is often the normal condition of psychoanalytic work" (p. 141). Even when the therapist is technically correct, the client can experience her as being wrong: she may talk when he wishes she would be silent or maintain silence when he wants her to talk; ask about his experience when he wants her to share her own (or vice versa); invite deeper exploration when the client wants to take a break. No matter how empathically skilled, the therapist cannot read the client's mind; occasionally she will miss him. Moreover, the client will organize those misses (and the "hits" as well) according to his own script beliefs; he expects to be treated as the world has always treated him, and he will filter and mold his interactions with the therapist to fit those expectations. Says Fosshage (1992), ". . . ruptures are inevitable because no analyst can understand perfectly or always be sufficiently available . . . and because an analysand will tend to perceive, organize, and construct the analytic experience by using problematic schemas that entail . . . failures" (pp. 37–38).

It can be frustrating to be misinterpreted by a client, to have our perfectly fine therapeutic behavior used to "prove" that we are uncaring or incompetent. We would rather our clients admire us; we would rather they followed our treatment plans and responded as our theories predict. But neither the world nor the people in it are perfect; and clients do sometimes behave in ways that are annoying, frustrating, or provoking to their therapists. Such behaviors are usually script-based: social patterns that have developed over time, patterns that were originally intended to be self-protective but now are so ingrained that they seem to the client to be the only possible way to respond. Although the therapist may be aware of this and do her best to avoid being irritated, or being drawn into a power struggle, or responding with her own self-protective patterns, she too is human. "Both client and therapist become partners in an interpersonal dance that, to varying degrees, reenacts unhealthy patterns that are characteristic for the client," say Safran and Muran (2000). Whatever unhealthy patterns the therapist may unknowingly be engaged in will also become a part of the mixture. Therapists are human; mistakes happen; and every client is an expert at using those mistakes to reinforce his self-protective life script system.

Recognizing the inevitability of errors should not make us complacent about them. We avoid them when we can; when we cannot, we attempt to use them therapeutically. Talking about the error, about what has happened and how it affected the client, is healing. Honest discussion of what one feels and thinks and apologies for one's errors are not what most clients are used to in their relationships. When the therapist responds in this way, she creates a "something different" experience that disrupts the client's old, set patterns. In the interchanges he is used to, breaches are likely to be resented, glossed over, or exaggerated but never discussed openly and respectfully. When he is encouraged to talk about his experience of feeling misunderstood or judged or not attended to—and when that experience is taken seriously—the client may begin to explore some of his deeper beliefs about and experiences in relationships.

Not only is it possible to turn an error into a therapeutically useful experience—such transformations may be actually necessary if the work is to be successful. Safran and Muran (2000) point out that "the exploration and resolution of therapeutic alliance ruptures also provides an important corrective emotional experience for the client. The experience of working through an alliance rupture can play an important role in helping the client to develop an interpersonal schema that represents the self as capable of attaining related-ness, and others as potentially available emotionally" (p. 237). Many clients have developed life scripts based on the belief that they must ultimately be alone, that others will never respond positively to them. For such clients, expe-riencing the therapist's readiness to acknowledge an error, to take responsibil-ity for a breach in the relationship and for healing that breach, challenges those basic beliefs and invites true contact. Bordin (1994) suggests that, the more severely disturbed the client is, the more he may need these episodes of rupture and healing to break through his well-established script patterns. Over the years, he has learned that trust leads only to pain and that expressing his needs drives others away; he has developed a protective shell that keeps him isolated from others, as well as from his own longing for relationship. A ther-apy in which everything went smoothly, in which the therapist made no errors, would have little chance of breaking through that shell. Interactions would be likely to remain superficial, and the basic script structure would not be altered. A therapeutic error invites the client to focus on his disappointment, to sink back into the familiarity of his old self-protective script pattern; while he is experiencing those reactions most intensely, the therapist's responsibility tak-ing and her attempt to repair the damage can significantly impact the client's script belief structure.

When a relationship rupture occurs, the first order of business is to heal the breach and reestablish contact. The most effective way to accomplish this is to talk about it—to talk about one's own part in creating what has happened and to ask the client what he thinks and feels and needs in order to get on with the work. "A central theme in working through alliance ruptures involves helping clients to learn that they can express their needs in an individuated fashion and assert themselves without destroying the therapeutic relationship" (Safran & Muran, 2000, p. 238). The therapist attunes herself to the client's affective expe-rience and responds with a reciprocal affect. If the client is angry, the therapist takes him seriously. If he is frightened, the therapist allows him to see her wish-to-protect. If he is sad, she is compassionate. Responding to his affect as his pres-ent reality, without concern for how he may have contributed to the problem himself or how mistaken his perception may be, and taking full responsibility for her own part in stimulating that affect, the therapist demonstrates that expressing one's feelings and needs—far from destroying the relationship—is the best way to restore it (Erskine, 1994/1997d).

## THE JUXTAPOSITION RESPONSE

Therapists most often are made aware of their errors by the client's response. When a client goes silent or persists in talking about trivial or superficial events, when he begins to arrive late for sessions or cancel sessions at the last minute, or when he frequently finds fault with the therapist's interventions, the wise therapist looks for ways in which she may have missed him, may have failed to respond to his therapeutic needs. Yet, while these client behaviors are frequently a signal of therapist error, they may also be a reaction to the contrast between the richness of the present therapeutic relationship, on the one hand, and the frustration and pain of previous relationships, on the other. We have termed such reactions *juxtaposition responses* (Erskine, Moursund, & Trautmann, 1999).

Modell (1991) describes such a juxtaposition response in the case of a client whose childhood relationship with her father was problematical: "Further, if she experiences within the therapeutic relationship a father love that she had lost or never had and experiences love in relation to the therapist as if he were a father, the gratification might lead to an acute sense of loss. Gratification of a father transference in current time may induce a mourning for what had been lost" (p. 26). To avoid re-encountering grief and mourning over that lost relationship (grief and mourning that have been pushed out of awareness because they were too painful to be experienced), she distances herself from the therapist by trivializing and/or criticizing the relationship.

Grief and mourning for a lost or never-was relationship are not the only reasons for a juxtaposition response. The experience of being understood, respected, and valued, an experience that most people find highly desirable, may be quite threatening to some clients. "What a child has repeatedly experienced as impossible and unreachable in relationships with key figures," say VanKessel and Lietaer (1998), "may have come to be seen, little by little, as unknown and hence unsafe, something that may have caused the longing to be no longer felt and thus be 'excommunicated.'" (p. 164). It is as if the client tells himself, "This is too good to be true; I must be misunderstanding what's happening; I mustn't let myself take it in or believe in it because I'll just get hurt and disappointed again."

Juxtaposition, then, represents a painful double bind for the client. He desperately wants and needs to experience a contactful relationship; it is the piece that may have been missing for him throughout his lifetime. Yet, to meet that need, he must not only risk further hurt but must also reawaken the pain of loss, the pain that he has spent that lifetime defending against. Moreover, major aspects of his life script have been organized around keeping the experience of loss out of awareness, and to deal with it now would require significant script change—more disruption, more confusion, more pain. No wonder he often chooses to reject the possibility of real contact in order to keep the old system intact!

It is easy for the therapist to underestimate the power of her therapeutic involvement to invoke a juxtaposition response. Orange (1995) points out that "many of our patients come to us with seriously disturbed attachment histories. The most ordinary emotional availability or responsiveness . . . may evoke the response of a starving person when offered ordinary food" (p. 132). What may seem like common courtesy, or simply friendliness—a smile, the touch of a hand, willingness to sacrifice one's own agenda and go with the client's—can be rich beyond belief to a client starved for relationship. In this sense, the juxtaposition response can, in fact, be thought of as signaling an error: the error of providing too much, too soon, before the client can handle it. Like other errors, this one can be used in the service of the work. Encouraging the client to talk about his experience, the contrast between what is being provided now and what was missing then, and how all this relates to his evolving therapeutic goals, will help him to bear the distress of reawakening his buried awareness and dissolving the script that has protected (and isolated) him for so long.

## SHAME

Another emotional reaction that can lead to a client's withdrawal from contact is that of shame. Clients may feel ashamed to have talked of forbidden things, to have displayed intense reactions, or even to have experienced the feelings engendered by their work. To deal with the shame, they pull back, retreat into the familiar patterns of their protective script, and the therapist is left wondering what happened—just when things seemed to be moving along so well.

Shame results from a complex combination of affective responses. One of these responses is sadness at not having been accepted as one was, of having one's behavior and even one's very self defined as wrong or not quite good enough—and believing that definition. The sense of being unaccepted and unacceptable translates into the present and can be projected onto the therapist, who is experienced as critical or rejecting of the client's current behavior. The next component is the fear of being abandoned in the relationship; when one is unacceptable, it makes sense that others will not stay in relationship with him once they know what he is really like. Finally, shame requires the disavowal of anger over the expected definition, criticism, or rejection (Erskine, 1994/1997d).

In its most basic form, this set of affects results in a lowering of self-esteem, an urge to hide or to go away, an intense desire to be and feel something other than what one is and is experiencing. It can lead to withdrawal behaviors similar to those seen in a juxtaposition response; indeed, the two are often paired, with the emotions engendered by relational juxtaposition triggering a sense of shame. For other clients, however, the defense against shame is to generate a fantasy of self-righteousness. This protects the client against the pain of loss of relationship, while at the same time providing a pseudotriumph over humiliation and rejection, and a temporary inflation of self-esteem. Baumeister and his colleagues (quoted by Izard, Ackerman, & Schultz, 1999) have noted this phenomenon among overly aggressive boys: "In this case, the root problem is not low self-esteem, but highly inflated self-esteem and favorable views of self that are relatively unstable" (p. 96).

Whether the experience of shame results in self-criticism and withdrawal, or in artificially inflated self-righteousness, it has the potential to distort or derail the course of therapy. The shame-filled client is likely to avoid contact with the therapist, either by berating himself and fantasizing the therapist's rejection or by denying fault, responsibility, or need for change. Says Hite (1996), "To feel . . . defective, isolated as unlovable, to crave for hidden solitude—all aspects of a shame experience—threaten the essential ingredient in all effective therapy: the empathic relationship" (p. 41).

The first step in dealing with a shame response is to recognize it. Understanding the basis for the client's withdrawal or his self-protective braggadocio gives the therapist permission to pause, organize her thoughts, and develop a plan for intervention. Whenever possible, that plan should (as usual) involve discussing the ongoing therapeutic interaction and the feelings that permeate it. Both shame and self-righteousness reflect the defenses used by the client to avoid experiencing the intensity of how vulnerable and powerless he is to the loss of relationship. Broucek and Ricci (1998) warn that while many clients will be able to talk about this vulnerability and will be helped by doing so, others "will react with more shame to any attempt to directly address their shame" (p. 435). When the client appears unable to tolerate direct discussion of his shame or unwilling to explore his sense of self-righteousness, it will do little good to press the issue. The defenses are in place, and battering at them will only drive his feelings farther out of awareness. It is more useful to continue building and talking about relationship, continue to work at whatever level the client can manage, and continue to offer him attunement and involvement. As the relationship strengthens, so will the client's ability to explore more deeply.

## THE MOMENT OF MEETING

Clear, clean, open discussion of the interaction between client and therapist is an important—perhaps the most important—intermediate goal of therapy. When we speak honestly to another person about our relationship, about what we experience from them and how we feel about it, and when the other person reciprocates with equal openness about his or her own experience with us, a very special sort of connection is created. Broucek and Ricci (1998) assert that a person can fully exist only in the context of relational connection. Reality, orientation, and creativity are born out of the communication between individuals; without this sort of contact, we cannot support our own becoming, can never be completely whole.

Whatever the specific problems a client may bring to therapy, his ultimate quest is for contact: for the ability to be fully aware of himself and to enter into a reciprocal sharing of that awareness with another human being. The absence of contact lies at the root of most long-standing emotional distress, and restoring contact is the beginning of healing. It is not surprising, then, that "early on [in therapy] we find that recognition between persons—understanding and being understood, being in attunement—begins to be an end in itself" (Benjamin, 1992, p. 47).

Authentic contact creates what Stern and colleagues (1998) have called a "moment of meeting." Such moments stand out from the ordinary give-and-take of our daily interactions, the social chitchat that fills most of our time with others. These moments of meeting are unique, fashioned out of the singular combination of needs, beliefs, thoughts, and feelings that each individual brings to this specific encounter. They can be moments of high excitement or of deep peace, of joy or fear or fulfillment. They are the moments in which the in-between is forged, the in-between that is the link between two individuals, separate, yet joined in this instant of time. They are the times of client accessibility, the times when old structures can be challenged and new awareness emerges. More importantly, they are precious and healing in and of themselves.

## SUMMARY

The therapeutic relationship itself is the therapist's most powerful intervention. It should be maintained through attending to three primary concerns: authenticity, therapeutic intent, and a constant attention to the relational context of all client behaviors.

Transference is a basic relational meaning-making process: people learn about relationships through having experienced them and bring those learnings into the present. A transference reaction is a description of the client's past relationships and always involves conflict because it has elements of both revisiting and resisting old memories. In addition, transference responses include current relational needs and expectations.

Countertransference, like transference, is an inevitable part of the therapeutic relationship; it is the sum of the therapist's reactions to the client. When these reactions are negative, the therapist must look to herself for their basis; consistently negative countertransference experiences may call for consultation and/or personal therapy for the therapist. Among the most harmful countertransference behaviors is sexual acting out with a client; there are no circumstances under which such behavior is acceptable. Touch is an important means of communication, especially with a regressed client. There are no formal rules for when and how to use touch; one's empathic sense provides the best guideline.

Therapeutic errors can be both harmful and helpful. They are harmful when they cause a breach in the therapeutic relationship and are not acknowledged but, rather, blamed on the client's "resistance." They can have therapeutic value when discussed openly and nondefensively. Encouraging the client to talk about his feelings and needs when the relationship is temporarily disrupted and taking full responsibility for our own contributions to the breach teaches the client valuable relational skills and challenges old script beliefs and patterns.

# Termination

# CHAPTER 11

The experience of ending is as common in one's life as the experience of beginning. Indeed, the two are inextricably connected, for beginning one thing must necessarily end something else. Learning something new ends forever the state of not knowing that thing. Every choice *for* is also a choice *not for* the other alternatives. Conversely, every ending is also a beginning, a beginning of life without that which has been left behind. The old-fashioned word for school graduation, "commencement," recognizes this relationship: the end of one's schooling commences a new set of challenges and opportunities. Endings are really not endings; they are transitions, passages, movements from one condition of being into another. We experience them in miniature every time we shift from one thought to the next, every time we bring a new set of perceptions into foreground and allow what had previously captured our attention to drift into background, every time we slip from waking to sleep or from sleep into wakefulness.

In psychotherapy, too, endings are ubiquitous. Every session comes to an end; within a session, the focus of the work may shift from one concern to another; over weeks and months, there are transitions in the pace and focus of the work; eventually, treatment terminates and the client moves on into the rest of his life. Yet, in spite of dealing with them so frequently, endings seem to be among the most difficult tasks for therapists—both to accomplish and to talk about.

In this chapter, we talk about therapeutic endings. We focus primarily on termination, the client's passage from being-in-therapy to no-longer-a-client; but much of what we say will also apply to the "little endings" that occur throughout the therapy process. One thing, though, is unique about therapy termination, uniquely different from all those other endings that client and therapist have experienced together: termination marks the end of the relationship. In all the other endings, the transition has been from one way or time of working together to another but the relationship has continued. Indeed, in a relationship-focused therapy, the relationship between client and therapist has been the ground upon which all the work has been based. Now that relationship will end; even if it is resumed in a new form at some future time, it will never be quite the same. Both therapist and client must deal with this often-painful reality. Says Yalom (1985), "Termination is a jolting reminder of the built-in cruelty of the psychotherapeutic process" (p. 373).

Western culture, as a rule, does not deal well with endings. We try not to think about them; when we do, we disguise them with euphemisms. We would rather say "I'll think about it" than "No"; "good-bye" is replaced with "see you soon" or "don't forget to write"; even death itself becomes "passing away." These sorts of expressions are a kind of deflection from what is really happening. In using them, we may spare ourselves some of the pain of the ending, but we also deprive ourselves of fully experiencing that which is now beginning. Clinging to the tattered shreds of the old, we cannot embrace the new; to the degree that we continue to look back, we do not see ahead. "Clients who do not say good-bye," say Goulding and Goulding (1979), "keep a part of their energy locked in yesterdays. They may refuse intimacy in the present and experience extreme difficulties with current 'hellos' and 'good-byes'" (p. 175). With the support of the therapist, the client can create a new and different "goodbye" experience. In this sense, the end of every session is a rehearsal for the end of therapy as a whole. As the client deals with each small good-bye, good-bye until the next time he and the therapist meet again, he learns how to experience fully both the end of this small segment of his life and the beginning of the next. He can begin to face the reality of transition, feeling both the discomfort of ending and the excitement of beginning, and can take that new way of ending (and beginning) out into all of the endings (and beginnings), large and small, of the rest of his life.

## TERMINATION CRITERIA

Unlike the end of each therapy session, which is usually determined by the clock rather than by a therapist's or client's sense that it is time to stop, termination must be consciously decided upon. Often, that decision is a difficult one; there are no clear and unmistakable signposts that say, "Now, it is time." There will always be more that could be done, new problems and issues that could be explored. The decision to terminate therapy does not mean that clients have worked out all their issues, that they have acquired all the skills and awareness necessary for a happy life. Termination should not be post-poned until everything is wonderful, until neither client nor therapist can find anything else to work on—if we waited for that, therapy would last forever. On the other hand, terminating as soon as an initial goal has been reached or as soon as the client reports that he doesn't know what to talk about may leave the most important issues untouched and set the client up for relapse and a sense of failure. Lankford (1980) points out that there is a difference between a client having reached a plateau (and needing some breathing space), being stuck, and being ready to terminate. A major challenge to therapists is to dis-tinguish among these events.

In theory, figuring out when to terminate should be simple. Therapy should end when the client has grown to the point at which he has more to gain from being independent of the therapeutic relationship than from contin-uing the work. That apparent simplicity often disappears, though, in the rough-and-tumble actuality of real work with real clients. How does the ther-apist know what the client will gain from being independent? How can she determine the relative benefits of leaving versus staying? What are the specific things that should be taken into account in making the decision to end a ther-apeutic relationship?

The first criterion for terminating therapy must, of course, be relief of the symptoms that brought the client to treatment in the first place. No matter what else he may have accomplished, if his painful feelings, his unproductive thinking, his self-hurtful behaviors have not changed, he will not have gotten what he came for. Yet, as Murdin (2000) reminds us, symptom relief is only a part of the picture: "My own conclusion is that relief of symptoms is an hon-orable goal and cannot be ignored by any therapist. Nevertheless, directly attacking the problem is not enough in the long term. A more complex view of the therapeutic process is needed if there is to be a profound change in an individual" (p. 16).

That "more complex view" must take into account not only surface, eas-ily observable changes in the client, but also a shift in the client's basic way of relating to himself, to the therapist, and to the world around him. The dis-comforts that brought him to therapy are, in fact, side effects of old and no longer useful problem solutions: script decisions and beliefs that do not work in the world in which he now lives. Until those decisions and beliefs have changed, he will continue to act out essentially the same self-limiting and mal-adaptive patterns that produced his symptoms in the first place. Browne (1990), speaking of clients who have experienced acute trauma, says, "The constricted patterns of living, attitudes, and behaviors, which have developed over the years in an effort to maintain the inibition and avoid the pain of expe-riencing the trauma that has been suspended, will also have to change. These do not automatically disappear because the original traumatic experience has now been fully resolved" (p. 31). The same is true for those whose trauma has been cumulative: until they have reevaluated and updated their script decisions and beliefs, until they no longer need to protect themselves in outdated ways against outdated dangers, they will be less than whole.

With changes in life script come new and more effective ways of dealing with the world. Contact with previously walled-off parts of self is restored, and the client can use all of that self in solving problems and developing relationships. His decisions become more integrated: he considers thoughts, feelings, and values, and he is prepared to take responsibility for the consequences of his behavior (Lankford, 1980). He has fewer unrealistic expectations of himself and of others, because he now bases his expectations on contact rather than on fear or fantasy. He may experience anxiety—everyone does, at some time or another—but he shows an "increasing ability to tolerate anxiety without the impatient and impetuous resort to all sorts of anxiety distracting or relieving ritualistic behavior" (Salzman, 1989, p. 225).

In a relationship-focused therapy, some of the major indicators of script change have to do with the way in which the client relates to the therapist. At the beginning of their work, most clients see the therapist as the person who will figure out what is wrong and will tell them what to do about it. Over time, the client begins to trust his own judgment, his own experiencing, and the therapist becomes more a consultant than an authority. The client begins to report experiences of success and of validation of what he has learned more often than he brings up problems or searches for new skills or awarenesses. He no longer needs protection and permission from the therapist, even though he still values the therapist's knowledge and insight. He is "experiencing the transition from reliance on the bond with the analyst to provide understanding and validation and is beginning to provide these functions for himself" (Stolorow & Atwood, 1989, p. 372).

As these changes take place, the therapist's experience of the client shifts, too. In the face of the client's increasing openness to contact, the therapist is likely to find herself feeling freer, more spontaneous and self-revealing (Geller & Nash, 1973). The client has changed, and the therapist, experiencing that change, can herself be different. Together, they are creating a new kind of in-between, a relationship between two whole adults rather than between patient and healer. It is at this point, says Mahrer (1998), that "the therapist and the new person face at least two wonderful possibilities. One is that this qualitatively new person can be the one who leaves the office and lives in the post-session extratherapy world. . . . The second is that this new world is essentially free of those scenes of bad feeling that had been in the old person's world" (p. 209). The changed person is ready to leave the therapist's office and walk out into a changed world.

## THE DECISION TO TERMINATE

What we have been describing in these paragraphs is the ideal termination situation: when both client and therapist feel that the work has been completed and agree to say good-bye. Sometimes, though, they will not agree: one will want to terminate while the other will not. Occasionally, termination will be necessary even though neither therapist nor client wants it. Figure 11.1 illus-

**Figure 11.1** | Choices to Terminate

|  | Client's Choice | |
|---|---|---|
|  | Terminate | Don't Terminate |
| **Terminate** | *Goals reached; script change has occurred -or- Therapeutic impasse has been reached* | *Client is "marking time"; no progress is occurring* |
| **Don't Terminate** | *Client fears making needed changes* | *Client can no longer pay -or- Client or therapist moving to another location* |

(Therapist's Choice labels the left axis)

trates these possibilities. Each of the four areas of the chart contains an example of what might be happening to bring about the situation. Unilateral and forced terminations are, unfortunately, not uncommon in the therapy world. Continuing to work together involves a commitment from both client and therapist; when either participant decides to quit, the work cannot continue. In our discussion of termination, we consider these less desirable sorts of terminations as well as those evolving out of a mutual decision that therapy should end.

## Opening the Termination Discussion

Therapists disagree about who should be the first to bring up the question of termination, client or therapist. Ideally, the client will sense when he is ready: his goals have been met, he no longer needs the support of the therapist to get on with his life, and he is comfortable in saying so. It is his decision, based on his awareness of himself and his needs, and he can experience a newly acquired confidence and independence in making it. Says Bond (1993), "I much prefer that the patient bring up the subject of termination first. Most of us have been weaned, toilet trained, sent to school, and so on when it suited our parents, instead of out of organic needs. . . . When the patient sets the date and the analyst makes sure the decision has grown out of an organic need, a repetition of the pathology may be at least partially averted" (pp. 51–52).

Many clients, however, are reluctant to suggest that it may be time to terminate. They may fear that the therapist will think they no longer value her help, that they are critical or ungrateful. They may expect the therapist to argue with them, to see them as "resistant." They may simply believe that the therapist knows best, and that, if she has not mentioned termination, she must see something more that needs to be done. Clients may be quite accurate in their assessment of themselves as not yet perfect—as still having unresolved issues—and may believe that therapy should not terminate until they are completely and permanently "cured." Waiting for such a client to mention termination can unnecessarily prolong therapy, as well as cause us to miss the chance to deal with whatever issues or mistaken ideas are preventing him from bringing up the subject.

Of course, talking about termination should not happen only at the close of treatment, any more than the end of a session should be abrupt and unanticipated. A conscientious therapist makes sure that the client knows when a session is about to end, and she also makes sure that the issue of termination is discussed at intervals throughout the work. The discussion of termination begins with the first session. When the client's insurance company or HMO designates a maximum number of sessions for which the therapist will be reimbursed, both therapist and client need to keep that limit in mind and tailor the work accordingly. Even when these constraints are not present, part of the information that clients need to have when they begin treatment is a sense of how long therapy will take and what it will cost—and this implies that it will eventually come to an end. Beyond these practical considerations, the therapist is still responsible for preparing the client for termination: after all, as Bond (1993) reminds us, the purpose of therapy is to finish. The therapist's job is not only to help the client to grow and change but also to do so in a way that progresses naturally toward the point at which therapy is no longer needed. Talking about that ending point, how it will be recognized, and how closely it is approaching, is an integral part of the therapeutic process.

## When the Client Wants to Terminate and the Therapist Does Not

Before we talk about termination of the whole of therapy against the therapist's better judgment, we need to go back to the idea of other, "mini" terminations: termination of the hour, curtailing discussion of a particular topic, ending a telephone call. Occasionally, clients will initiate these kinds of endings, wanting to leave the session early or closing off a discussion by changing the subject or by becoming silent. While these disruptions may be simply a matter of the client's not knowing what to say or where to explore next, they are more likely to be a signal of some relational need not being responded to appropriately. The need is usually underground, out of the client's awareness; what he does feel is discomfort, a sense of being missed or misunderstood by the therapist, or a sense that going on may be too uncomfortable or dangerous. Dealing with such situations explicitly is always important; overlooking them can reinforce the client's avoidance and strengthen his old, script-bound patterns of behavior. Murdin (2000) describes it like this: "Because desire is perceived as a source of pain it is repressed, and a symptom or neurotic problem will arise. The relation to the therapist will be distorted by this attempt to avoid pain but the distortion shows the place where the wound is. The avoidance causes many small endings. Some patients stop talking before the end of a session. Some try always to end a session before the therapist does. Some patients will exercise control, not only at the end of the session but also by ending their therapy abruptly" (p. 33).

"Little endings" within a session, then, can be both helpful and hurtful. They are helpful in that they point to what needs to be looked at: by his very closing down, the client is saying, "This is where it hurts." They are hurtful in that, if not remedied, they can create a growing rupture in the therapeutic relationship. If the ending is truly "little," there will be opportunities to return to the issue, to talk about what happened, and to repair the damage. Allowing the pattern of avoidance and contact disruption to escalate into a premature termination, in contrast, does not allow for remediation; and the client leaves with his problems unsolved and his pain unrelieved.

As indicated earlier, psychological functioning can be roughly divided into thoughts, feelings, behaviors, and physical sensations; if any of these aspects are neglected, the work is likely to be hollow and unsatisfying and the client may withdraw. Focusing only on behaviors, for instance, may bring about some temporary symptom relief, but the underlying life script system out of which the symptoms grew remains intact and the client remains constricted in his ability to deal with future problems. Working only with physical sensations is a "go-nowhere" strategy; focusing on physical sensations is most often an introduction to dealing with behaviors, cognitions, or emotions. Overemphasis of feelings, encouraging emotional catharsis with no cognitive follow-up, can have the same effect: "If underlying beliefs contributing to the excessive affect levels are not uncovered and understood, a therapeutic focus on isolated affects runs the danger of premature termination because of affective overstimulation, disappointment because the changes do not last, or an addictive therapeutic relationship without changes in those underlying beliefs" (Lee, 1998, p. 144). And dealing exclusively with the client's belief system may help him to understand his behavior but is unlikely to change it in any lasting way; his emotions are an integral part of his way of relating to self and others, and these must be attended to if he is to fully reclaim and integrate all the parts of himself that he has closed off over the years.

Wherever the client begins, with cognition or affect or behavior or physiology, the work, for most clients, must eventually touch on all four or it will not be complete. Neglecting any one of them is likely to result in the client's feeling unsatisfied, missed, not getting what he needs. This sense of not getting what one needs is perhaps the most common reason for ruptures in the therapeutic relationship and for premature termination. The therapist, because of her own blind spots, lack of skill, poor timing, or limited theoretical orientation, may not have been sufficiently attuned to the client's communication; or the client may simply have been too fearful, too guarded, or too closed to his internal experience, to let his needs be known and dealt with.

Even when the therapist is conducting a well-balanced integrative therapy, conscientiously attending to her client's behavior, affect, cognition, and physical sensation, and maintaining the therapeutic relationship with skill, the client may nevertheless decide to not continue in treatment. In such situations, the therapist's responsibility is to manage the termination in such a way that the client will not be driven even farther into his old dysfunctional relationship patterns. "There are three emotional states which predominate when patients leave therapists without agreement," says Murdin (2000): "they leave in anxiety, they leave aggressively, and they leave in silence. Each of these endings present the therapist with a different problem to solve, because each is a different version of the refusal of the awareness that therapy offers" (p. 61). Why does a client refuse this awareness? Because, at this moment, he is not ready for it. The discomfort, inconvenience, or perceived dangers of continuing outweigh, in his mind, the possible benefits of further work. Arguing with him or coaxing him to stay is likely to make him even more resistant, to feel misunderstood, and to erode the sense of respect and validation so necessary in a relationship-centered therapy. Instead, the therapist can acknowledge the client's decision and compliment him for being clear about his wants and needs (and for his strength in doing so, even in the face of the therapist's disagreement). The function of the client's anxiety, his anger, or his silence can be validated: they are each protective in some way, and each serves an important psychological function. At some time in the future, the client may decide that he wants to find a different and better way to live his life; when that happens, he may return to treatment. Until then, he leaves with the therapist's best wishes.

One exception to this rule of "blessing the inevitable," and that is the situation in which the client, by leaving treatment, puts himself or others in serious jeopardy. The therapist must assess carefully the possible risks the client incurs in terminating therapy. Her first duty is to the client's welfare, and she must take whatever action is needed to protect him. If the client's immediate safety or that of others around him is endangered (fortunately, an unlikely circumstance), she is legally and ethically obligated to break confidentiality and report her concerns to the appropriate authorities and/or to the other people involved. She will, if possible, also talk with the client about those concerns and tell him what she intends to do.

More often, a premature termination involves no such dramatic action. The client is simply choosing to deal with his problems on his own; and, while his choice may be unwise, it is not immediately dangerous. The therapist will encourage the client to talk about his decision. She will want to understand what (if anything) went wrong, how it is that she and the client could differ so much in their sense of what is best for him. She will help him to explore his reasons for quitting, to understand and appreciate what he has accomplished in his work and what is yet to be done, and to anticipate what all this will mean as he goes on about the business of being in the world. If his choice to leave does not change as a result of this discussion, the therapist will support the decision in such a way that the client can return to treatment (with her or with someone else) at a later date, should he decide to do so, not as someone who terminated and then could not make it on his own but as a person who has respected his own pacing and timing and is now ready to begin another chapter of his work.

Just because the therapist is surprised or dismayed by a client's decision to terminate does not necessarily mean that the client is wrong. Before assuming that the therapist has failed him or that the client is too defended, we must consider another possibility: the client may be correct in wanting to terminate, and the therapist mistaken in wanting to continue. The many reasons for this sort of therapist error range from practical and financial (this client pays his bills on time; the therapist's appointment schedule is not full) to emotional (the client is enjoyable to work with, the sessions are stimulating, there are many more issues that would be interesting to explore). The therapist may be insecure about her professional competence or unable to see that the client really has benefited from the work (Bordin, 1968). Or she may be unconsciously using the client to meet her own relational needs. Murdin (2000) describes, for example, the therapist whose reluctance to terminate resembles "the emotional exploitation of the mother who cannot let her child go and who exercises all sorts of emotional manipulation to keep the patient who fulfills her narcissistic needs" (p. 67). Just as letting go of the therapist can be difficult for many clients, so letting go of the client—even when it is time for him to leave her care—may be a challenge to the therapist.

## When the Therapist Wants to Terminate and the Client Does Not

Sometimes a disagreement about termination can work in just the opposite way: the therapist believes that termination is in the client's best interest, but the client wants to continue. This can happen when a time for termination has been agreed upon earlier and, as the time approaches, the client balks. According to Kramer (1990), even Freud—who proposed that the therapy process may in fact never be terminable—suggested that at times it may be useful to set a fixed date to end the work, in order to accelerate the treatment process. However, when the date arrives, the client may protest: "I'm not done yet; I have more issues to deal with; I've just begun to get to the real stuff."

As with every other therapeutic issue, the therapist's course of action must first be based upon the needs of the client. Why is he now arguing a decision that he agreed upon earlier? Does he really need to continue, or is he engaged in an "illusory, magical quest for eternal happiness and perfection, a fragment of childhood narcissism that we never completely surrender" (Arlow, 1991, p. 51). Would the benefits of extending his work outweigh the consequences of giving in to his unrealistic demands and, possibly, fostering therapeutic dependency? If therapy does continue, will he make good use of his time or will he drag his feet, fearing that if he "gets well" he will lose this relationship that means so much to him?

When therapy becomes an end in itself rather than a means to a more fulfilling life in the outside-of-therapy world, it may begin to do more harm than good. While the relationship with the therapist may temporarily become more important than other relationships in the client's life, that exaggerated importance must not continue indefinitely. The client, though, may not cooperate in reassessing and realigning the therapeutic relationship. Just as some infants resist being weaned, rejecting solid food in favor of the warmth and comfort of the mother's breast, some clients resist being weaned from therapy. While both client and therapist may find a great deal of pleasure in the intimacy of the therapeutic hour, pleasure is not the primary goal; when the client has outgrown therapy but is unwilling to move into the weaning process, it is the therapist's responsibility to initiate that process.

If a client has made little or no progress over a period of several months, if he appears content to deal only with superficial topics or insists on focusing on the behavior and problems of others rather than himself, and if confronting these nonuseful behaviors does not change them, it may well be time to begin discussing termination. Such a discussion should include careful inquiry as to the client's sense of what is being accomplished (much more may be going on than the therapist is aware of) and his reasons for wanting to continue. What the client reveals here may confirm the therapist's suspicion that continued therapy is no longer advisable, or it may point to the area in which further work is needed. "There are certain patients," says Yalom (1985), "for whom even a consideration of termination is problematic. These patients are particularly sensitized to abandonment: their self-regard is so low that they consider their illness to be their only currency in their traffic with the therapist. . . . If they were to improve, the therapist would leave them; therefore, they must minimize or conceal progress" (p. 371). For such a client, the work of termination, including developing a sense of self-worth sufficient to survive the loss of the therapeutic relationship, *is* the needed therapy.

Even in situations in which client and therapist have agreed that therapy is done, that the client's goals have been reached and he is ready to move on, the approach of the actual moment of good-bye may be an anxious time for the client. Maybe he was wrong; maybe just a few more sessions. . . . "I've changed my mind," he says. "I don't want to terminate after all." Salzman (1989) advises: "The therapist should not be trapped into postponing or abandoning his plans to terminate because the patient experiences renewed anxiety. It should be clearly understood by both patient and therapist that anxiety . . . will occur throughout the patient's life and that therapy is not a permanent guarantee against disturbed living" (p. 229).

## Forced Terminations

At times, sadly, therapy must terminate in spite of the wish of both client and therapist to continue. Most common among these are terminations required by the policies of the agency or institution within which the therapy is being done or by the limitations of the client's insurance or HMO. Occasionally, but not often, third-party payers or agency supervisors will allow exceptions to their usual rules; occasionally, clients are willing to continue therapy at their own expense when their insurance benefits have been exhausted. Kramer (1990) says of these arrangements, "Those therapeutic disciplines that work with specific and identifiable symptoms, contractual agreements, or predetermined time limits do not have the same confusion as the open-ended psychotherapies about how and when to stop treatment. They may have the opposite problem: when to continue" (pp. 4–5). In other words, before seeking an exception to the rules or encouraging the client to pay out of pocket for additional sessions, the therapist should make certain that this *is* an exception: that the client's situation has turned out to be different from what either therapist or client anticipated, and that more therapy is actually needed rather than simply desirable. To do otherwise may send a signal to the client that he is unable to function without the therapist's help.

Life changes—for either therapist or client—may also force an undesired termination of therapy. For example, the client's career may require him to move to another location or to work hours incompatible with the therapist's schedule. The therapist may change jobs, or move, or leave her practice temporarily for further training. Illnesses can make it impossible for the therapist or the client to continue the work. Sometimes these problems can be worked out with sessions scheduled at a different time or in a new location or less frequently than before, and sometimes they cannot. When a forced termination becomes a possibility, the focus of the work should shift immediately to that termination—what it will mean to the client, how he will deal with it, whether he will transfer to another therapist, and what he can accomplish in the time remaining. Shifting the focus in this way does not mean that his other issues will be ignored; these issues are the background that will shape and color his reaction to termination.

Ending therapy, particularly a therapy in which the relationship between client and therapist is of central importance, always carries with it some sadness. Something that has been very important is ending; the special bond that has grown between these two people is being severed. When therapy ends prematurely, forced by circumstances beyond client's and therapist's control, the sadness can be complicated by anger and resentment. Dealing with these feelings and their relationship to both past and future endings is the next-to-last task of therapy. The last task of all is actually saying good-bye.

## PREPARING FOR TERMINATION

"Termination," says Salzman (1989), "should be gradual and rarely absolute. Nor should it be done at the moment the issue is raised either by the patient or by the therapist. The topic should first be considered, evaluated, and discussed" (p. 228). As we have said earlier, these considerations, evaluations, and discussions should not be postponed until it is close to the time for termination. The eventual end of treatment should be discussed at its outset and should be referred to at intervals throughout the work. Mahoney (1991) reminds us that psychotherapy is a special form of human relationship, one that becomes quite significant in the life of the client (and perhaps of the therapist as well). It offers the client a kind of psychological comfort and safety that he is unlikely to experience anywhere else, a comfort and safety that he can come to accept as a necessary part of life. To avoid his slipping into the expectation that this situation will go on indefinitely, it is important that the therapist "reiterate that the secure base provided by optimal psychotherapy is a base and not a permanent home" (p. 334).

Preparing for termination would be much easier if there were clear and unmistakable guideposts to let both client and therapist know when the end of the work is coming. Unless the number of sessions has been agreed upon beforehand, however, this kind of clarity seldom exists. Much may have been done—many objectives reached and goals accomplished. But therapeutic goals shift and change as clients rediscover parts of themselves; increased contact with self and others leads to new challenges and new areas of growth. As new issues open, clients often find that their original goals are not enough; possibilities exist that they never dreamed of when they began their work. There is always more that could be done, new worlds that could be explored.

With such clients, instead of a rational we-did-what-we-agreed-to-and-now-we're-done, client and therapist may simply sense that an ending is near. Therapy is becoming a luxury rather than a necessity. The therapist suspects that the client may gain more from being on his own than from continuing the work; the client wonders about the same thing. If the client does not bring up the subject, the therapist must; it is not in the client's best interests to drag out the work while each participant waits for the other to open the issue of termination.

Nor is it in the client's best interests to pretend that termination is no more important than the completion of a business arrangement. It may be tempting to treat it this way; endings that involve emotional ties to another person are often uncomfortable, and most of us do not enjoy going through them. However, denying the client an opportunity to talk about his feelings—or even to fail to encourage him to talk about them if he does not do so spontaneously—is to leave him vulnerable to the pain of both past and future endings. Working through issues of loss, grief, and abandonment is one of the last tasks of therapy, a task that can only be completed as the client deals with the loss of the therapeutic relationship itself. Separation, says Bond (1993), "whether by natural or unnatural causes is an intrinsic part of life and must be dealt with throughout therapy to immunize the patient against eventual termination as well as other separations he or she will inevitably experience" (pp. 46–47).

## Feelings About Termination

The most obvious feeling that clients may experience at termination time is sadness. Something they have valued is ending. A relationship that has been important to them will no longer be a part of their lives. It is natural to feel sad about losing someone who knows you so well, has been so understanding and so supportive. Along with sadness, there is likely to be some resentment, especially if the client experiences the therapist as less concerned about termination than he himself. "Why doesn't she tell me I should continue? Why isn't

**Figure 11.2** | Correspondence Between Kubler-Ross Stages and Tasks of Psychotherapy Termination

| Kubler-Ross Stages | Tasks of Grieving | Termination Tasks |
|---|---|---|
| Denial and isolation | To accept the reality of loss | To remind the client of the ending and its link with the contract |
| Anger | To experience the pain and grief | To accept the client's feelings, to deal with any unfinished business |
| Bargaining | | To validate the function of the bargaining and bring to the client's awareness any transferential elements |
| Depression | To experience the pain and grief | To maintain contact with the client |
| Acceptance | To adjust to an environment in which the deceased is missing | To consolidate script cure, to review the contract |
| Hope | To withdraw emotional energy and reinvest it in other relationships | To affirm the client's reorientation, relearning, and self-support strategies |
| | | To end |

(Source: Adapted from "What Do You Say About Saying Good-bye?: Ending Psychotherapy," by K. Tudor, 1995, *Transactional Analysis Journal, 25,* pp. 228–233. Copyright © 1995 International Transactional Analysis Association. Adapted by permission.)

she sad about quitting? Maybe she doesn't care . . . she's got lots of other clients. Maybe she's even glad to get rid of me! It's not fair that I should be so upset, while she doesn't even feel a thing!" Old fears and resentments over having been left or abandoned may be aroused and old defenses against those fears triggered. The client may become withdrawn, may begin to come late or cancel sessions, may even want to terminate immediately (thus leaving the therapist before the therapist can leave him). All of this must be talked about if it is not to continue to fester long after the termination is done.

Tudor (1995) has pointed out the remarkable similarity between the emotional issues of dealing with death and dying, as introduced in the work of Kubler-Ross, and the issues of therapy termination. Figure 11.2 shows the correspondence between these issues. Notice that, for each of the grieving tasks that must be accomplished by the client, a reciprocal response for the therapist facilitates the client's work. Notice, also, that one of the Kubler-Ross stages, *Bargaining,* has no corresponding grieving task, although there is a therapeutic task. (We have taken liberties with Tudor's conceptualization of this issue, choosing to focus on the importance of the client's becoming aware of his own experiencing rather than on the need for confrontation.)

Bargaining involves an activity as well as an emotional experience: the "if you'll do this, I'll do that" activity and its accompanying sense of false hope. Its most common manifestation in psychotherapy is the attempt to establish a new kind of relationship with the therapist in the future. The client may suggest meeting the therapist for lunch, for instance, or offer to babysit or provide some other service. If the client is not helped to understand his process—and to value it for the functions it serves—he may continue to deny the reality of parting and thus deprive himself of the chance to work through the remaining stages.

In thinking about the end of therapy and the sadness that the client may feel over what he is losing, we tend to focus on the loss of the therapist and of the opportunity to experience this kind of unique relationship. But there is another loss as well, one that is perhaps not as obvious. In making the changes that occur in successful therapy, the client must let go of old strategies, old ways of being, old patterns of expectation. The therapist has been the temporary holder of these aspects of the client's self; she has been the one who understood them, tolerated them, validated their function. With her, the client could be all of himself, even those parts that he will eventually outgrow and give up. Now, as therapy ends, that outgrowing time has arrived, and he may experience "a deep reluctance to bid farewell to these wild and childish parts of the self" (Coltart, 1996). Ending therapy means saying good-bye, not only to the therapist and to the therapeutic relationship but also to one's oldest friend of all, one's former self.

Fear, too, can be a part of the termination experience. "Will I be able to make it on my own?" "What will I do if I start falling back into the same old stuff?" "Who will there be to understand me and help me when I need it?" "Things will feel so empty for me, without this relationship; I'm scared of what that will be like." As with all of the other emotions of parting, fear and anxiety should be met head-on: explored, talked about, validated. It makes sense to be afraid of termination, especially if the therapy has been long term and the client has come to rely on the therapist's presence. It makes sense to experience that fear rather than to try to bury it out of awareness. It also makes sense to move ahead, through the fear; new beginnings nearly always carry some portion of anxiety, and the client can handle it.

Some clients become angry as termination nears. Anger can be a defense against fear and sadness, or it can be a genuine response to the frustration and unfairness of having to say good-bye to a valued relationship. The client may be embarrassed by his tender or loving feelings toward the therapist and use anger to cover those feelings; or he may feel that the therapist is abandoning him; or he may be angry because his own discomfort seems so much greater than that of the therapist. "I'm feeling terrible, and it doesn't seem to bother her very much. Maybe she doesn't really care about me after all—I probably should never have trusted her. . . ." With all of these reactions, the therapist's job is to help the client to talk openly about his feelings, to accept them nondefensively, and to take them seriously. Anger can be energizing and empowering, and termination can provide an opportunity for the client to be angry while still maintaining—or even enhancing—contact with the person who is the target of his anger.

While sadness, grief, anger, and fear all have their part in the client's experience of termination, focusing only on these uncomfortable emotions would be wrong. There can be joy and triumph in termination as well. It is a time for congratulations on a job well done, for celebration of a new beginning. It is a time for appreciation of all that has been accomplished, by both therapist and client. Says Bond (1993), "It is essential that a healthy person be able to express gratitude and feelings of love to the analyst before termination can occur. After all, theirs has been the most intimate relationship of which human beings are capable" (p. 59). Expressing love is one of the eight relational needs that we have identified (Erskine, Moursund, & Trautmann, 1999; see also chapter 3); and this need can emerge strongly toward the end of a relationship. Strangely, it is often more difficult for therapists to accept expressions of gratitude and love than to deal with the client's more negatively toned emotions. Therapists are trained, after all, to help their clients work through all sorts of frightening and uncomfortable feelings; unfortunately, many are also trained to be suspicious of such things as love or gratitude, labeling them as "transference" or "manipulative." In so doing, they deprive their clients of the opportunity to end their work with a contactful and loving expression of what that work has meant to them.

## The Therapist's Feelings

"More than any other phase of the treatment process," says Kramer (1990), "the ending calls upon therapists to examine and understand their own needs and feelings. It is a time to look deeply inside and honestly confront one's dependence, anxieties, and fears" (p. 2). The therapist who has no feelings about ending her work with a client has not developed an authentic relationship with that client. Relationship requires involvement, and ending an involved relationship is always an emotional experience. In therapy, unlike other relationships, parting is built in. Ending, dissolving this relationship that has been constructed so carefully and (occasionally) with such effort, is inevitable; and often it seems that the end must come at precisely the point when the therapist might have come to enjoy it most. The worst of the struggles are over; the client is becoming more and more the person he wants to be; client and therapist know each other well and communicate freely. Contact between them is full and mutually rewarding. And now, just when everything is going so well, it all must end.

Of course, when therapy terminates because the client has achieved his goals, the therapist will experience pleasure and satisfaction. The purpose of parenting is to usher a healthy adult into the world, and the purpose of therapy is similar; when those purposes have been accomplished, parents and therapists alike feel a sense of satisfaction with a job well done. But they feel sad as well; this new and healthy adult has just gotten to the point where he would be a delightful friend, and now he is leaving.

It is highly appropriate that the therapist share with the client some of her own ambivalence around termination. Not only does such sharing keep the relationship authentic, without cover-up, but it is also another marker in the gradual shift from one-up-one-down (that inevitably characterizes the beginning of treatment) to a more balanced way of relating. Geller and Nash (1973) have found that "clinicians representing diverse points of view seem to agree that towards the end of treatment, therapists need not strive for as much neutrality and objectivity, but may be freer, more spontaneous and self-revealing. Essentially a shift in the direction of an egalitarian relationship is regarded as the most therapeutically efficacious" (p. 5). The therapist would be unlikely to discuss her feelings toward the client during the first few sessions of therapy, but here, as therapy is ending, she can be a (nearly) equal partner in exploring how both she and the client are experiencing their last few hours together. In fact, this sharing models perhaps the last significant therapeutic experience for the client: saying good-bye honestly and openly, without hiding one's sadness from oneself or from the person from whom one is parting.

## TASKS OF TERMINATION

We have used the phrase "termination process" a number of times in these paragraphs. Termination *is* a process, not an event. It is a process that involves a number of tasks; and, while the exact nature of these tasks will differ from client to client, there is a core of similarity among all planned therapy terminations, a set of tasks that need to be attended to if the therapy is to be complete. All of these tasks involve exploring the client's internal experience: his thoughts, feelings, and fantasies about ending therapy. "To ensure that separation is not experienced by the patient as a catastrophic loss or as abandonment, the therapist needs to actively engage the patient in the separation experience. The therapist does this by making the feelings and thoughts associated with termination explicit. His job is to enable the patient to talk about the apprehension and sadness, as well as the exhilaration, that the patient feels" (Cashdan, 1988, p. 144).

The first issue likely to be raised is the client's readiness to terminate. With some clients, this is relatively straightforward: they have (with the therapist's support) decided that it is time to end their work, and they are ready to explore their mixed feelings about their decision. Indeed, they have been doing so all along, for these feelings have been an important part of the decision process. Clients for whom termination is likely to be more difficult, in contrast, tend to fall into two extremes: either they protest, bring up new issues, relapse into previously outgrown behaviors; or they shrug off termination as unimportant, something about which they have no strong feelings.

The client who acknowledges no particular feelings about termination, whose attitude seems to be "I came to do a job, I did it, what's the big deal?"

may be sliding back into an old pattern of disavowal in which uncomfortable feelings are simply papered over rather than dealt with openly. Bond (1993) advises, "When leave-taking is too comfortable, the experienced [therapist] will get suspicious and seek to help the patient find and experience the hidden grief beneath his defenses. If he leaves without experiencing a mourning period, he is in line for trouble later" (p. 47). The therapist needs to inquire patiently about the client's feelings and may need to go back to strategies used earlier in treatment to help the client recognize and own his feelings—for instance, using exploration of body sensations as an avenue into emotional awareness.

The client who protests termination, who pleads for additional sessions, brings up old issues (or new ones), or relapses into symptomatic behavior, is not denying his reluctance to terminate; if anything, he is exaggerating it. These kinds of behaviors may be a kind of bargaining, a way of hanging on to a relationship that the client is afraid to give up. The therapist's first task with such a client is to carefully reevaluate the termination decision: Is it really in the client's best interests to quit now? What impact is the client trying to make, and upon whom? Is it possible that the client is right, that further therapy is needed at this time? Consultation can be quite helpful in these situations, and the consultation should always include a consideration of the therapist's feelings and motivations too: if she was wrong in suggesting or agreeing to termination, why did she allow herself to make that error? What is happening in the therapeutic relationship that makes her so ready to end it?

If, after careful consideration, the therapist concludes that termination is in fact the best course, she must inquire about the client's experience, memories, and relational needs. The most effective way of dealing with self-hurtful behavior (and exaggerating one's need for therapeutic help is, ultimately, self-hurtful) is likely to be *validation:* confirming and validating the function of the behavior. Talking about what is happening and what needs the client is attempting to meet, allows him to feel understood even as he is invited to be honest with himself about what he is doing. It is seldom experienced as critical or belittling; rather, the client becomes a partner in the business of discovering what his behavior is intended to accomplish and how those goals can be met in more appropriate and effective ways.

Clients who attempt to cajole or coerce their therapist into prolonging the work are likely to use the same kinds of techniques with other people in their lives. They have learned over and over again that asking straight out does not work, so they wheedle or threaten instead. Often they are not consciously aware that they are being manipulative; nor are they aware of the effect that this sort of behavior has on their friends, family, or coworkers. The therapist's sharing of her own internal response to his actions can not only help him realize what he is doing but can also point out the costs of such behavior in his other relationships. Says Cashdan (1988), "A major goal in the . . . final stage of treatment is to provide patients with vital information about the way they are perceived by others. Patients need to learn in a very direct and immediate way how their interpersonal manipulations affect those about them. This is accomplished by providing patients with feedback about what it is like to be the recipient of their projective manipulations" (p. 133). Again, though, the therapist must take care to couple this feedback (which is a kind of confrontation) with validation of the underlying function of the behavior. To end therapy without such confrontation and validation would deny the client one of the most important aspects of treatment: the experience of being accepted, valued, and understood even when behaving in ways that seem hurtful or inappropriate.

Since termination of therapy marks the end of a relationship, it is a natural time to explore other endings, other good-byes. Lankford (1980) describes her termination work: "I also encourage people to look at their past and consider if they have unfinished business with people. Might they wish to resolve this with the people directly, or do they prefer to resolve it within themselves so they can leave it in the past?" (p. 176). This kind of discussion can lead to the client's literally going out to people who have been important in his life and talking with them about issues that have been left unfinished, or it can lead into pieces of therapeutic work in which the client deals with the fantasy image of someone who is no longer physically available to him. In either case, the process works in two directions: working through old unfinished issues allows the client to deal with ending therapy more clearly, unentangled by the threads of past guilts and resentments; and the experience of talking openly about the end of therapy helps him find the courage and the skill to resolve those old and often painful relationship issues.

Resolving old issues means letting go: letting go of the anger, the resentment, the fears and regrets that characterize unsuccessful relationships. It means giving up the dream that the past can somehow be changed and everything be made all right again. Dealing with feelings toward the person or persons who have failed the client in the past—who have abused, neglected, or abandoned him—clears the way for forgiveness: "The patient does not have to forgive these objects for what they did, but rather for their inability to appreciate the devastating psychological legacy it would leave behind" (Cashdan, 1988, p. 140). What they did to him may indeed be unforgivable; but they can at least now be understood as people who were too ignorant, or too caught up in their own needs, to understand the full import of what they were doing. Knowing this, the client can also recognize how far he has come, how different he now is from both himself back then and from the significant others on whom he was once dependent. No longer needing to protect or distance himself from them, he can walk away free of the emotional burden he has been carrying for so long.

Pistole (1999) emphasizes the shifting role of the therapist and the client's need to accept that shift as therapy moves toward termination. At many times throughout therapy, the therapist has assumed the role of the nurturing, caring other who was not available in the past when the client needed relational support: in other words, the therapist has acted so as to respond to the client's archaic needs as expressed in the transference. At other times—and increasingly often toward the close of the work—the therapist acts "so as to promote security in the here-and-now relationship" (p. 440). Behavior aimed at prolonging the therapy may be a signal that the client does not yet feel able to function as an autonomous adult and fears that he will fail without the support of a parental figure. Working through such issues is a significant facet of the termination process. Therapy cannot be completely successful until the therapeutic transference has been recognized and is replaced—at least for the most part—by a relationship between two contactful and fully present individuals.

As he prepares to end the therapy that has been such a central part of his life, the client will begin to shift his focus from what he is leaving behind to what he is moving toward. Relationships outside of therapy will become increasingly important and the relationship with the therapist less so. This shift must be supported. The therapist must help the client to anticipate the challenges of dealing with his world on his own, to anticipate the problems he may face and develop strategies for solving them. She needs to affirm clients' "reorientation and relearning, [their] withdrawal from therapy, and [their] (re)investment in themselves, in others, and in the social world beyond therapy" (Tudor, 1995, p. 232).

Before shifting entirely into that out-of-therapy world, though, the client needs to take a long look back at what he has accomplished. He needs to develop a cognitive frame that will give structure to the affective work he has done and the changes he has made. Greenberg and Paivio (1997) suggest that "the final phase of this work involves the creation and consolidation of new meaning by reflecting on what has occurred and developing a narrative of how the experience one has been through fits, or changes, one's identity" (p. 128). To the degree that therapy has been a worthwhile investment, the client has made significant shifts in his patterns of thinking, feeling, and behaving. He needs to be grounded in these new ways of being, feeling the connection between old self and new, integrating all that he has been with what he is now becoming.

## TAKING NEW BEHAVIORS OUT INTO THE WORLD

The phrase "new ways of being" implies that what the client has learned to do in the context of the therapeutic relationship must generalize into the extratherapeutic world. In a real sense, this generalization is the whole purpose of therapy: learning to be different in the therapist's office is of little value to the client unless those differences can be translated into new ways of dealing with the rest of his life. Ensuring that therapeutic learnings do generalize to other situations is not only a task of termination; it is the therapist's responsibility throughout the work. We have chosen to discuss it here not so much because it uniquely characterizes termination work but, rather, because it is one more aspect of therapy that must be attended to before the work can be completed.

The anticipation of generalization and transfer of learning is a background for any therapeutic work, but it moves to foreground as each major piece is completed. Discussions of how the work will generalize typically occur at the close of a session; they are essential at the close of the entire therapy process. "How will what you have done today (or in these weeks or months of therapy) make a difference in your life?" "How will other people know that you have changed?" Mahrer (1998) suggests that the client be encouraged to imagine himself as a new person going out into his old world. He invites the client to think of "several prospective scenes and situations in which the new person can be, exist, live. These can occur right after the session is over, or in the next few days or so, rather than weeks or months from now. You ought also to think of a number of behaviors that the new person can carry out, ways for the new person to undergo the new experiencing" (p. 210). Anticipating and describing specific things that may happen as a result of therapy can become a self-fulfilling prophecy: opportunities for new responses that might otherwise have gone unnoticed will be attended to and utilized because the client has sensitized himself to them.

Even more effective in promoting extratherapy changes is experimenting in the therapy session with how one might be different "out there." Role-play work like this has a number of advantages: it does not involve other real people, so errors do not create new problems; it can be stopped and redone as many times as needed; and it can begin with fantastic and unrealistic scenarios, working gradually toward something that might actually happen. Mahrer (1998) suggests five steps in developing this sort of work: (a) think of scenes, and imagine being in them as this new, changed person; (b) make sure that the scenes are playful, caricatures, not realistic; (c) gradually create and imagine oneself in more realistic scenes; (d) rehearse and refine ways of being in the realistic scenes; (e) make a commitment to follow through and actually try out the new behaviors.

Beginning the role play with a highly unrealistic scene ("You'd probably never actually do this, but just let yourself imagine what it would be like") can allay the client's performance anxiety; adding humor allows both client and therapist to have fun with the exercise. Says Mahrer (1998), "To make things safe, the context is playful unreality. Make it exceedingly clear that this is not for real. Instead, the atmosphere is one of sheer nonsense, silliness, outrageousness, caricature. Make it clear that the aim is just to gain a sense of what it could be like to be this whole new person out in the extratherapy world" (p. 213). A client who first acts out kicking his boss around the parking lot like a football, for instance, can experience his newfound strength and assertiveness. He may then express his anger by just shouting at his imagined boss, still with a sense of strength. Eventually, he can take his angry feelings into a role play of setting clear and effective limits at work, and this behavior may be one he is ready to actually try out in reality.

One of the things the client leaves behind as therapy ends is the opportunity to face himself, to be con-fronted in a supportive and positive way. Therapeutic confrontations, as we have described them, involve not just calling some response to the client's attention, but doing so in order that client and therapist together can explore the psychological function of that response.

This kind of confrontation requires that the client observe himself, that he stand back and ask what it is he is needing, what he is trying to accomplish. Learning to develop this kind of self-awareness is an important generalization task: clients need to be able to step back from problematic situations, observe themselves and their responses, and open their awareness not only to what they are doing but also to the needs that they are experiencing and how their behavior is related to those needs. This is one area in which the client can usefully take the therapist's voice with him into the post-therapy world. "The collaborative aspects of the therapeutic relationship," say Glickauf-Hughes, Wells, and Chance (1996), "strengthen the client's capacity to observe and reflect upon his/her experiences in the presence of the therapist and to gradually extend these observing functions to situations outside of the therapeutic situation" (p. 433).

## THE LAST SESSION

Sooner or later, all the preparation has been done and client and therapist find themselves beginning their last session together. This last session, like the first, is qualitatively different from all the others. The fact that it is the last colors everything that is said. It is not a time to bring up new issues, or even to rework old ones. It is a time to finish and to say good-bye.

Good-bye-saying is an opportunity to look forward to what things will be like when therapist and client have gone their separate ways and to look backward at what has been done and at what the relationship has become. Looking forward to what will happen for the client during the coming weeks, months, and years has probably been going on to some extent during the last few sessions; it is an important part of preparing for termination. The last session's forward-looking is essentially a review of this work: what sorts of situations are likely to be difficult for the client and how will he manage them? How will the work he has done over the course of therapy help him to handle those difficulties in a new and more effective way? Under what circumstances is he likely to relapse into his old patterns, and how will he recognize a relapse, and what will he do about it? How will he know if he needs to return for more work, either a therapeutic "booster shot" or for more extended treatment?

The backward-looking of the final session should be a review of what has been accomplished and, perhaps more importantly, of how the client's relationships (with the therapist and with others) have changed. Salzman (1989) takes a rather businesslike view of this retrospective process: "Before termination, the therapist should review the work done and also what has been left undone. Introspection, not preoccupation, should be encouraged, and a closing statement of the history of treatment and assessment of progress should be made before the therapeutic relationship is brought to an end" (p. 228). Salzman is correct, of course; these things do need to be done. However, in a relationship-focused therapy, there is much more to consider than an objective "assessment of progress." Here are two people who have created, between themselves, something unique and precious, something that will never be exactly repeated. The special quality of their working relationship, of the openness they have developed and the struggles they have shared, must also be acknowledged and celebrated.

Along with acknowledging the relationship they have created, therapist and client will need to acknowledge each other, to share their sense of appreciation for what the other has done. The client has changed in ways that would not have been possible without the therapist's guidance, and he is grateful. He is grateful for the therapist's patience, for her support, and for her skill. He needs to express this gratitude, and the therapist needs to accept it graciously. This is not the time to explore the hidden meaning of a gift or a thank-you, to be concerned about manipulation or unresolved transference; this is the time to simply accept with thanks.

The therapist too may choose to share her appreciation of the client, of what the client has done and of what being a part of the client's journey has meant to her. She may have her own reasons for gratitude: she too has had her off days, has occasionally misunderstood or been too focused on her own agenda, and the client has been willing to move past her errors. Cashdan (1988) suggests that the therapist may wish to thank the client for putting up with "some of the therapist's idiosyncrasies or occasional lapses. The therapist might want to acknowledge the patient's forbearance in the face of trying episodes that occurred during the course of treatment" (p. 146).

Both client and therapist have done well; and both could have done things differently, perhaps with even better results. Termination can bring a sense of regret for lost opportunities, for work not done, and for possibilities not realized; and this too should be acknowledged. Murdin (2000) comments, "Both the patient and the therapist will have ideas about what has been missed, although they may be different. Patients can be encouraged to say what they have missed or not been able to change. Therapists are less likely to say what they think has not been done unless it relates to what the patient has already said" (p. 146). The old guideline for therapeutic credit and blame—that the client gets credit for what goes well and the therapist takes responsibility for what goes badly—is perhaps most critical at the end of treatment. One of the cardinal objectives in termination is that the client should leave with a sense of accomplishment, both in order to engage in posttherapy pursuits with confidence and to be able to return to treatment, if necessary, without having to lose face or feel that he has failed. The therapist may choose to comment on areas for future work but must be careful to avoid any sense of criticism of how the client has used their time together.

After all this—the reviews, the appreciations, the regrets—comes, at last, the moment of good-bye. This is a moment, says Tudor (1999), "in which the psychotherapist models in his or her behavior, thinking, expression of feeling, attitude (posture), and social and transpersonal awareness an integrated Adult relationship which allows him or her to let go of the client, thus ultimately promoting the client's autonomy" (p. 233).

But must the therapist let go completely? Must the relationship truly and forever end? Is there no possibility of some new kind of coming-together, some new basis for relationship? After all, these two people have been through so much together and know each other so well—what a loss to let all of that disappear. Yes, it is difficult, but to do otherwise would prevent the client from doing what he most needs to do at this point: end the work. Termination with the hope of continuing in some other way is not real termination. Coltart (1996) lists a number of reasons why termination should be a true parting: "the reinforcement of the strength of internal objects; a refusal to expose, and perhaps *im*pose, too much of the therapist's real self on vulnerable ex-patients; and granting them a freedom to work through and resolve final transferences, in fact, all remaining problems, on their own. It also allows patients to be sad and to manage their own mourning for the loss" (p. 125).

And so the work ends. The client leaves, perhaps to seek therapy again sometime in the future, perhaps not. Even if he does return, to this therapist or to someone else, it will not be the same. This therapy, this unique experience of being and working and growing together, is done. The growing together is over, but the growing is not: both therapist and client, in their separate lives, will continue to grow and change. It is their continued growth that prevents either from returning to this relationship that has now ended. There is an old saying, "One cannot step twice in the same river." The river flows on, continually changing; it can never again be exactly as it is now. As therapy ends, two lives that have joined for a time now flow apart; they can never rejoin in exactly the same way.

## SUMMARY

Endings are an inevitable and often difficult part of life. Psychotherapeutic termination can be particularly difficult because it marks the end of a highly valued relationship.

Criteria for termination include symptom relief, changes in the client's underlying script, improved problem-solving and relationship skills, and a shift in the client-therapist relationship. Client and therapist may not agree about when to terminate. If the client chooses to leave prematurely, the therapist should allow him to do so in a way that will facilitate his returning to treatment at a later time. If the client is overly reluctant to terminate, it is important to discuss his reasons fully; dealing with termination issues may be the major therapeutic work that needs to be accomplished.

Sometimes circumstances force termination against the wishes of both client and therapist. These circumstances include restrictions on the part of insurance or agency, or client's or therapist's life changes.

Preparing for termination involves a thorough discussion of feelings. The client may feel sadness, fear, anger, or joy and satisfaction. The therapist, too, may feel both pleasure and regrets and will want to share some of these feelings

In the preceding chapters, we have presented a great deal of theoretical material, as well as some highly practical suggestions about how to conduct an effective relationship-focused integrative psychotherapy. To show how these ideas are actually used, we have prepared an annotated transcript of a therapy session. The transcript is taken from a recording of a session conducted in the offices of the Institute for Integrative Psychotherapy; it is a verbatim record of the full session, changed only to protect the identity of the client.

Annotations, particularly when they occur frequently, can interrupt the reader's sense of the flow of therapeutic work. To avoid this kind of interruption, we have chosen to insert the annotations as footnotes; the reader is then free to read transcript and annotations together or to first read through the transcript without interruption and then re-read it in connection with the annotations. In most cases, annotations contain a reference to a page or pages in previous chapters where the issue in question is discussed. The reader will also notice that the transactions between therapist and client are numbered to make referencing them easier.

The client, in this session, Ellin, is a tall, attractive woman in her late 40s. This is her fourth session with this therapist (she also was in treatment with another therapist for several months, some years earlier), and she is familiar with the setting in which the work will take place. She enters, makes herself comfortable, and waits for the therapist to speak first:

1   **THERAPIST:** Where would you like to start today?

2   **ELLIN:** Um, I've got an idea, but I'm not quite sure where it will lead. And, um . . .there's so much I've been thinking about, like when I wake up at 4 A.M. and can't go back to sleep; I think I've gone about as far as I can go with it on my own. And I want to know where else it can go. And, um, it's, um, it's to do with not feeling safe around my dad.[1]

3   **THERAPIST:** Ouch . . . What a constant tension that must bring to you. Not so much like an ouch, but more like just a heaviness.

4   **ELLIN:** Yeah, and I've felt that way for so long, and I've talked about it before, but now I don't want to, you know, I can see that's no point in it still being around. So I want to really try and get rid of it.[2]

5   **THERAPIST:** (pause) What kinds of things do you think about at 4 in the morning?

6   **ELLIN:** Well, I was thinking about the times when I, when I haven't trusted my dad. Or I haven't respected him. Um . . . but it's all tied up with my mother, and my mother's, um, well partly my mother's jealousy, and partly expectation of my dad, um, cheating on her. Which he did, all the way through their marriage. And they now live separately, um . . . (pause) so it's partly like there was a real reason for her to feel jealous; which I was aware of when I got older. And there was a real reason for me to feel on guard around my dad. Because . . . (pause) it's like, because he, he couldn't show affection, he didn't know how to be affectionate, it all got tied up in sexual innuendos, and sort of inappropriate language . . . (pause) Well, what I was thinking this morning is, um. . . well, there are hundreds of things, but one is that I recently went up to Chicago and joined my family for a kind of reunion. And, um, there's a tension between my mother, my father, and my aunt. Because my mother feels jealous of my aunt, and anybody who's affectionate to her. And my dad clearly prefers my aunt to my mother, even though there isn't anything sexual, cause they're sort of in their 70s and 80s. And it's, um, it's that, that is a sort of continuation of years and years. But, um, it's like . . . yeah. Um . . . well like one time I wanted to go through Chicago to my mother's house, and I decided to stay the night at my dad's apartment. And that, that felt risky, because I don't really know whether I can trust him, cause that

---

[1]Although this is not an initial session, and the overall therapeutic contracting work was done earlier, the therapist still invites Ellin into a contract. Both Ellin and the therapist know, by now, that this session contract is likely to be a springboard, a starting place rather than a statement of what will actually be accomplished, and the therapist's question acknowledges this. Ellin, too, acknowledges that she doesn't know where the work will take her; what she does know is that she wants to deal with unfinished business with her father. Saying that she has "gone about as far as I can go on my own" is a request to be taken further by the therapist. (See chapter 7, p. 140; chapter 9, p. 163.)

[2]Ellin has worked with this therapist for three previous sessions and has learned to move into her work with little or no warm-up. The therapist, recognizing Ellin's readiness to work, waits a moment (to allow her to elaborate if she will) and then asks a question that will move her quickly from her rather vague statement to a specific starting point. (See chapter 6, pp. 107–108)

would be me alone with him. But it was also sort of added to by my mother's reaction: "Oh, he won't like that. He doesn't like people staying at his place." And it was this kind of "keep off"—you know, it's like, I think there's always been that element of "don't get close."

7  **THERAPIST:** You think the message was "don't get close," rather than her attempting to protect you from his rebuff.[3]

8  **ELLIN:** Definitely. Yeah. I didn't have a sense of her being protective.

9  **THERAPIST:** The way you describe her, she sounds so critical.[4]

10  **ELLIN:** Yeah. She is. Yeah . . .

11  **THERAPIST:** What just happened to you there?[5]

12  **ELLIN:** (voice is breaking) Well it's just like, her old relationship with me and to the world is critical. . . . And it's kind of like one of these, um, like you finish a phone call and you realize you feel worse afterwards. But I'm getting better at picking it up. I mean, the most recent example is, I went to this wedding. And she asked me, "How did the wedding go? Did you look nice? You tried your best to look nice." And it's that kind of . . . you know, it's like "why bother?" That's how I hear it, anyway. Sort of like . . .[6]

13  **THERAPIST:** Why bother? What's that mean?

14  **ELLIN:** (tearful) It's a waste of time.

15  **THERAPIST:** You mean, you tried your best and you still can't look nice?

---

[3]Throughout this whole, rather rambling statement of Ellin's, the therapist has not only listened respectfully, but has maintained cognitive attunement, following both the content of her discourse and the way in which she organizes and frames that content. He has put himself into her frame of reference, adjusting his thinking pattern to hers, following her process of moving from one idea to the next. It is this attunement that allows him to extract the most important feature of her story, that mother was rejecting rather than protective. As we shall see, this lack of protection has been a critical element in forming the script pattern that is now so troubling to her. (See chapter 6, p. 102)

[4]This is one of many empathic interventions in this transcript in which the therapist's tone of voice conveys even more than his words. With the addition of body language, his response goes beyond simply reflecting what the client has said: he has "listened from within," attending to his own reactions to Ellin's description of her mother as well as to Ellin's. His short statement includes both his sense of Ellin's experience and an acknowledgment of his own emotional response to mother. (See chapter 5, p. 91)

[5]The therapist's affective attunement sensitizes him to a subtle shift in Ellin's affective state, and he makes a phenomenological inquiry. Does the question predict or create Ellin's immediate emotional response? Or does her behavior predict/create the therapist's intervention? The therapeutic process has already become a mutually regulated process, a dance between two fully involved individuals, each responding to the subtle cues given by the other. (See chapter 6, pp. 99, 116)

[6]Thinking and feeling are intertwined throughout life. Ellin's thoughts about her appearance are shaped by her feeling about herself (which, in turn, have been twisted and toxified by Mother's criticisms). Her feelings are triggered and directed by the beliefs—the cognitions—that accompany them. (See chapter 3, p. 38)

<sup>16</sup> **ELLIN:** (nods) And, um . . . sort of like, um, it's all (sigh) . . . it's all tied up with being attractive. It's sort of like feeling it was dangerous to be attractive in my, in my childhood. (sigh)[7]

<sup>17</sup> **THERAPIST:** (pause) And that's in reference to both mother and father.

<sup>18</sup> **ELLIN:** Yeah. Yeah.

<sup>19</sup> **THERAPIST:** Mother would be jealous, and father . . . you couldn't be sure what he'd do.

<sup>20</sup> **ELLIN:** That's right.

<sup>21</sup> **THERAPIST:** And mother says "You *tried* your best." Meaning no matter how much you try, you still won't look good?[8]

<sup>22</sup> **ELLIN:** Yeah. It's little things, like, that stick in my mind. Like, when I was two they had a picture taken of me. And she said, you know, that, there's this theory that you double your height. That by age two you're half your future height. And the sort of thing she would say was, "If I'd of realized then what you would have been . . ." you know, it would have been like a disaster.[9]

<sup>23</sup> **THERAPIST:** So you're not even accepted in the size of your bones.

<sup>24</sup> **ELLIN:** Not at all. (deep sigh)

<sup>25</sup> **THERAPIST:** Are you unusual in your family, with your height? Or are others tall also?[10]

<sup>26</sup> **ELLIN:** Um, oh, my mom was tall for her generation. You know, she kind of started small and worked her way to the top of the line (chuckle). And, um, my dad is about 6 foot. And my brothers are taller than I am; one is about 6′2 and the other is about 6′4.

<sup>27</sup> **THERAPIST:** Well, that's basic biological structure. You didn't *make* yourself tall? (Ellin chuckles ruefully.) You laugh at that. That was a serious question.

---

[7]Every child needs attention and approval. But Ellin's early efforts to satisfy these needs met with criticism from Mother and sexualized responses from Father. No wonder the need to be approval-worthy had to go underground! Feelings involving a desire to be close and to be admired were transformed into feelings of wariness and anxiety, and her perception of herself as lovable was buried beneath a protective belief in her own unattractiveness. (See chapter 3, pp. 39–40, 50)

[8]In this and the several preceding transactions, the therapist is using phenomenological inquiry to explore both the client's early experience and her current thoughts and feelings about those experiences. He is respectful and interested; he does not interpret Ellin's words or add to her story but, rather, uses clarifying questions (and implied questions) to help both of them understand how past and present interact for her. (See chapter 6, p. 116)

[9]The earlier a script pattern is established, the more firmly set it becomes within one's overall way of being in the world. Here is evidence that events shaping her script belief that she is unattractive were occurring at least as early as 2 years. No wonder that belief is so well entrenched, so capable of withstanding the evidence of her own eyes! (See chapter 2, p. 22)

[10]Unlike the previous inquiries, which have been primarily phenomenological—that is, having to do with Ellin's internal experience—this question asks about an external reality. Its purpose is to place the client's description of the problem, and her affect around it, in the context of what her family was like, and so to evaluate its objective significance.

28   **ELLIN:** Yeah.

29   **THERAPIST:** You think you went and made yourself tall?

30   **ELLIN:** No, I don't. I, I'm always, when I come in here I don't feel tall. But every-where else I do. (cries)[11]

31   **THERAPIST:** Hm. I was watching you walk down the hall last week and thinking about why you don't look unusually tall to me. And I think it's because of the almost perfect shape of your body, that fits your tallness. You're just perfectly proportioned. (Ellin looks uncomfortable.) What happens when I say that?[12]

32   **ELLIN:** It's that, yeah, I'm sort of overwhelmed. I'm remembering back to playing volleyball back at school, and being in the front row. And, um, people just, like freaking out, when I stood in front of the net. (sigh)[13]

33   **THERAPIST:** What age are you talking about, as a volleyball player?[14]

34   **ELLIN:** Anywhere from 11 to 16.

35   **THERAPIST:** So in some ways that's the age you're reexperiencing right now. Somewhat under 16.[15]

36   **THERAPIST:** (continuing) So if I tell you that you look good . . .

---

[11]In the context of an antagonistic relationship, one in which the child does not feel accepted or respected, criticism interferes with the development of a sense of self-worth and creates, instead, a sense of shame. The therapist's authentic respect and involvement in the therapeutic relationship allow Ellin, in his presence, to temporarily set aside her feelings of physical wrongness, even though the rest of the time Mother's criticisms continue to distort her sense of self. (See chapter 3, p. 44; chapter 4, p. 66; chapter 10, p. 197)

[12]The therapist's matter-of-fact reference to Ellin's figure is worlds away from her father's sexual suggestions; Ellin is being given an experience that runs directly counter to the experiences with Father on which her script beliefs and decisions are based. The therapist's question is designed not only to elicit information (useful to both Ellin and the therapist) but also to ensure that Ellin notices and remembers this new way of being in relationship. (See chapter 5, p.79)

[13]Appreciation of her physical beauty, unaccompanied by any sexual invitation or innuendo, does not fit Ellin's life script. According to her script, people will either find her unattractive or will sexualize their interactions with her. Since the therapist's comments cannot be assimilated into her pattern of script expectations, she defends against them by quickly moving on to another memory, rather than staying with the here-and-now experience. (See chapter 3, p. 44)

[14]The therapist suspects that Ellin may be not only relating what happened but actually reexperiencing it: a spontaneous (though partial) regression. His question is designed to assess that regression, as well as to give Ellin permission to continue it. (See chapter 9, p. 177)

[15]Even though Ellin's description of her volleyball experience was given in the past tense, her body language, voice tone, and vocabulary were that of a teenager. At this moment, an archaeopsychic (Child) ego state may be in charge. Developmentally attuned, the therapist recognizes the partial regression: although Ellin was experiencing the world at that moment from a Child ego state, her neopsychic (Adult) ego is still accessible and can respond to the therapist's question. The script information Ellin needs, though, will not be found in the answers of an Adult; it lives and operates in a Child ego state. Through much of the rest of this piece of work, the therapist will focus on helping Ellin to continue to access that young ego state so as to recover the emotions, cognitions, and decisions that are distorting her ability to function in the world as a creative and contactful adult. To do so, and to take advantage of the regression when it occurs, he will need to maintain a constant developmental attunement with her. (See chapter 4, p. 74; chapter 6, p. 104; chapter 9, p. 175)

37   **ELLIN:** I go back to the horrible place.[16]

38   **THERAPIST:** Do I threaten your sexual security, like Dad's sexual innuendos threatened your security? (Ellin nods a "yes.") So you're in a real double bind. (Ellin begins to sob.) Needing to be seen by us guys as not the gawky kid to laugh at, and yet needing not to be seen as a sexual object. And with boys you usually get one or the other.[17]

39   **ELLIN:** (sigh) (long pause) (sigh) You know, the, the double bind is, I expect, um, I expect to be rejected for the way that I look, and if I'm not then I reject that person.[18]

40   **ELLIN:** (continuing, after a long pause), I have this sort of image, I just became aware of it about a month ago. That, um, if anybody touches me, even a woman, like a friend or my daughter, I'm wary. I'm wary: what will other people think? It's like, you know, this worry . . .[19]

41   **THERAPIST:** What will my mother think if someone likes me?

42   **ELLIN:** No, it's like . . . touch equals sex. And they will think I'm doing something wrong . . . (sigh) It's, that's how my dad has contaminated my thoughts. You know, everything had a sexual slant, and nothing could be natural.[20]

---

[16]The partial emotional regression continues: Ellin's early experiences with Father have led her to form a script belief that admiration from a man will always lead to a sexual advance. She now plays out that expectation in her response to the therapist's compliment, going back to the "horrible place" of having to deal with father's abuse. (See chapter 8, p. 159)

[17]Reading Ellin's body language, the therapist recognizes that her sense of security with him is threatened: his compliments have triggered a transference reaction, and she is responding to him in the same way that she responded to her father's sexual innuendos. Simply acknowledging her need for relational security, giving words to the tension between wanting to be attractive, yet not wanting to be a sex object, does far more to meet the need for security than would any facile reassurances. His comment is an interpretation, but it resonates so exactly with Ellin's experience that it feels to her more like a reflection of what she is saying, a confirmation that the therapist does understand—a demonstration of his cognitive attunement. (See chapter 6, pp. 109–110; chapter 9, p. 165; chapter 10, p. 187)

[18]The constant barrage of verbal and nonverbal criticism, and the constant need to be wary of Father, constitute a severe cumulative trauma. Not only the verbal criticisms from mother, that Ellin remembers, but much earlier relational patterns as well have probably been a part of her script-forming process. Mother didn't suddenly decide, when Ellin was 13 or 14 years old, to disapprove of her; hints of that rejection must have been present throughout most of Ellin's life. Ellin's processes of implicit relational knowing organized these hints into something that made sense: "I'm not lovable." "Unlovable people get rejected." "If someone doesn't reject me, there's something wrong and I'd better keep my distance." (See chapter 3, p. 56; chapter 8, p. 159)

[19]Ellin's script belief is that she will be rejected because of her physical unattractiveness. This belief shapes her behavior: she is "wary" and rejects people who don't fit her expectations. It's easy to see how this script belief-behavior system is self-perpetuating: when people don't reject her, she treats them in such a way that they *will* reject her the next time they meet. Her wariness and expectation of rejection are thus confirmed. (See chapter 2, p. 20)

[20]What a wonderful description of an introject: "dad has contaminated my thoughts." The introjected father is present in Ellin's cognition, injecting his sexuality into all of her relationships. The defenses are softening, however, in response to the therapist's attentive and respectful inquiry. The very fact that Ellin realizes that these are Father's responses, not her own, suggests that she may be ready to dissolve the introject and rid herself of the contamination. (See chapter 2, p. 29)

43    **THERAPIST:** We need to talk to him here about that. How he contaminated you. And continues to contaminate your life.

44    **ELLIN:** (sigh) What, just talk to him?

45    **THERAPIST:** Well, listening to myself I wonder if *I* started to talk to him. Listening to my voice tone here, I suspect *I* have something to say to him.[21]

46    **ELLIN:** What are you saying?

47    **THERAPIST:** Could you hear my voice tone?

48    **ELLIN:** Yeah.

49    **THERAPIST:** What did you think of my voice tone, when I brought up talking to him?[22]

50    **ELLIN:** Well . . . angry.

51    **THERAPIST:** Yeah, I was feeling angry. And you heard the anger in my suggestion.[23]

52    **ELLIN:** I'm feeling a bit scared now. (sigh) I'm remembering the other thing I thought this morning, in bed, was that he was very, um, he was very strong. And, um, you know in some ways I wanted to rely on him. You know, like, he was, he *was* there when I was really . . . say in danger, or—you know, he was reliable in that way. And I just had this image of, um . . . (crying) what happened one time, I couldn't get home, and we lived in a very small place, with no bus route. And something went wrong that I didn't get home, and I remember telephoning, and my dad walking all this—about two miles, to meet me. And I was waiting under this tree. (cries) And I just think, "Why couldn't he be there the rest of the time?"[24]

[21]The therapist is involved, emotionally active, in this relationship. He is not sitting back in some cognitively remote place. He attends to his own emotional response, not only as he experiences it phenomenologically but also through listening to his own voice tone and body language. Here, his voice has been rather harsh, and he realizes that he has grown angry with Ellin's father—angrier, probably, than Ellin can yet allow herself to be. He shifts his focus to Ellin and how she is responding to his angry sounding voice; his choice of intervention is based both on her experience of him (as he understands it) and on his own feelings. That intervention, acknowledging his own anger and implicitly inviting Ellin to do the same, will help her to reclaim her own genuine anger, just as it helps the therapist to maintain and enhance his contact with her. (See chapter 4, p. 64; chapter 5, p. 84)

[22]One of the most important areas of inquiry is that of the therapeutic relationship itself. The therapist's question here invites Ellin to talk about how it is between them, but she doesn't hear it that way; she responds with a description of his voice rather than of what it was like for her to hear it. The therapist does not press the point; Ellin's choice of answer suggests she is not yet ready for a discussion of their relationship. (See chapter 6, p. 117)

[23]The therapist has responded emotionally and does not try to hide his emotional response from himself or from Ellin. He is providing a model of internal and external contact. More important, he is continuing to build relationship by bringing his whole self to the interaction. (See chapter 5, p. 82; chapter 6, p. 118)

[24]As Ellin allows herself to reenter the psychological world that she lived in as a young girl, she begins to experience the phenomenology of that younger person, feelings and thoughts that she successfully barricades herself against when she is in her normal, adult state. (See chapter 9, p. 173)

53    **THERAPIST:** Yeah. Say that to him, Ellin. Just look at him here (gestures toward an empty chair). "Why couldn't you be here?"[25]

54    **ELLIN:** I wanted to feel safe.[26]

55    **THERAPIST:** Yeah. Tell him.

56    **ELLIN:** (talking to the "father" chair) I didn't like the way you talked. I wanted you to listen, when I said I didn't want to hear those jokes.

57    **THERAPIST:** Keep going.[27]

58    **ELLIN:** (sigh, long pause; then, to the chair) I wanted you to be faithful to the family . . .[28]

59    **THERAPIST:** (pause) And tell him what you mean by that.

60    **ELLIN:** (to the chair) I just wanted an ordinary dad.

61    **THERAPIST:** Faithful to the family . . . (Ellin sobs) An important phrase. Not just to your mother. The *family.* (Ellin sighs deeply) Keep going, Ellin. Keep telling him about that pain inside.

62    **ELLIN:** (long pause) Yeah, it's almost like, with his behavior, like he aggravated the difficulty between me and my mom. You know, he kind of, because . . .

63    **THERAPIST:** Tell him that.[29]

64    **ELLIN:** Right. (long pause)

---

[25]Openness to one's own feelings, concern for the client's welfare, and the skillful use of therapeutic technique are all demonstrated in this single, short intervention. The therapist's initial "Yeah" is said with voice tone and feeling that clearly convey his involvement, his frustration with Ellin's father's behavior and his strong support for her beginning to demand what she needs. That involvement helps him to select and introduce a technique—empty-chair work—that will help Ellin to re-create the psychological state in which she experienced her relationship with Father in childhood: the state in which her early memories were laid down, and which may need to be reexperienced if those memories are to be brought back into awareness. Speaking "to" Father, rather than talking about him, not only supports the regression but also allows Ellin to experience in fantasy the kind of contact that was denied her in reality. (See chapter 5, p. 82; chapter 9, p. 169)

[26]Ellin goes simply and directly to the heart of her problem with father: the most basic relational need, that for security in the relationship, was not met. (See chapter 3, p. 44)

[27]"Keep going" is an inquiry, even though it is not formally a question. It is a request that Ellin explore further, expanding her internal awareness. It is completely neutral: it does not suggest what Ellin should be discovering or where her exploration should lead. This neutrality respects Ellin's ability to discover her own answers. (See chapter 6, p. 114; chapter 9, pp. 164–165)

[28]The open-ended "keep going" has yielded something new. Even though the therapist does not yet fully understand what Ellin means, he is alerted by the unexpectedness of her response and quick to follow up on it. (See chapter 6, p. 116)

[29]Ellin has not fully immersed herself in the fantasy of talking to Father; she breaks off and addresses her comment to the therapist. But talking *about* her father, to someone else, will not be as useful as interacting *with* him. To bring her back into that interaction, the therapist simply requests that she tell Father what she has just told him. (See chapter 9, p. 174)

65   **THERAPIST:** "You . . ."[30]

66   **ELLIN:** (bursts into sobs; then, to "Father") I was going to say, you made it impossible for her to like me.

67   **THERAPIST:** Mmmm. Tell him how he did that.

68   **ELLIN:** (pause) It's like even, even in her own home, she couldn't, she couldn't trust him. So we all had to be on guard. (sobs again, then looks up at the therapist)

69   **THERAPIST:** It's really hard to talk to your dad, isn't it?[31]

70   **ELLIN:** (cries again, then more calmly) I know I don't like the way he's behaving now. (looks toward the "father" chair) I don't like the way you're behaving with your new girl friend.

71   **THERAPIST:** Talk to that younger man, who was around when you were just getting into your teens.[32]

72   **ELLIN:** (long pause; then, to "Father") I know you meant well. But it was like, your comments to me were, your appreciation of me was always, with sex. Like, it seemed, it didn't seem like a father talking.[33]

73   **THERAPIST:** (also talking toward the "father" chair) Father, I want to talk to you too. She just let you off the hook, when she said she knew you meant well. It is not your well-meaningness alone that counts. It is your behavior towards her that affects her. You can mean well, and I think she said that to keep you a good guy. But she is always tense, and you've—*got—to—stop*—what you're doing! Stop the sexual innuendos! . . . Stop that screwing around behavior! Mom is critical of her, and she needs to come to you for support. (Ellin begins to cry) She needs to rely on you and relax up against you, and she can't if you keep making sexual innuendos. And she can't even tell you how terrible it is with Mom's criticism . . . Now you gotta stop it and make it safe for her to

---

[30]Although Ellin agreed to talk to Father, she found it difficult to begin again. The therapist "primes the pump," encouraging her to extend and expand on the thought that she had begun to express.

[31]The therapist responds empathically to Ellin's emotional discomfort. Rather than insisting that she continue the dialogue with Father, he reflects how hard it is for her to do so, even in fantasy. The warmth and kindness in his voice, his forward-leaning body, his facial expression, and his willingness to abandon his agenda in order to acknowledge her distress are further evidence to her that he does understand, that he is fully present and aware of her internal experience. (See chapter 5, pp. 93–94; chapter 9, p. 179)

[32]As soon as she feels heard, understood, protected, Ellin is willing to return to the empty-chair exercise. Taking advantage of her willingness to deal with Father directly, the therapist invites her to do so within a regression: through imaging and talking to her young father, Ellin will herself be pulled back to the time when her father was that age—her own early adolescence. (See chapter 9, p. 177)

[33]Children (and adults as well) often try to protect their parents, even when those parents have behaved badly. The relationship with parents is needed and must be maintained. Ellin excuses her father because he "meant well," thus preserving the image of a good daddy. In order to do so, she must deny her own knowing, her ability to be fully aware of her internal and external experience. The denial allows her to stay in relationship with him even though he has been sexually inappropriate with her. In his response, the therapist picks up on this dynamic and makes it explicit. (See chapter 3, p. 42)

come close to you. You are damaging your daughter, because now she has neither parent. . . . Now listen to her, and change!³⁴

74    **ELLIN:** No, it's too late. Too late.

75    **THERAPIST:** Tell your father that.

76    **ELLIN:** (sigh) (pause) Yeah . . .

77    **THERAPIST:** Tell him, "It's too late, Dad."

78    **ELLIN:** Yeah. It's too late.

79    **THERAPIST:** And tell him what that means.³⁵

80    **ELLIN:** (sigh; pause; then, to "Father") Yeah, it's like when I wanted to, when I was a child I needed you there. It's no use saying you love me. I know you say you love me . . .

81    **THERAPIST:** Which isn't the same as "I know you love me." "I know you say you love me."³⁶

82    **ELLIN:** Oh, yeah . . .

83    **THERAPIST:** (talking again to the chair) Father. Loving, to a child, is always in behavior. Not in abstract concepts. And this daughter of yours needs you to love her by stopping all of the sexual innuendos, (Ellin sighs loudly) and stopping the sex outside—with other people—She's begging you to be faithful to the family. (Ellin weeps) Take her seriously, Father!³⁷

84    **ELLIN:** (deep sigh) It hurts . . .

---

³⁴The therapist is attending to a number of things in this relatively long intervention. He is modeling the effective use of the empty-chair technique, showing Ellin how to make Father's presence psychologically effective. He is demonstrating his attunement to Ellin's needs: his understanding of her emotional experience, and his own emotional response to that experience. Finally, by demanding—in Ellin's presence—that Father behave appropriately, he is allowing Ellin to at last be in relationship with a strong, protective, trustworthy man. Since such a relationship is not possible in the context of Ellin's script system, the experience constitutes a strong challenge to that script. (See chapter 6, pp. 99–100)

³⁵"It's too late" is almost a sign-off statement: "It's too late, so I won't talk to you about it." The therapist's intervention encourages Ellin to stay in contact with Father rather than withdrawing. Equally important, it is a form of phenomenological inquiry: "what is happening, inside you, as you say those words?"

³⁶One's sense of self is shaped by the experience of loving and being loved. But the love Father offered was not love at all but, rather, a way of using Ellin for his own gratification. Ellin collaborated with Father in maintaining the illusion of his loving her, in order to preserve the needed relationship. But that illusion must be identified and reevaluated if Ellin is to regain her ability to be fully contactful with self and with others. (See chapter 3, p. 50)

³⁷The therapist has become the Child's advocate, interposing himself between Ellin and her father. He says what may be impossible for Ellin—for any child—to say to a parent who is loved and needed and simultaneously feared and disliked. The therapist senses that Ellin's relational need, as she confronts her powerful father, is to be in the presence of someone who is strong and protective: a need that her mother did not meet when Ellin was small. (See chapter 3, p. 44)

85    **THERAPIST:** (still talking to "Father") She doesn't dare get angry at you because you're all she's got . . . and she doesn't really have you, when she's so tense.

86    **ELLIN:** What's coming through my head now is, um, it is, it's important, because it's like, um, it confirms the feeling I've had all these years, like, when I was sitting on the bus with my dad, we were heading back to my dad's apartment. And my dad started to get off the bus, like, it was one stop ahead. And then he kissed me on the lips—it felt like an intrusion. It felt like that wasn't needed. I didn't want it! And it's like . . . it's like he snuck in—you know, he kind of, it's like he was pouncing. When I didn't expect it. And I don't want it.[38]

87    **THERAPIST:** (repeating Ellin's words) "I don't want it. I *don't* want it." Try those words again.

88    **ELLIN:** (bursts into loud crying)

89    **THERAPIST:** (to "Father") Father, listen to her. She said "I don't want it." "I don't want it," she said, Father. Now listen to her, and respect that. (pause) And she still wants you.[39]

90    **ELLIN:** (to "Father") I want to be able to be close. (cries loudly again)

91    **THERAPIST:** "I want . . ."

92    **ELLIN:** (to "Father") I want to feel just safe . . . I want to feel loved without being frightened.

93    **THERAPIST:** "And what I want you to do is . . ."

94    **ELLIN:** Oh, yeah . . . (to "Father") I want you to keep the boundary. (cries)

95    **THERAPIST:** "So that . . . (pause) You keep the boundary, Father, so that . . ." (long pause) Say it, Ellin.

96    **ELLIN:** I don't know!

97    **THERAPIST:** "So that I don't have to." See if those words fit your experience. "You keep the boundary, Father, so that I don't have to. Just try it out, see if those words fit your experience. If not, change them.[40]

---

[38]We have no way of knowing whether Father's sexual advances went beyond what Ellin is reporting here—nor does she. Her relationship with her father is a classic example of a situation in which repression of trauma is likely to occur: knowledge of the trauma would damage her relationship with both parents, relationships that are, in spite of everything, still very important to her. If some traumatic memory has been repressed, it may reemerge spontaneously as the work progresses. There is no need for the therapist to probe for it; Ellin can continue her work on the basis of what she does know about Father's behavior. (See chapter 2, p. 26)

[39]Closely attuned to Ellin's process, the therapist is able to put into words the two polarities that represent Ellin's pain around her relationship with her father: she doesn't want his sexuality, but she does want him. (See chapter 6, p. 98)

[40]Attuned to what Ellin herself cannot yet articulate, the therapist suggests an experiment. His suggestion is an interpretation—it goes beyond what Ellin has put into words—but it is qualified by an invitation to see if it fits her experience. If it doesn't fit, if the interpretation was off the mark, she is free to change it. Either way, she is supported in deepening her awareness of her long-unexpressed needs and wants. (See chapter 9, p. 170)

⁹⁸  **ELLIN:** (still to "Father") It's like, I want you to see it from my point of view.⁴¹

⁹⁹  **THERAPIST:** Tell him what would happen, Ellin, if *he* would take the responsibility for keeping the boundaries. What would be different for that teenage girl, if he was the responsible one for keeping the boundaries?⁴²

¹⁰⁰  **ELLIN:** Then it would have been safe to be attractive.

¹⁰¹  **THERAPIST:** Keep going.

¹⁰²  **ELLIN:** (cries softly)

¹⁰³  **THERAPIST:** Safe to be attractive . . . (pause) but there's even more . . .⁴³

¹⁰⁴  **ELLIN:** (long pause) And then I wouldn't have needed to be the enemy. For my mom.⁴⁴

¹⁰⁵  **THERAPIST:** Ummm. You lost both parents. (Ellin sighs deeply) You lost all security.⁴⁵

¹⁰⁶  **ELLIN:** I remember them calling me a, a shrew. And a school-marm. All those years . . . I remember sweating and stinking, just being so uncomfortable . . . I just felt wrong, in everything.⁴⁶

¹⁰⁷  **THERAPIST:** They didn't help you be beautiful, to let your own beauty come forward? Did they help you be beautiful?

¹⁰⁸  **ELLIN:** No. It was like, for my mom it was like I needed, I needed false, I needed, you know, like I couldn't do it; I had to have bras with false, additions, you know. To try and compensate.

---

⁴¹While her longing for father's understanding is not new—Ellin has felt it for as long as she can remember—she has never before conceptualized it in quite this way. Enactment of an interaction with Father, this time with the therapist's support and with the skills and life experience of an adult, has allowed her to frame her feelings in a new way, a way that may allow her to go even more deeply into the pain of the old need-not-met. (See chapter 9, pp. 169–170)

⁴²This is an inquiry about Ellin's fantasy of what could have been. Her response will help her to reconnect with the fears and dreams of the young girl who so badly needed an appropriately loving father. (See chapter 6, p. 117)

⁴³The pauses here and in Ellin's response reflect the therapist's rhythmic attunement to Ellin's pace and tempo. She needs to stop, cry, experience the feelings that have been hidden away for so long. The therapist speaks gently, softly, slowly, allowing her time to explore her internal experience while at the same time encouraging her to go even farther. (See chapter 6, p. 107)

⁴⁴With Mother, too, the relational need for security was not met. How can you feel safe with someone who regards you as the enemy? Moreover, Mother did not meet Ellin's need for acceptance and validation in relationship. Yet the relationship with Mother was still needed, and Ellin had to find a way to protect herself without destroying that relationship. One way in which she does this is by introjecting Mother's perception of her; she has come to experience herself as unattractive, too tall, and masculine-looking. (See chapter 2, p. 28; chapter 3, p. 44)

⁴⁵This is more than a reflection, different from an interpretation. The therapist's voice tone is perhaps more important than his actual words; it is deeply compassionate. He enfolds Ellin in his concern and caring, much as a parent would respond to his child's pain. (See chapter 10, p. 185)

⁴⁶One of the indications of the presence of an introject is self-criticism: "I just felt wrong in everything." Ellin's self-critical inner dialogue probably involves an introject of Mother, whom Ellin has reported as being a constant critic. (See chapter 2, p. 30)

109    **THERAPIST:** (somewhat incredulous) As a teenager?

110    **ELLIN:** Yeah. (pause) It was like the message was like, um, "you're just so unattractive, it's unbelievable." (cries)

111    **THERAPIST:** That hurts so much . . . (pause) In some ways having your dad appreciate how you looked might have felt nice, if you didn't have to be scared. If *he* would have been responsible for maintaining appropriate boundaries.

112    **ELLIN:** I remember, I just remembered something. When I went to school, and I was walking—see, this was another mistake that they didn't realize; they, they sent me to this school that was, like, two miles away. When I was 5—I had to walk there on my own. And I used to get so scared, walking past these woods. And um, one time I was walking up this street. A guy pulled up in a car and exposed himself. And, uh (her voice sounds frightened), I remember—I remember (crying) thinking "I can run into these houses if he follows me." And I remember when I got home (crying again) I didn't tell my mom. I told my aunt, who was visiting, cause I didn't think mom would be there. I didn't think she would support me.[47]

113    **THERAPIST:** What did you imagine Mother would do?

114    **ELLIN:** (loud sigh) Uhhh, she would twist it somehow. (breathing heavily)

115    **THERAPIST:** Would Mother criticize you, in that twist? Would she make it your fault?

116    **ELLIN:** Ohhhh . . . just that she wouldn't sympathize . . . I didn't trust her to . . . it's like the message has always been, "Oh, you can cope. You don't need support."

117    **THERAPIST:** She was wrong.[48]

118    **ELLIN:** (pause) You don't need affection. You're just like your dad. (crying)

119    **THERAPIST:** What's that mean, "you're just like your dad"?

---

[47]This passage exemplifies a number of developmental principles. First, it is an example of how social learnings give meaning to the events of our lives. To an infant or young child, the sight of a man's genitals is not threatening; the child may be curious, but hardly frightened. Ellin has learned from others (parents, siblings, schoolmates, books, or television) that when someone exposes himself he is dangerous. Moreover, she has learned not to expect protection from her mother, protection that she needs in order to develop effective strategies for dealing with her fears. The fearful experience remains in her memory as an effective "hot spot," capable of triggering the same sense of fear and pain now as it did when she was a schoolchild. Finally, the intensity of her current feelings about the event clearly indicate that it constituted trauma—and the trauma lay not so much in seeing a man exposing himself as in the absence of support and comfort from mother. (See chapter 2, p. 18; chapter 3, pp. 51–52).

[48]Much of Ellin's story reflects an intense need for support and acceptance, and the therapist chooses to respond to that need. He will be a strong, dependable, caring other (like Ellin's aunt) who can be counted on to understand and value this young girl, even—especially—when her parents do not meet that need. (See chapter 3, p. 44)

120   **ELLIN:** I'm cold. And I don't like hugs.[49]

121   **THERAPIST:** That's wrong. I imagine that you like the right kind of hug . . . one that's genuine, and just for you. Right?

122   **ELLIN:** You know, you remember when I first called and asked if you had any openings, and when you said yes, I said that I wanted to work with you and you said Okay—you know, I didn't want to get my hopes up and then be disappointed, and you said "I won't let that happen." I just (crying) . . . you were there for me. . . .

123   **THERAPIST:** Mmmm. Someone you could really depend on.[50]

124   **ELLIN:** With them, it's like I had to do it on my own.

125   **THERAPIST:** Well, the feeling I get, Ellin, with you is that you were so beaten down by this, that your self-esteem is so shattered by this—

126   **ELLIN:** (sobs; gestures toward floor) It's down there!

127   **THERAPIST:** Yeah. So far down that you can't even stand up for yourself.

128   **ELLIN:** I do. I do stand up, but I do it aggressively.

129   **THERAPIST:** That's sort of like holding your breath. Bet you don't stay aggressive, do you? You burst something out, and then you shut up again.[51]

130   **ELLIN:** Uh-huh . . .

131   **THERAPIST:** It's even hard to face your dad and talk to him. Did you notice that here? You kept talking *about* him. . . . How was it for you when *I* talked to him? I was aggressive.

132   **ELLIN:** I just felt the damage has been done. It's like, I couldn't undo it. (sigh) I needed it then.

---

[49]Ellin's early expressions of affection were met with criticism by Mother and by inappropriately sexualized responses from Dad. No wonder she sent her affectionate feelings underground: the consistent message to her was that such feelings were either inappropriate or dangerous. Over the years, her ability to behave affectionately was repressed again and again until it became split-off, no longer available to her. She experienced herself as "cold," and probably was experienced that way by others as well. (See chapter 3, p. 50)

[50]All her life, Ellin has longed for this kind of compassion and protection; finally, with the therapist, she is experiencing such a relationship. She needs to express her appreciation, her sense of connectedness with the therapist. He has been there for her; now she wants to tell him how meaningful that was. The therapist doesn't shrug off or minimize what she says, nor does he treat it as a manifestation of transference; he simply reflects what was important to her and accepts her gratitude. (See chapter 6, pp. 110–111; 113–114; chapter 8, p. 150)

[51]The therapist is commenting on Ellin's script-bound behavior, her substitution of withdrawal for anger. This substitution serves all the functions in the PICS acronym: it keeps life *predictable* (she knows what to expect from people when she shuts down and withdraws); it preserves her *identity* (as a person who doesn't get angry); it provides *continuity* (she acts, and is seen as acting, in pretty much the same way from day to day, and others therefore treat her in the same way); and *stability* (to behave differently would make her feel uncomfortable, frightened, maybe even out of control). She will need a great deal of support and encouragement from the therapist if she is to break through the old response pattern. (See chapter 2, pp. 21–22)

133    **THERAPIST:** Yes, you did.

134    **ELLIN:** (pause) But I want to take something away so I don't go on doing it. You know, as an adult, I don't spoil my relationships . . .

135    **THERAPIST:** "So I don't go on doing *it*"? What's the *it?*

136    **ELLIN:** Sense of, um, dread, really.

137    **THERAPIST:** Have you ever gotten angry with your father?

138    **ELLIN:** Um . . . (pause) I remember getting angry with him, in a therapy session when I was working with Dr. Johnson.

139    **THERAPIST:** How was that?

140    **ELLIN:** Well, it was angry. (laughs) Yeah. But it wasn't angry about me. It was angry about the way he was treating my brother.[52]

141    **THERAPIST:** I mean angry about you.

142    **ELLIN:** No, I haven't done that.

143    **THERAPIST:** It seems to me like that's what might give you some of your self back. That you're not just subject to his damage. That you can retrieve yourself from this. But not alone. With my support.[53]

144    **ELLIN:** Yeah, I could do that.

145    **THERAPIST:** So how about talking to him directly about how he damaged you, and what you feel about that.

146    **ELLIN:** What I'm thinking now is it, it . . . it wasn't anything big.

147    **THERAPIST:** (loudly) It *was* big! (more calmly) Look how it's affected you. That's big![54]

148    **ELLIN:** (sighs)

---

[52]Ellin has felt sad about her relationship with Father and has been frustrated by his unwillingness to change. Her deep desire to maintain the possibility of a better relationship, though, has led her to close off awareness of how angry she has been at his inappropriate behavior. She literally cannot feel her own anger (and her laugh is a way of defending herself against becoming aware of it), so it is no wonder that she cannot express it. (See chapter 8, p. 146)

[53]This is an interpretation in the form of a suggestion of how to proceed: almost, but not quite, a directive. The therapist is saying that Ellin needs to experience being angry with Father on her own behalf, to use that anger to protect herself and to learn that she does not have to be a frightened victim. Again, the interpretation follows so smoothly from Ellin's own discoveries that there is no break in Ellin's process, no sense that she has been interrupted and set upon another path. (See chapter 9, p. 167)

[54]The therapist, in this initial comment, allows his own strong feelings to emerge. His response is almost an outburst, a spontaneous expression of indignation and outrage. As such, it not only validates her experience, and its long-term significance, but it also demonstrates his involvement, letting Ellin know that she has made an impact on him and thus meeting another of the primary relational needs. (See chapter 3, p. 45; chapter 6, pp. 112–113)

149   **THERAPIST:** What an important desire you have, to protect him like that. To protect him from all criticism. And you do want me to know that he's not a totally bad man.[55]

150   **ELLIN:** He's not.

151   **THERAPIST:** That you still love him and feel loyal to him, even with what he's done. And that he still loves you. He's still your dad, and he's still there in important ways sometimes.

152   **ELLIN:** Yeah. That's the part that—I don't want to have a sort of, um, well, I don't want to have a barrier between me and him if it's not needed.

153   **THERAPIST:** Great. This is about having what you want with him in the way of relationship. Not about getting rid of him.

154   **ELLIN:** Yeah. I don't want to do that. (Her voice breaks) I *really* don't . . .[56]

155   **THERAPIST:** Okay. I've got the message. I'm not going to trash your dad. (pause) Now, talk to him.[57]

156   **ELLIN:** (gusty sigh, then turns again toward the empty chair) Oh, I do want you to be different.

157   **THERAPIST:** Keep going. "I want you to be different, Dad . . ."

158   **ELLIN:** (to "Father") I want you to reform. It's like, kind of like, I want you to get rid of those thoughts.

159   **THERAPIST:** (pause) Um-hm. Keep going.

160   **ELLIN:** (to "Father") It's like, we went all the way to the West Coast so that it would be safe to come back, but it wasn't. So you let my mum down. And I was seven then, and from then on it was still bad. And it could have been a new beginning. You could have, (sigh) you could have committed yourself to . . . (sigh) to being moral.

---

[55]Ellin minimizes the damage done to her by her father's behavior, and the minimizing is part of what keeps her fragmented, within herself and in her relationships with others. Minimizing her own feelings is not helpful to her, not something that the therapist wants to encourage. Yet it has an important function: it protects Father, and thus sustains the illusion/possibility of a warm and supportive relationship with him. The therapist, in validating and valuing the function of the behavior, expresses his involvement and attunement without supporting the behavior itself. (See chapter 6, p. 120)

[56]As we have seen, Ellin still clings to the possibility (the illusion?) of a relationship with her father. What she had with him was painful, but it was nevertheless important. Even painful relationships are still relationships, still meet our need to be in contact with others. The therapist will need to allow Ellin to express *all* of her feelings toward her father—not just the anger—so that she does not experience herself as destroying the connection entirely. (See chapter 3, p. 42)

[57]Ellin's fear of losing her father has threatened to overwhelm her. Rather than inviting her to explore that fear (which could be too much for her to deal with right now, and could cause her to throw up her old defenses again) the therapist is calm and matter-of-fact as he states his own intentions. He lets Ellin know that he heard and understood how important Father is, and that he will not try to take that relationship away from her. He does so at a pace, and with a tone, that also conveys his own calm, his own comfort that the work is moving along as it should. (See chapter 8, p. 148)

161    **THERAPIST:** Um-hm. That says a lot. Go ahead, Ellin. "You could have . . ."

162    **ELLIN:** (to "Father") If only I could have respected you!

163    **THERAPIST:** Here comes the harder part. You ready? (Ellin cries) "I'm angry with you, Dad . . ."[58]

164    **ELLIN:** (to "Father") I'm angry with you for letting me down . . .

165    **THERAPIST:** Yes! (pause) Keep going. "And I'm angry . . ."

166    **ELLIN:** (to "Father") Angry at you . . . always slipping that sexual thing into every relationship.

167    **THERAPIST:** "I'm angry!"

168    **ELLIN:** (to "Father") I'm angry for having been on guard for so long! I'm tired! I don't want to be on guard any more! (sobs)

169    **THERAPIST:** Right! . . . (loudly) "I'm angry!"[59]

170    **ELLIN:** (slightly louder, to "Father") I'm angry at your behavior. At the way you think. The way you speak.

171    **THERAPIST:** "I'm angry that you didn't take care of *me!*"

172    **ELLIN:** (to "Father") I'm angry that you didn't listen.

173    **THERAPIST:** Yeah. You didn't listen to me, and you didn't listen to my mom. Keep going: "I'm angry that . . . I'm angry . . ."

174    **ELLIN:** (more softly) Just thinking when I was little . . . I worshiped him . . .[60]

175    **THERAPIST:** Keep talking to him. "I worshiped you, Dad . . ." (Ellin sighs several times) "And you corrupted that."

176    **ELLIN:** Yeah . . . (softly, to "Father") You corrupted . . . my love.

---

[58]The therapist is helping Ellin to access feelings that will be painful and hard to bear, and Ellin's anxiety level is rising again. Yet, even though she is very uncomfortable, she continues to follow his direction. She understands what he is doing and trusts that he will not let her get lost in her feelings. (See chapter 8, p. 149)

[59]The therapist is not neutral here, nor even simply supporting what Ellin is doing. He is a part of the dialogue, letting his own emotion show as he, too, expresses his anger toward Father even as he is speaking for Ellin. He models the free access to feelings that Ellin needs to achieve, and in so doing he gives both permission for and impetus to Ellin's own emerging anger. (See chapter 6, p. 118; chapter 9, p. 171)

[60]Although impossible to convey in a written transcript, the above several exchanges involve a great deal of rhythmic attunement on the part of the therapist. As Ellin begins to allow herself to feel her frustration and anger toward her father, her rhythmic pattern changes: she speaks more quickly, without long pauses between sentences. The therapist picks up on this shifting pattern and responds quickly as well, not allowing pauses between her statements and his that could break the rhythm. Voicing, and even exaggerating, her rhythm and voice tone, helps Ellin to maintain the regression and access the forbidden feelings. Eventually, however, her need for a good daddy, her need to keep Father in that role, overcomes her anger; she returns, sadly, to her longing for Father's uncontaminated support and approval. (See chapter 6, p. 106)

177   **THERAPIST:** Um-hm. . . . Keep going, Ellin . . . Tell him . . . about protecting his children.[61]

178   **ELLIN:** Yeah . . . He, he could have protected me. (turning to "Father") And instead, I felt you, uh, abusing me.

179   **THERAPIST:** More concerned about himself . . .

180   **ELLIN:** You don't know how right that is. That is him. (to "Father") Always concerned about what suited you.[62]

181   **THERAPIST:** "And I feel . . ."

182   **ELLIN:** I feel damaged. . . . That, that's just another thought that I had in bed this morning. I thought, when we went to a restaurant, there were five of us round the table. We'd be looking at the menu. Before we'd finished ordering, he would say, "Five of the so-and-so's please." What he'd decided to have.

183   **THERAPIST:** Regardless of what *you* wanted.

184   **ELLIN:** He still does that. If I'm at a restaurant, and I say "I like white wine," he will order red.

185   **THERAPIST:** Tell *him* about that, Ellin. "You—don't listen! You don't care!

186   **ELLIN:** You don't care. You're just thinking about yourself and your own needs.

187   **THERAPIST:** Now keep—let your energy get higher, Ellin. So that he can feel the impact of you. Let him hear you! Let him feel you![63]

188   **ELLIN:** (a bit louder) I want—my—needs—to count.

189   **THERAPIST:** Yes! Now louder. (shouting) "Listen to me!"

190   **ELLIN:** (sigh) Listen to my therapist![64]

---

[61]Ellin's rhythm has shifted again; she now speaks more slowly, reflectively. The therapist shifts with her, softening his voice and pausing between phrases, just as Ellin is doing. (See chapter 6, p. 106)

[62]At this point, it is as if we are observing family therapy: Father's presence is almost palpable, and there is no sense of strangeness in either Ellin's or the therapist's addressing the empty chair. Each of them moves easily between talking to each other and talking to "Father." Creating this situation in fantasy gives the added advantage of a "Father" who does not fight back, does not defend himself in the familiar ways that might have propelled Ellin back into her old script behaviors. She is free to deal with him in a new way and experience her strength and wholeness in doing so. (See chapter 9, p. 170).

[63]Much of the work with the image of Father involves behavioral interventions, inviting Ellin to experiment with new behaviors and to discover what those new behaviors lead to. Encouraging Ellin to increase the intensity of her demands will help her to experience the depth of her feelings, the anger and frustration that she has kept locked away. The therapist frames his urging as a way to let Father hear and feel Ellin's anger, but the primary therapeutic purpose is to bring to awareness the parts of herself—her feelings, belief, and decisions—that have been hidden away since early childhood. (See chapter 9, pp. 171–172)

[64]Ellin tried, but she couldn't bring herself to be fully open to her father about her anger—and was probably unable to be fully open with herself either. Her response is a slip-of-the-ear; perhaps she misunderstood the focus of the therapist's last three words. Such slips are often an expression of an unconscious need—does she want the therapist to speak for her? She cannot ask more directly, because she also needs the therapist to offer on his own, rather than simply acquiesce to her request. She needs him to be her voice, and she also needs him to step in, take over, so that she can feel protected. The two primary relational needs at this moment are that the therapist be strong and protective and also initiate what comes next—and he does. (See chapter 6, pp. 110–111; 113)

191   **THERAPIST:** Hm . . . that's what I said before. I guess I do want to talk to him. Is that okay?

192   **ELLIN:** I wish you would.

193   **THERAPIST:** (shouting) Listen to your daughter! She's got things to say. What she thinks and what she feels matters. Not just you. And not just your satisfaction.[65]

194   **ELLIN:** That makes sense, "not just your satisfaction." That's like my whole childhood. I want to feel protected. What I had to do as a child is think round corners. I had to . . . I wanted to protect myself from the jokes, cause I didn't want to be sexualized by them.

195   **THERAPIST:** Yes! (to "Father") Keep *your* satisfaction and *your* sexual needs private and in *your* bedroom! It doesn't belong in the living room, and it doesn't belong in the dining room, and it doesn't belong in the kitchen.

196   **ELLIN:** That's right. I remember a secretary coming to our house. I must have been about 14 . . . and I remember her tidying herself up, cause my dad hadn't come back from work, and I remember her putting on lipstick, making her hair look nice . . . (cries) I just realized that she's another one that he . . . (cries hard) And it was in my house . . . It's like, I always had to be on guard . . . (cries)[66]

197   **THERAPIST:** (to "Father") Keep your sexual contacts out of her space. You don't bring your secretaries that you've had sex with into your house, where she has to encounter it! It's too confusing!

198   **ELLIN:** Ahhhhhhh. . . .

199   **THERAPIST:** So that she can be beautiful because she's beautiful, not for your pleasure!

200   **ELLIN:** Ahhh! (cries) Ahhh . . .

201   **THERAPIST:** Not so that you can wonder what she's like! But because *she's* beautiful! For *her*self![67]

202   **ELLIN:** It's like nobody was safe. Like everybody, everybody had been contaminated.

---

[65]This is more than simply mirroring, or even exaggerating, Ellin's feelings. The therapist's words, voice tone, and body language convey his own emotions, his genuine indignation and outrage at what Ellin's father has done. The therapist is not sitting back and reflecting what Ellin experiences; he is fully present and involved in the interaction. The intensity of his commands may have an impact on Ellin's introjected father—the aspects of her father that she has taken into herself and that continue to contaminate her thinking—and it also continues to provide her with the experience of a strong and protective relationship. (See chapter 2, p. 28; chapter 4, p. 69; chapter 6, p. 118).

[66]Until this moment, Ellin had been able to keep herself from conscious awareness that her father was having an affair with this secretary. All of the pieces were there—she hasn't learned any new facts during this therapy session—but she kept those pieces unconnected, frozen, unassimilated. Now, with the therapist's support, the pieces are beginning to come together, and along with those connections come the painful feelings that have been festering away for so many years. (See chapter 8, p. 154)

[67]As the therapist joins Ellin in her demands, he expresses his own anger resonating with hers. Ellin does not have to deal with Father alone; she has a powerful ally who feels much as she does. With the experience of support and of being emotionally joined, she is able to take the next step in discovering her blocked off memories. (See chapter 4, p. 72)

203    **THERAPIST:** Right. It's too confusing! And so it's hard to be a woman and enjoy your own beauty in the midst of all that.[68]

204    **ELLIN:** I couldn't.

205    **THERAPIST:** No! (to "Father") And *you*, Father, were responsible for keeping that safe for her!

206    **ELLIN:** But even my aunt . . .

207    **THERAPIST:** (still to "Father") Even her aunt, whom she so much loves and trusts . . . (Ellin cries hard) Even that was contaminated! And when she's angry with you about it, you listen to her! (Ellin cries more loudly) You have corrupted her life, and she has to tell you about it! Cause that's how she can know herself: as she hears herself tell you!

208    **ELLIN:** Ohhhh! Ohhhhhh! I wanted to feel safe! (sobbing loudly)

209    **THERAPIST:** (to "Father") She needed you in order to feel safe with her mother! To make sense out of her mother! And when you go and get screwy on her, where does she go? . . . She needs you! And she needs you to be strong, and she needs you to be safe! And she needs you to be a father. (pause, then to Ellin) Now you use your words with him. Your words. Your energy.

210    **ELLIN:** (to "Father") Ohhh, I wanted to feel safe!

211    **THERAPIST:** Yes. Again. Scream it at him![69]

212    **ELLIN:** (more quietly, still to "Father") Oh, I wanted to feel safe, to be close . . . I can't get close, cause it's not safe . . . I don't want you to die without me feeling safe!

213    **THERAPIST:** Yes.

214    **ELLIN:** And close.

215    **THERAPIST:** Um-hm.

216    **ELLIN:** He should have protected me. I shouldn't have needed to be on guard. (sigh)

217    **THERAPIST:** (pause) Is there more you need to say to him?[70]

218    **ELLIN:** I'm just trying to remember something . . . I don't know, but I think it must have been a dream. . . . It's all it was like . . . just contaminated everything.

---

[68]By inference, the therapist is saying that anyone would have been confused in Ellin's situation, anyone would have found it difficult to feel and act like a beautiful, sexual woman. He is normalizing Ellin's behavior—one of the elements of therapeutic involvement. (See chapter 6, pp. 120–121)

[69]The therapist is encouraging Ellin to increase the intensity of her demands: as one's intensity increases, one is able to access more and more of the buried emotion of past experiences. Ellin needs to recover that experience so that she can deal with it in awareness rather than having it fester underground and contaminate her ways of being with people in the present. (See chapter 9, pp. 171–172)

[70]Recognizing that Ellin has spontaneously emerged from the regression (she has partly done so several times already, but this time she seems more completely in the present, speaking as an Adult ego), the therapist acknowledges the shift. The end of the session is approaching, and it would be helpful for Ellin to reach some sort of closure before she leaves. (See chapter 9, pp. 179, 180)

219   **THERAPIST:** Yes. What else . . .

220   **ELLIN:** It's like . . . I've always had to be, I felt I've always had to be on guard. (sigh)

221   **THERAPIST:** Okay. We have just a little time left. May I take you one step further? (Ellin nods) Will you look at me? (Ellin cries) And say, "I need to feel safe with you."[71]

222   **ELLIN:** That feels scary . . .[72]

223   **THERAPIST:** Um-hm.

224   **ELLIN:** I'm just aware of you. And that feels good.[73] (Long pause; Ellin's head is down. Then she bursts into loud tears) Keep me safe!

225   **THERAPIST:** I will.

226   **ELLIN:** You didn't! No! (crying hard)

227   **THERAPIST:** What did I do, Ellin?

228   **ELLIN:** Ohhhh. . . . (gradually calms)

229   **THERAPIST:** What did I do, Ellin? Or what did I not do?[74]

---

[71]The therapist sees an opportunity to deal with what is happening between himself and Ellin: to use their ongoing process as a kind of laboratory, in which Ellin can learn more about how she keeps herself out of contact with others and how much she wants to have a different sort of relationship. There are two inquiries in his intervention: the first requests Ellin's permission to proceed (a kind of mini-contract), and the second, in the form of a directive, invites Ellin to explore her feelings about him. Note, too, that the therapist uses this transition as a time to remind Ellin that the session will soon end: part of his trustworthiness lies in his commitment to keep her safe, and part of safety is not being caught unaware by the end of their time together. (See chapter 6, pp. 114–115; chapter 11, p. 206)

[72]Ellin's feelings toward the therapist are mixed with her feelings (current and past) toward her father. Both Father and therapist are strong; both are important to her; she would not want to damage either relationship. Telling the therapist "I need to feel safe with you" is scary partly because it would have been scary—perhaps even dangerous—to make that statement to Father, but it is also frightening to risk her current relationship with the therapist by suggesting that she might not feel safe with him. This is the essence of transference: feelings and responses experienced toward significant people in the past are transferred onto and combined with current feelings in current relationships. Behaving in this new and contactful way with the therapist—expressing her needs clearly and strongly—is a way to practice a new behavior that she needs to carry out into her out-of-therapy world. (See chapter 4, p. 67; chapter 10, p. 187; chapter 11, p. 219)

[73]Ellin and the therapist have been searching deeply into experiences that Ellin has kept buried away for a long time. In doing so, Ellin has experienced a sense of genuine contact. She has let her barriers down and has remained safe. And it feels good. But, even in the feeling good, another piece is about to emerge. (See chapter 4, p. 71)

[74]In this response, and in the preceding one, the therapist mistakenly believes that Ellin's sudden and intense need for relational safety has to do with what is happening here, in the therapy session: that he has missed something and has created a break in the contact between them. Rather than asking first about her feelings (which would subtly shift the responsibility back to her), he immediately owns his therapeutic responsibility and asks her to tell him where he went wrong. What he does not realize is that Ellin has again regressed, and is reexperiencing the need for protection from her mother. When he does understand what is happening, the therapist moves to support her demands: confronting Mother's lack of protection is a new behavior, inconsistent with Ellin's script beliefs and decisions, and may lead to dissolving some of those old restrictions. (See chapter 5, p. 81; chapter 10, p.193)

230  **ELLIN:** (frantically) I don't know, you didn't, you didn't keep me safe! . . . Can't remember . . . (breathing very hard)[75]

231  **THERAPIST:** It's Mother you're talking to now, huh? (Ellin nods) Keep telling Mom. Say that again to Mom. "You didn't keep me safe, Mom." . . . (pause) Keep talking to Mama. "You didn't keep me safe."

232  **ELLIN:** (breathes hard for several seconds, then cries)

233  **THERAPIST:** Let it come, Ellin. Say the words. It's all right.

234  **ELLIN:** Ohhh. . . . There's something missing. It's like, it's like, uh, I felt she was jealous for a reason . . .[76]

235  **THERAPIST:** (pause) She knew about your father. . . . And she knew that you might be . . .

236  **ELLIN:** It's like she didn't, she didn't keep me safe . . . I couldn't relax.

237  **THERAPIST:** She didn't talk to you about it. She didn't say, "These are some things you can do." And most of all, by talking about it, to say "You can talk with me, because I know."

238  **ELLIN:** I couldn't talk to her.

239  **THERAPIST:** She just got angry at you. As though you were the problem.

240  **ELLIN:** Yeah . . . (pause) That was, I was dreaming about it. I couldn't tell her, because she would be angry. She was the last person I could tell.

241  **THERAPIST:** And you needed to be able to tell her.

242  **ELLIN:** (crying) I think that's, why I, it's like . . .

243  **THERAPIST:** Even the man who exposed himself . . .

244  **ELLIN:** (sobs loudly) I couldn't tellllll. . . .

245  **THERAPIST:** Like you were somehow responsible?

246  **ELLIN:** Yeah!

247  **THERAPIST:** For a pervert?

248  **ELLIN:** Yeah!

---

[75]This is hard, frightening work for Ellin, and her body language shows how frightened she feels. The crux of her problems with Mother was not only Mother's criticism, but also Mother's lack of protection—and this was the part she could not let herself know about. Had she allowed herself to recognize what she needed from Mother, she would also have had to be aware of how unsafe she felt with Father. And that lack of safety (along with her anger) had to be kept out of awareness in order to hold onto some semblance of relationship with him. Her resistance is an automatic self-protective reaction: her heightened affect and frantic speech allow her to be confused, to not know, using fear to avoid the pain. She knows that she needs to open this dark area and look inside—but she still doesn't want to do it. (See chapter 8, pp. 146, 150)

[76]Another hint that Father's behavior may have gone beyond the things that Ellin has been describing. Again, though, the therapist does not press for details. If there was more, and when she is ready to talk about it, Ellin will do so. In the meantime, the therapist follows her lead. (See chapter 2, p. 25)

249    **THERAPIST:** At 5 years old?[77]

250    **ELLIN:** It would be turned against me.

251    **THERAPIST:** So say that to your mother. "I need *you* . . ."

252    **ELLIN:** To protect me.

253    **THERAPIST:** Um-hm!

254    **ELLIN:** To be there for me.

255    **THERAPIST:** Um-hm!

256    **ELLIN:** It's like, I'm slipping away now. It's, I'm remembering . . . I don't know if I dreamed it. It's like, I don't have the protection. Wasn't safe . . . Something I saw on TV triggered something off for me that . . . I had to do it all on my own. Um . . . that's what I've been dreaming about all night.[78]

257    **THERAPIST:** Tell me the dream.

258    **ELLIN:** I couldn't go for help. Because if I did it was, it was me that caused it. My mother would have blamed me (crying). (pause) I had to be on guard against them both. Against her accusations as well. It's like it's all mashed around in my head.

259    **THERAPIST:** Yes.

260    **ELLIN:** That's . . . cause I was bad.

261    **THERAPIST:** (turning back to the chair, that now stands for "Mother") No, Mother. She was not bad. You were the one who felt unwanted and unloved. It's your feelings of being unwanted and unloved that are the problem. And you experienced that when you were growing up, you experience it with your husband, and you imagine it with your daughter, although it's not true.[79]

---

[77]In these last two comments (and earlier, as well), the therapist's voice tone expresses his indignation. He is not merely reflecting Ellin's story—he is resonating to her pain and feeling fiercely protective of her. He will not try to take the pain away—Ellin needs to deal with it herself, and the therapist recognizes that—but he wishes he could, wishes it had never happened, is angry at Ellin's mother for her treatment of Ellin. His involvement gives Ellin the courage she needs to go even farther into her painful memories. (See chapter 8, p.147)

[78]A report of "slipping away," especially from someone who has been articulate and willing to explore unknown areas, is often a signal of heightened resistance. Long-buried thoughts and feelings are being stirred, broken connections are being remade, and Ellin's script system is under siege. Closing down, becoming confused, not communicating—these are the last-ditch strategies of a defensive system that can no longer contain repressed memories and ideas. Ellin's dream was likely a preview of her work today, rising out of her knowledge that she would be seeing the therapist and would be moving into frightening material; repressed ideas and feelings often emerge in dreams, when the mechanisms of defense relax their vigilance. Now, those mechanisms are snapping back into place, but at a more primitive level. (See chapter 8, p. 152)

[79]The therapist recognizes Ellin's "I was bad" as a child's response to Ellin's introjected critical mother. This child cannot defend herself, can only accept Mother's toxic criticisms and apologize. To forestall Ellin's retraumatization and a reinforcement of her script system, the therapist speaks for her, confronting Mother's displacement of her own pain onto Ellin. In doing so, he also meets Ellin's relational need for other-initiation (which she never got from Mother) and for safety and acceptance from a strong and dependable other. He also (here and in his next remarks to Mother) demonstrates his continued involvement: he is not neutral but is genuinely angry with Mother on Ellin's behalf. (See chapter 3, pp. 44, 45; chapter 6, pp. 110–111, 113)

262    **ELLIN:** I was, I was a threat.

263    **THERAPIST:** (to Mother) Don't blame her! She is not the problem! If your husband isn't desiring you, it's not your daughter's fault! If your daughter doesn't nurse from you as soon as she's born, it's not her fault! It doesn't mean she doesn't love you. It means she's weak from a long birth process.

264    **ELLIN:** Yeah, it's like I was cast as the enemy. . . . . There's so many thoughts rushing through my head, I can't untangle them all . . . But it's like I, I felt I deserved her hatred.

265    **THERAPIST:** You didn't.

266    **ELLIN:** I thought I must have done something . . . but that something was all tied up with my dad. And I think that's why I had to be masculine. So I wasn't a threat.

267    **THERAPIST:** Do you think you're masculine?

268    **ELLIN:** Yeah.[80]

269    **THERAPIST:** One of the few clients I have who wears dresses for her sessions? You're beautiful! I don't see you as being masculine.[81]

270    **ELLIN:** (cries) It wasn't safe to be a daughter. (continues to cry) It wasn't safe to be feminine . . .

271    **THERAPIST:** And you are. And you may try to hide it. I believe that. Cause you don't feel safe.

272    **ELLIN:** I still don't. I sit on a bus at the age of 49 and I still don't feel safe next to my dad.[82]

---

[80]As we have seen, Ellin has introjected her mother's perception of her as being unattractive and too tall. At the time she was introjecting this self-description, she translated 'unattractive' and 'too tall' into 'masculine'. She now carries this view of herself, believing that it is an accurate reflection of reality; she is unaware that it is Mother's perception, not her own. Just as with her introjection of Father's way of sexualizing relationships, this introjection acts like a piece of Mother residing within Ellin's psyche, a foreign presence that Ellin nevertheless believes to be part of herself. (See chapter 2, p. 28)

[81]A confrontation calls attention to a discrepancy, in this case between Ellin's perception of herself and her actual appearance and behavior. It invites her to look more closely at the contrast between the two and at the possible purpose served by maintaining the distortion. (See chapter 6, p. 120)

[82]Here is the pervasiveness of script: Ellin, a mature and competent adult, still finds herself reacting like a frightened child in the presence of her father. (See chapter 2, p. 32)

273  **THERAPIST:** I want you to be safe with me. And that's *my* responsibility. It's up to *me,* when people are telling jokes before our group sessions start, to choose which jokes I'm gonna tell, and which jokes I won't tell, so that you can be among us. (pause) It's up to me to know when and how and with appropriate permission, about touching you. And if I don't do that, I bear the responsibility. And it's up to me to make sure that *I* get my own needs met elsewhere, so that I don't look lustfully at you.[83]

274  **ELLIN:** (whispering) Oh, God . . . Ohh . . . that's beyond my wildest dreams . . . (crying)[84]

275  **THERAPIST:** (pause) You don't have to dream about it; you have it. Right here. So that you can be safe to do the therapeutic work you need to do. (pause) Is this a good stopping place for you?

276  **ELLIN:** (still very softly) Yes . . . I want to go home, and just think about this, and feel what it's like . . . to feel safe . . . (cries again)[85]

277  **THERAPIST:** I think that's a good idea. How about sitting here quietly for a few minutes, to reflect on what you've learned this morning? And I'll see you again, next week, same time.

278  **ELLIN:** Yes. Thank you.

---

[83]Hearing this response, it is hard to imagine anything that could be more different from Father's way of relating to Ellin. The therapist has been open about his appreciation of Ellin's physical appearance, but he is equally clear about the boundaries he will keep. She can enjoy his admiration without fearing what may come next—exactly what she needed, and didn't get, from her father. The explicitly verbalized experience of this new way of being with a man is a direct challenge to her script beliefs that she is unattractive, and that it would be unsafe to be physically desirable. (See chapter 4, p. 70; chapter 5, pp.79, 85; chapter 9, p. 163)

[84]The ultimate quest of all human beings is contact: being aware of self, and being in relationship with another who has that same awareness. Ellin's life script has never allowed her such a relationship. Her father's sexuality and her mother's criticism, and the absence of needed protection provided by either parent, have led her to protect herself by not trusting, by holding herself aloof and apart. Yet she longs for what she has never had and could never really put into words. What the therapist promises has created a moment of meeting, a moment of relationship that is, indeed, beyond her wildest dreams. (See chapter 10, p. 199)

[85]As Ellin thinks about what she has experienced emotionally, she will create a cognitive framework that anchors her therapeutic gains. Over a series of similar pieces of work, she will begin to understand—both cognitively and emotionally—how her old script beliefs were protective for her at one time but are no longer needed in the present. This kind of processing may either precede or follow actual behavioral changes outside of therapy, but it nearly always occurs at some time or other as the client begins to reestablish a coherent sense of self. (See chapter 4, p. 70; chapter 11, p. 219)

## POSTSCRIPT

This session exemplifies a number of principles of relationship-focused integrative psychotherapy, as can be seen from the many annotations we have added. The two threads that run through the work have to do with Ellin's father's sexual inappropriateness and her mother's criticism, rejection, and lack of protection. Ellin's life script has developed as a way to protect herself against both Mother and Father, while still maintaining a semblance of relationship with them. She has learned to think of herself as masculine and unattractive (thus simultaneously preempting Mother's criticism and protecting herself from Father's sexual come-ons) and to be wary and untrusting in relationships. By providing her with a new relational experience, in which she is respected, accepted, and admired for her beauty, while at the same time maintaining clear and strong sexual boundaries, the therapist challenges Ellin's script system.

It is unlikely that one such therapeutic experience would bring about long-lasting changes in Ellin's life script or in the behavior patterns that the script has dictated. Over time, however, with more opportunities to feel what this kind of relationship can be like, and what *she* can be like as she begins to change her script beliefs and behaviors and to recover the softer, more feminine parts of herself, changes will occur. Ellin is on the way to becoming a whole person, spontaneous and creative, contactful in her relationships, freed from the constrictions of an outgrown life script.

# Transcript Linkage Index

In this index, we provide links between the content of the first 11 chapters and the verbatim transcript found in chapter 12. Number signs (as in "#5") refer to transactions in the transcript itself; "note" refers to associated footnotes. We have attempted to select examples that typify the client reactions and characteristics and the therapist activities described in the text. Often, though, we have found that the "example" is spread throughout large sections of transcript; indeed, our awareness of the interrelationship between the whole transcript and each of the individual excerpts was a major factor in our decision to provide you with an entire session of therapeutic work.

Whether you use the following material to find transcript examples as you read the chapters for the first time, or whether you use it later—after you have already read through the whole transcript—you may well find segments that illustrate our ideas better than the ones we have chosen. That can happen if we have not found the very best examples, but it can also be a function of a kind of synergy: you, the reader, have now become a part of creating the process reflected in our transcript. You will invest the printed words with your own meanings, your own history, your own emotional response. In a very real sense, each reader will discover a different transcript, because each reader (like each client and each therapist) understands the work through the lens of his or her unique personal history.

At any rate, we have enjoyed preparing this set of links. It has allowed us to appreciate once again the fact that our work does, indeed, reflect our theory—that we do practice what we preach. We hope that the section will be useful and enjoyable for you, as well.

# CHAPTER 2

p. 17, the importance of relationships to human functioning: #12 & note 6; #30 & note 11

p. 17, others' reactions to us shape our emotional responses: #12 & note 6; #16 & note 7

p. 20, scripts provide rules for managing our lives: #39, 40, & notes 18, 19

p. 21, reasons for staying in script: #129 & note 51

p. 22, tension between illusory safety of script and problems created by script-bound behavior: #40 & note 19

p. 24: example of repression: #196 & note 66

p. 28, example of an introject: #104 & note 44; #266–68 & note 79

p. 29, nature of introject: #257–260

p. 31, the script spiral: #40–42; #106; #258

p. 32, people create life experiences that further reinforce script: #39

# CHAPTER 3

p. 36, self is shaped by relationship experiences: #106 & note 46, #110

p. 38, cognition and emotion are intertwined: #12 & note 6

p. 40, importance of significant other's responses: #12

p. 40, script is self-perpetuating aspect of personality: #40–42 & notes 19, 20

p. 40, script perpetuates the belief that one's needs won't be met: #39 & note 18

p. 43, response to an adult relational need being met: #122

p. 44, relational need for security: #52

p. 49, two parents give different messages to child: #16–19

p. 50, script results in beliefs about the self: #260–261 & note 79

p. 55, recollection of cumulative trauma: #106

# CHAPTER 4

p. 59, client has thought about problems: #2

p. 60, clients' emotional experience interferes with everyday life: #39–42 & notes 18, 19; #168

p. 62, cognitive aspects of memories easy to recall: #52

p. 65, healing is experienced through mutually experienced emotional connection: #270–274 & notes 83, 84

p. 66, therapist's involvement helps client to feel cared for: #30 & note 11

p. 67, contactful relationship feels good: #224 & note 72

# CHAPTER 5

# CHAPTER 6

# CHAPTER 7

# CHAPTER 8

# CHAPTER 9

# CHAPTER 10

## CHAPTER 11

p. 206, therapist warns client when session is about to end: #222
p. 220, discuss how work will generalize: #276–277 & note 85

# References

Agosta, L. (1984). Empathy and intersubjectivity. In J. Lichtenberg, M. Bornstein, & D. Silver (Eds.), *Empathy* (Vol. 1, pp. 43–61). Hillsdale, NJ: The Analytic Press.

American Psychiatric Association. (2000). *Diagnostic and statistical manual of mental disorders* (text rev.). Washington, DC: Author.

Andrews, J. (1991). Integrative psychotherapy of depression: A self-confirmation approach. *Psychotherapy, 28,* 232–250.

Ansbacher, H. L., & Ansbacher, R. R. (1956). *The individual psychology of Alfred Adler.* New York: Atheneum.

Arlow, J. (1969a). Fantasy, memory, and reality testing. *Psychoanalytic Quarterly, 38,* 28–51.

Arlow, J. (1969b). Unconscious fantasy and disturbances of conscious experience. *Psychoanalytic Quarterly, 38,* 1–27.

Arlow, J. (1991). A new look at Freud's 'Analysis terminable and interminable.' In J. Sandler (Ed.), *On Freud's "Analysis terminable and interminable"* (pp. 43–55). New Haven: Yale University Press.

Aron, L. (1991). The patient's experience of the analyst's subjectivity. *Psychoanalytic Dialogues, 1,* 29–51.

Atwood, G. E., & Stolorow, R. D. (1984). *Structures of subjectivity: Exploration in psychoanalytic phenomenology.* Hillsdale, NJ: The Analytic Press.

Atwood, J. D. (1999). Social construction theory and therapy assumptions. In J. D. Atwood (Ed.), *Family scripts*. Washington, DC: Accelerated Development.

Bacal, H. (1997). The analyst's subjectivity—How it can illuminate the analysand's experience. Commentary on Susan H. Sands's paper. *Psychoanalytic Dialogs, 7*(5), 669–681.

Bandler, R., & Grinder, J. (1975). *The structure of magic I: A book about language and therapy*. Palo Alto, CA: Science and Behavior Books.

Barrett-Lennard, G. T. (1997). The recovery of empathy—Toward others and self. In A. Bohart & L. Greenberg (Eds.), *Empathy reconsidered* (pp. 103–121). Washington, DC: American Psychological Association.

Basch, M. (1976). The concept of affect: A reexamination. *Journal of the American Psychoanalytic Association, 24,* 759–777.

Basch, M. (1988). *Understanding psychotherapy: The science behind the art*. New York: Basic Books.

Beck, A. (1991). Cognitive therapy: A 30-year retrospective. *American Psychologist, 46,* 368–375.

Benjamin, J. (1992). Recognition and destruction: an outline of intersubjectivity. In N. Skolnick & S. Warshaw (Eds.), *Relational perspectives in psychoanalysis* (pp. 43–60). Hillsdale, NJ: The Analytic Press.

Bergner, R. (1999). Status enhancement: A further path to therapeutic change. *American Journal of Psychotherapy, 53*(2), 201–214.

Berne, E. (1961). *Transactional analysis in psychotherapy: A systematic individual and social psychiatry*. New York: Grove Press.

Berne, E. (1963). *The structure and dynamics of organizations and groups*. New York: Grove Press.

Berne. E. (1966). *Principles of group treatment*. New York: Oxford University Press.

Berne, E. (1972). *What do you say after you say hello?: The psychology of human relationships*. New York: Grove Press.

Billow, R. M. (2000). Self-disclosure and psychoanalytic meaning: A psychoanalytic fable. *Psychoanalytic Review, 87*(1), 61–79.

Blackstone, P. (1995). Between the lines. *Transactional Analysis Journal, 25,* 343–346.

Bohart, A. C., & Tallman, K. (1998). The person as active agent in experiential therapy. In L. S. Greenberg, J. C. Watson, & G. Lietaer (Eds.), *Handbook of experiential psychotherapy* (pp. 178–200). New York: The Guilford Press.

Bond, A. H. (1993). *Is there life after analysis?* Grand Rapids, MI: Wynwood Press.

Bordin, E. S. (1968). *Psychological counseling*. New York: Appleton-Century-Crofts.

Bordin, E. S. (1994). Theory and research on the therapeutic working alliance: New directions. In A. O. Horvath & L. S. Greenberg (Eds.), *The working alliance* (pp. 13–37). New York: John Wiley & Sons.

Bornstein, R. F., & Bowen, R. F. (1995). Dependency in psychotherapy: Toward an integrated treatment approach. *Psychotherapy, 32,* 520–534.

Bower, G. H. (1981). Mood and memory. *American Psychologist, 36* (2), 129–148.

Bowlby, J. (1969). *Attachment and loss: Vol. I. Attachment*. New York: Basic Books.

Bowlby, J. (1973). *Attachment and loss: Vol. II. Separation: Anxiety and anger.* New York: Basic Books.

Bowlby, J. (1980). *Attachment and loss: Vol. III. Loss: Sadness and depression*. New York: Basic Books.

Breggin, P. R. (1997). *The heart of being helpful*. New York: Springer.

Bromberg, P. M. (1998). *Standing in the spaces*. Hillsdale, NJ: The Analytic Press.

Broucek, F., & Ricci, W. (1998). Self-disclosure or self-presence? *Bulletin of the Menninger Clinic, 62,* 427–438.

Brown, G. W., & Harris, T. (1978). *Social origins of depression: A study of psychiatric disorders in women*. New York: Free Press.

Browne, I. (1990). Psychological trauma, or unexperienced experience. *ReVision, 12* (4), 21–34

Buber, M. (1958). *I and Thou* (R. G. Smith, Trans.). New York: Scribner.

Buirski, P., & Haglund, P. (1999). The self object function of interpretation. In A. Goldberg (Ed.), *Pluralism in self-psychology: Progress in self-psychology* (Vol. 15, pp. 31–50). Hillsdale, NJ: The Analytic Press.

Callaghan, G. M., Naugle, A. E., & Folette, W. C. (1996). Useful constructions of the client-therapist relationship. *Psychotherapy, 33,* 381–390.

Cashdan, S. (1988). *Object relations therapy*. New York: W. W. Norton.

Cervone, D., & Shoda, Y. (1999). Social-cognitive theories and the coherence of personality. In D. Cervone & Y. Shoda (Eds.), *The coherence of personality: Social-cognitive bases of consistency, variability, and organization* (pp. 3–33). New York: The Guilford Press.

Chamberlain, D. B. (1990). The expanding boundaries of memory. *ReVision, 12* (4), 11–20.

Chevalier, A. J. (1995). *On the client's path*. Oakland, CA: New Harbinger Publications.

Clocksin, W. F. (1998). Artificial intelligence and human identity. In J. Cornwell (Ed.), *Consciousness and human identity* (pp. 101–121). Oxford, England: Oxford University Press.

Cloitre, M. (1997). Conscious and unconscious memory: A model of functional amnesia. In D. J. Stein (Ed.), *Cognitive science and the unconscious* (pp. 55–88). Washington, DC: American Psychiatric Press.

Coltart, N. D. (1996). Endings. In L. Rangell & R. Moses-Hrushovski (Eds.), *Psychoanalysis at the political border* (pp. 117–132). Madison: International Universities Press.

Coyne, J. C. (1999). Thinking interactionally about depression: A radical restatement. In T. Joiner & J. C. Coyne (Eds.), *The interactional nature of depression* (pp. 365–392). Washington, DC: American Psychological Association.

Crick, N. R., & Dodge, K. A. (1994). A review and reformulation of social information-processing mechanisms in children's social adjustment. *Psychologyical Bulletin, 115,* 74–101.

Efron, J. S., Lukens, M. D., & Lukens, R. J. (1990). Language, structure, and change: Frameworks of meaning in psychotherapy. New York: W. W. Norton.

Ellis, A. (1997). *The practice of rational emotive behavior therapy* (2nd ed.). New York: Springer.

Erikson, E. (1968). *Identity: Youth and crisis.* New York: W. W. Norton.

Erskine, R. G. (1997a). Therapeutic intervention: Disconnecting rubberbands. In R. G. Erskine, *Theories and methods of an integrative transactional analysis: A volume of selected articles* (pp. 172–173). San Francisco: TA Press. (Original work published 1974)

Erskine, R. G. (1997b). Transference and transactions: Critique from an intrapsychic and integrative perspective. In R. G. Erskine, *Theories and methods of an integrative transactional analysis* (pp. 129–146). San Francisco: TA Press. (Original work published 1991)

Erskine, R. G. (1997c). The process of integrative psychotherapy. In R. G. Erskine, *Theories and Methods of an Integrative Transactional Analysis: A Volume of Selected Articles* (pp. 79–95). San Francisco: TA Press. (Original work published 1993)

Erskine, R. G. (1997d). Shame and self-righteousness: Transactional analysis perspectives and clinical interventions. In R. G. Erskine, *Theories and methods of an integrative transactional analysis: A volume of selected articles* (pp. 46–67). San Francisco: TA Press. (Original work published 1994)

Erskine, R. G. (1998a). Attunement and involvement: Therapeutic responses to relational needs. *International Journal of Psychotherapy, 3,* 235–244.

Erskine, R. G. (1998b). Psychotherapy in the USA: A manual of standardized techniques or a therapeutic relationship? *International Journal of Psychotherapy, 3,* 231–234.

Erskine, R. G. & Moursund, J. P. (1988/1998). *Integrative psychotherapy in action.* Newbury Park, CA: Sage. (Republished by The Gestalt Journal Press, Highland, NY).

Erskine, R. G., Moursund, J. P., & Trautmann, R. L (1999). *Beyond empathy: A therapy of contact-in-relationship.* Philadelphia: Brunner/Mazel.

Erskine, R. G., & Trautmann, R. L. (1997). Methods of an integrative psychotherapy. In R. G. Erskine, *Theories and methods of an integrative transactional analysis: A volume of selected articles* (pp. 20–36). San Francisco: TA Press. (Original work published 1996)

Erskine, R. G., & Zalcman, M. (1997). The racket system: A model for racket analysis. In R. G. Erskine, *Theories and methods of an integrative transactional analysis: A volume of selected articles* (pp. 156–165). San Francisco: TA Press. (Original work published 1979)

Feierstein, R. (2001, Spring). Experiential psychotherapy with children: The relationship of the child and the therapist. *Voices: The Art and Science of Psychotherapy, 23.*

Fosshage, J. L. (1992). Self-psychology: The self and its vicissitudes within a relational matrix. In N. Skolnik & S. Warshaw (Eds.), *Relational perspectives in psychoanalysis* (pp. 21–42). Hillsdale, NJ: The Analytic Press.

Frank, K. A. (1991). Action, insight, and working through: Outlines of an integrative approach. *Psychoanalytic Dialogues, 1,* 535–577.

Frank, K. A. (1997). The role of the analyst's inadvertent self-revelations. *Psychoanalytic Dialogues,* 7(3), 281–314.

Freud, A. (1937). *The ego and the mechanisms of defense.* London: Hogarth Press.

Freud, S. (1938). The interpretation of dreams. In A Brill (Ed. & Trans.), *The basic writings of Sigmund Freud.* New York: Random House. (Original work published 1900)

Freud, S. (1955). Beyond the pleasure principle. In J. Strachey (Ed. & Trans.), *The standard edition of the complete works of Sigmund Freud* (Vol. 18, pp. 3–64). London: Hogarth Press. (Original work published 1920)

Freud, S. (1958a). The dynamics of transference. In J. Strachey (Ed. & Trans.), *The standard edition of the complete psychological works of Sigmund Freud* (Vol. 12, pp. 97–108). London: Hogarth Press. (Original work published 1912)

Freud, S. (1958b). Observations on transference-love: Further recommendations on the technique of psychoanalysis, III. In J. Strachey (Ed. & Trans.), *The standard edition of the complete psychological works of Sigmund Freud* (Vol. 12, pp. 157–173). London: Hogarth Press. (Original work published 1915)

Freud, S. (1959). Recommendations for physicians on the psycho-analytic method of treatment. In E. Jones (Ed.), *Sigmund Freud: Collected papers.* New York: Basic Books. (Original work published 1912)

Freud, S. (1963). Repression. In P. Rieff (Ed.), *General psychological theory: Sigmund Freud's papers on metapsychology* (pp. 104–115). New York: Collier Books. (Original work published 1915)

Freyd, J. (1996). *Betrayal trauma.* Cambridge, MA: Harvard University Press.

Gehrie, M. (1999). On boundaries and intimacy in psychoanalysis. In A. Goldberg (Ed.), *Pluralism in self-psychology: Progress in self-psychology* (Vol. 15, pp. 83–94) Hillsdale, NJ: The Analytic Press.

Geller, J., & Nash, V. (1973). Untitled, unpublished manuscript.

Gelso, C. J. & Hayes, J. A. (2001). Countertransference management. *Psychotherapy,* 38, 418–422.

Glassman, N. S., & Anderson, S. M. (1999). Streams of thought about the self and significant others: Transference as the construction of interpersonal meaning. In J. A. Singer & P. Salovey (Eds.), *At play in the fields of consciousness: Essays in honor of Jerome L. Singer* (pp. 103–140). Mahwah, NJ: Erlbaum.

Glickauf-Hughes, C., Wells, M, & Chance, S. (1996). Techniques for strengthening clients' observing ego. *Psychotherapy,* 33, 431–440.

Gold, J. R. (1996). *Key concepts in psychotherapy integration.* New York: Plenum.

Goleman, D. (1985). *Vital lies, simple truths.* New York: Simon & Schuster.

Goulding, M., & Goulding, R. (1979). *Changing lives through redecision therapy.* New York: Brunner/Mazel.

Greenberg, J. R., & Mitchell, S. A. (1983). *Object relations in psychoanalytic theory.* Cambridge, MA: Harvard University Press.

Greenberg, L. & Elliott, R. (1997). Varieties of empathic responding. In A. Bohart & L. Greenberg (Eds.), *Empathy reconsidered* (pp. 167–186). Washington, DC: American Psychological Association.

Greenberg, L., Elliott, R., Watson, J. C., & Bohart, A. C. (2001). Empathy. *Psycotherapy, 38*, 380–395.

Greenberg, L., & Paivio, S. C. (1997). *Working with emotions in psychotherapy.* New York: The Guilford Press.

Greenberg, L., & Pascual-Leone, J. (1991). A dialectical constructivist approach to experiential change. In R. A. Neimeyer & M. J. Mahoney (Eds.), *Constructivism in psychotherapy* (pp. 169–191). Washington, DC: American Psychological Association.

Greenson, R. (1967). *The techniques and practice of psychoanalysis.* New York: International Universities Press.

Grove, D. (1989) *In the presence of the past.* Eldon, MO: David Grove Seminars.

Guidano, V. F. (1991). Self-observation in constructivist psychotherapy. In R. A. Neimeyer & M. J. Mahoney (Eds.), *Constructivism in psychotherapy* (pp. 155–168). Washington, DC: American Psychological Association.

Guistolese, P. (1997). Failures in the therapeutic relationship: Inevitable *and* necessary? *Transactional Analysis Journal, 4*, 284–288.

Haines, B. A., Metalsky, G. I., Cardamone, A. L., & Joiner, T. (1999). Interpersonal and cognitive pathways into the origins of attributional style: A developmental perspective. In T. Joiner & J. C. Coyne (Eds.), *The interactional nature of depression* (pp. 65–92). Washington, DC: American Psychological Association.

Haley, J. (1986). *Uncommon therapy: The psychiatric techniques of Milton H. Erikson, M.D.* New York: W. W. Norton.

Hammen, C., & Goodman-Brown, T. (1990). Self-schemas and vulnerability to specific life stress in children at risk for depression. *Cognitive Therapy and Research, 14*, 215–227.

Hanna, F. J. (1996). Precursors of change: Pivotal points of involvement and resistance in psychotherapy. *Journal of Psychotherapy Integration, 6*, 227–264.

Harlow, H. F. (1958). The nature of love. *American Psychologist, 12*, 673–685.

Hegel, G. (1976). *Science of logic* (A. Miller, Trans.). New York: Humanities Press. (Original German edition 1812–1816)

Heisenberg, W. (1952). *Philosophic problems of nuclear science.* New York: Pantheon. (Original work published in 1934)

Henry, W. P., & Strupp, H. H. (1994). The therapeutic alliance as interpersonal process. In A. O. Horvath & L. S. Greenberg (Eds.), *The working alliance* (pp. 51–84). New York: John Wiley & Sons.

Hirt, E. F., Lynn, S. J., Payne, D. G, Krackow, E., & McCrea, S. M. (1999). Expectancies and memory: Inferring the past from what must have been. In I. Kirsch (Ed.), *How expectancies shape experience* (pp. 93–124). Washington, DC: American Psychological Association.

Hite, A. (1996). The diagnostic alliance. In D. L. Nathanson (Ed.), *Knowing feeling* (pp. 37–54). New York: W. W. Norton.

Horvath, A. O. (2001). The alliance. *Psychotherapy, 38*, 365–372.

Izard, D. E., Ackerman, B. P., & Schultz, D. (1999). Independent emotions and consciousness: Self-Consciousness and dependent emotions. In J. A. Singer & P. Salovey (Eds.), *At play in the fields of consciousness: Essays in honor of Jerome L. Singer* (pp. 83–102). Mahwah, NJ: Erlbaum.

Jack, D. J. (1991). *Silencing the self: Women and depression.* Cambridge, MA: Harvard University Press.

Jack, D. J. (1999). Silencing the self: Inner dialogues and outer realities. In T. Joiner & J. Coyne (Eds.), *The interactional nature of depression* (pp. 221–246). Washington, DC: American Psychological Association.

James, M., & Goulding, M. (1998). Self-reparenting and redecision. *Transactional Analysis Journal, 28,* 16–19.

James, W. (1890). *The principles of psychology.* New York: Henry Holt & Co.

Janoff-Bulman, R. (1993). *Shattered assumptions: Towards a new psychology of trauma.* New York: The Free Press.

Janov, A. (1970). *The primal scream.* New York: G. P. Putnam.

Johnson, M. H., Dzuirawiec, S., Ellis, H., & Morton, J. (1991). Newborns' preferential tracking of face-like stimuli and its subsequent decline. *Cognition, 40* (1–2), 1–19.

Kainer, R. (1999). *The collapse of the self and its therapeutic restoration.* Hillsdale, NJ: The Analytic Press.

Kelly, G. A. (1955). *The psychology of personal constructs.* New York: W. W. Norton.

Khan, M. M. (1963). The concept of cumulative trauma. *The Psychoanalytic Study of the Child, 18,* 286–306.

Kramer, S. A. (1990). *Positive endings in psychotherapy.* San Francisco: Jossey-Bass.

Lambert, M. J. & Barley, D. E. (2001). Research summary on the therapeutic relationship and psychotherapy outcome. *Psychotherapy, 38,* 357–361.

Lankford, V. (1980). Termination: How to enrich the process. *Transactional Analysis Journal, 10,* 175–177.

Lazarus, A. A. (1989). *The practice of multimodal therapy.* Baltimore: Johns Hopkins University Press.

Lee, R. R. (1998). Empathy and affects: Towards an intersubjective view. *Australian Journal of Psychotherapy, 17,* 126–149.

Lister, E. D. (1981). Forced silence: A neglected dimension of trauma. *American Journal of Psychiatry, 139* (7), 872–876.

Lourie, J. (1996). Cumulative trauma: The nonproblem problem. *Journal of Transactional Analysis, 26,* 276–283.

Lowen, A. (1976). *Bioenergetics.* New York: Penguin. (Original work published 1975)

Lyons-Ruth, K. (1995). Broadening our conceptual frameworks: Can we reintroduce relational strategies and implicit representational systems to the study of psychopathology? *Developmental Psychology, 31,* 432–436.

MacIsaac, D. S. (1997). Empathy: Heinz Kohut's contribution. In A. Bohart & L. Greenberg (Eds.), *Empathy reconsidered: New directions on psychotherapy* (pp. 245–264). Washington, DC: American Psychological Association.

Mahler, M., Pine, F., & Bergman, A. (1975). *The psychological birth of the human infant: Symbiosis and individuation.* New York: Basic Books.

Mahoney, M. (1991). *Human change processes: The scientific foundations of psychotherapy.* New York: Basic Books.

Mahoney, M. J., & Norcross, J. C. (1993). Relationship syles and therapeutic choices: A commentary on the preceding four articles. *Psychotherapy, 30,* 423–430.

Mahrer, A. R. (1998). How can impressive in-session changes become impressive post-session changes? In L. S. Greenberg, J. C. Watson, & G. Lietaer (Eds.), *Handbook of experiential psychotherapy* (pp. 201–223). New York: The Guilford Press.

Maslow, A. (1987). *Motivation and personality*. New York: Harper & Row. (Original work published 1954)

Meltzoff, A. N., Gopnik, A., & Repacholi, B. M. (1999). Toddlers' understanding of intentions, desires, and emotions: Explorations of the dark ages. In P. Zelazo, J. Astington, & D. Olson (Eds.), *Developing theories of intention: Social understanding and self-control* (pp. 17–41). Mahwah, NJ: Erlbaum.

Midgely, M. (1998). Putting ourselves together again. In J. Cornwell (Ed.), *Consciousness and human identity* (pp. 160–177). Oxford, England: Oxford University Press.

Miller, G., & DeShazer, S. (2000). Emotions in solution-focused therapy: A re-examination. *Family Process, 39*(1), 5–23.

Mitchell, S. (1988). *Relational concepts in psychoanalysis: An integration*. Cambridge, MA: Harvard University Press.

Mitchell, S. (1992). True selves, false selves. In N. Skolnik & S. Warshaw (Eds.), *Relational Perspectives in Psychoanalysis* (pp. 1–20). Hillsdale, NJ: The Analytic Press.

Mitchell, S. (1993). Hope and dread in psychoanalysis. New York: Basic Books.

Modell, A. H. (1991). The therapeutic relationship as a paradoxical experience. *Psychoanalytic Dialogues, 1*, 13–28.

Moreno, J. L. (1964). *Psychodrama* (3rd ed.). New York: Beacon House.

Morton, J., & Johnson, M. (1991). The perception of facial structure in infancy. In G. Locikhead & J. Pomerantz (Eds.), *The perception of structure: Essays in honor of Wendell R. Garner* (pp. 317–325). Washington, DC: American Psychological Association.

Murdin, L. (2000). *How much is enough? Endings in psychotherapy and counselling*. London: Routledge.

Nathanson, D. L. (1993, October). *Toward a new psychotherapy*. Paper presented at conference "Toward a New Psychotherapy," Philadelphia.

Nathanson, D. L. (1996). About emotion. In D. L. Nathanson (Ed.), *Knowing feeling* (pp. 1–21). New York: W. W. Norton.

Neimeier, G. J. (1995). The challenge of change. In R. A. Neimeyer & M. J. Mahoney (Eds.), *Constructivism in psychotherapy* (pp. 111–126). Washington, DC: American Psychological Association.

Nichols, M. P. (1986). Catharsis: History and the theory. In M. P. Nichols & T. Paolino (Eds.), *Basic techniques of psychoanalytic psychotherapy* (pp. 79–101). New York: Gardner Press.

Norcross, J. C. (1990). Eclectic-integrative psychotherapy. In J. K. Zeig, & W. M. Munion (Eds.), *What is psychotherapy? Contemporary perspectives* (pp. 218–220). San Francisco: Jossey-Bass.

Norcross, J. C. (1995). Dispelling the dodo bird verdict and the exclusivity myth in psychotherapy. *Psychotherapy, 32*, 500–519.

Norcross, J. C. (2001). Purposes, processes, and products of the task force on empirically supported therapy relationships. *Psychotherapy, 38*, 345–356.

Norcross, J. C., & Newman, C. F. (1992). Psychotherapy integration: Setting the context. In J. Norcross & M. Goldfried (Eds.), *Handbook of psychotherapy integration* (pp. 3–45). New York: Basic Books.

Ohlsson, T. (1998). Two ways of doing regressive therapy: Using transactional analysis proper and using expressive techniques. *Transactional Analysis Journal, 28,* 83–87.

Olson, D. R., & Askington, J. W. (1999). Introduction: Actions, intentions, and attributions. In P. Zelazo, J. Astington, & D. Olson (Eds.), *Developing theories of intention: Social understanding and self-control* (pp 1–13). Mahwah, NJ: Erlbaum.

Orange, D. (1995). Emotional understanding: Studies in psychoanalytic epistemology. New York: The Guilford Press.

Patterson, C. H. (1985). *The therapeutic relationship: Foundations for an eclectic psychotherapy.* Monterey, CA: Brooks/Cole.

Perls, F. (1944). *Ego, hunger, and aggression: A revision of Freud's theory and method.* Durban, South Africa: Knox Publishing.

Perls F. (1969a). *Gestalt therapy verbatim.* New York: Bantam Books.

Perls, F. (1969b). *In and out the garbage pail.* Moab, UT: Real People Press.

Perls, F. (1973). *The Gestalt approach and eyewitness to therapy.* Palo Alto, CA: Science & Behavior Books.

Perls, F., & Baumgardner, P. (1975). *Legacy from Fritz: Gifts from Lake Cowichan.* Palo Alto, CA: Science & Behavior Books.

Perls, F., Hefferline, R. F, & Goodman, P. (1951). *Gestalt therapy: Excitement and growth in the human personality.* New York: Julian Press.

Perls, L. (1978). An oral history of Gestalt therapy, Part I: A conversation with Laura Perls, by Edward Rosenfeld. *Gestalt Journal* (Winter), 8–31.

Pistole, C. M. (1999). Caregiving in attachment relationships: A perspective for counselors. *Journal of Counseling and Development, 77,* 437–446.

Plakun, E. M. (1998). Enactment and the treatment of abuse survivors. *Harvard Review of Psychiatry, 5,* 318–325.

Polster, E., & Polster, M. (1973). *Gestalt therapy integrated.* New York: Brunner/Mazel.

Poppell, E. (1988). *Mindworks: Time and conscious experience.* Boston: Harcourt Brace Jovanovich.

Querlu, D., Lefebre, C., Renard, S., Titran, M., Morillion, M., & Crepin, G. (1984). Perception auditive et reactive du nouveau-ne de moins de deux herus de vie á la voix maternelle (Eng. trans.). *Journal de Gynecologie, Obstetrique et Biologie de la Reproduction, 13,* 125–134.

Racker, M. (1968). *Transference and countertransference.* New York: International Universities Press.

Rhinehart, J. W., (1998). Touching and holding during regressive therapy. *Transactional Analysis Journal, 28,* 57–64.

Rogers, C. R. (1951). *Client-centered therapy.* Boston: Houghton Mifflin.

Rossi, E. L. (1990). Psychobiological psychotherapy. In J. K. Zeig, & W. M. Munion (Eds.), *What is psychotherapy? Contemporary perspectives.* San Francisco: Jossey-Bass.

Rowe, C. R. Jr. (1999). The self-object transferences reconsidered. In A. Goldberg (Ed.), *Pluralism in self-psychology: Progress in self-psychology* (Vol. 15., pp. 15–30). Hillsdale, NJ: The Analytic Press.

Safran, J. D. (1993). Breaches in the therapeutic alliance: An arena for negotiating authentic relatedness. *Psychotherapy, 30,* 11–24.

Safran, J. D., & Muran, J. C. (2000). Resolving therapeutic alliance ruptures: Diversity and integration. *Journal of Clinical Psychology, 56,* 233–243.

Safran, J. D., Muran, J. C., Samstag, L. W., & Stevens, C. (2001). Repairing alliance ruptures. *Psychotherapy, 38,* 406–412.

Salzman, L. (1989). Terminating psychotherapy. In F. Flach (Ed.), *Psychotherapy* (pp. 223–230). New York: W. W. Norton.

Sands, S. H. (1997). Self-psychology and projective identification—Whither shall they meet? A reply to the editors (1995). *Psychoanalytic Dialogs, 7*(5), 651–668.

Schneider, K. J. (1998). Existential processes. In L. S. Greenberg, J. C. Watson, & G. Lietaer (Eds.), *Handbook of experiential psychotherapy* (pp. 103–120). New York: The Guilford Press.

Schwaber, E. (1992). Countertransference: The analyst's retreat from the patient's vantage point. *International Journal of Psycho-Analysis, 73,* 349–362.

Shlien, J. (1997). Empathy and psychotherapy: A vital mechanism? Yes. Psychotherapist's conceit? All too often. By itself enough? No. In A. Bohart & L. Greenberg (Eds.), *Empathy revisited: New directions in psychotherapy* (pp. 63–80). Washington, DC: American Psychological Association.

Sigmund, E. (1998). The conscious natural child. *Transactional Analysis Journal, 28,* 20–30.

Slap, J. (1987). Implication for the structural model of Freud's assumptions about perception. *Journal of the American Psychoanalytic Association, 35,* 629–645.

Snyder, M. (1994). The development of social intelligence in psychotherapy: Empathic and dialogic processes. *Journal of Humanistic Psychology, 34* (1), 84–108.

Socor, B. J. (1989). Listening for historical truth: A relative discussion. *Clinical Social Work Journal, 17,* 103–115.

Spiegler, M., & Guevremont, D. (1993). *Contemporary behavior therapy* (2nd ed). Pacific Grove, CA: Brooks/Cole.

Spitz, R. A. (1945). Hospitalism: An inquiry into the genesis of psychiatric conditions in early childhood, Part I. *Psychoanalytic Studies of the Child, 1,* 53–74.

Stein, D. J., and Young, J. E. (1997). Rethinking repression. In D. J. Stein (Ed.), *Cognitive science and the unconscious* (pp. 147–175). Washington, DC: American Psychiatric Press.

Steiner, C. (1974). *Scripts people live.* New York: Grove Press.

Stern, D. N. (1985). *The interpersonal world of the infant: A view from psychoanalysis and developmental psychology.* New York: Basic Books.

Stern, D. N., Sander, L. W., Nahum, J. P., Harrison, A. M., Lyons-Ruth, K., Morgan, A. C., Bruschweiler-Stern, N., & Tronick, E. Z. (1998). Non-interpretive mechanisms in psychoanalytic therapy: The 'something more' than interpretation. *International Journal of Psycho-Analysis, 79,* 903–921.

Stolorow, R. D. (1992). Closing the gap beween theory and practice with better psychoanalytic theory. *Psychotherapy, 29,* 159–166.

Stolorow, R. D., & Atwood, G. E. (1989). The unconscious and unconscious fantasy: An intersubjective-developmental perspective. *Psychoanalytic Inquiry, 9,* 364–374.

Stone, A. (1996). Clinical assessment of affect. In D. L. Nathanson (Ed.), *Knowing feeling* (pp. 22–36). New York: W. W. Norton.

Strupp, H. (1969). Toward a specification of teaching and learning in psychotherapy. *Archives of General Psychiatry, 21,* 203–212.

Strupp, H. H. (1996). Some salient lessons from research and practice. *Psychotherapy, 33,* 135–138.

Tansey, M. J., & Burke, W. F. (1989). *Understanding countertransference: From projective identification to empathy.* Hillsdale, NJ: The Analytic Press.

Terr, L. C. (1991). Childhood traumas: An outline and overview. *American Journal of Psychiatry, 148* (1), 10–20.

Terr, L. C. (1994). *Unchained memories: True stories of traumatic memories, lost and found.* New York: Basic Books.

Tropp, J. L., & Stolorow, R. D. (1997). Therapeutic empathy: An intersubjective perspective. In A. Bohart & L. Greenberg (Eds.), *Empathy reconsidered: New directions in psychotherapy* (pp. 279–291). Washington, DC: American Psychological Association.

Tudor, K. (1995). What do you say about saying good-bye? Ending psychotherapy. *Transactional Analysis Journal, 25,* 228–233.

VanKessel, W., & Lietaer, G. (1998). Interpersonal processes. In L. S. Greenberg, J. C. Watson, & G. Lietaer (Eds.), *Handbook of experiential psychotherapy* (pp. 155–177). New York: The Guilford Press.

Wachtel, P. L. (1990). Psychotherapy from an integrative psychodynamic perspective. In J. K. Zeig & W. M. Munion (Eds.), *What is psychotherapy? Contemporary perspectives* (pp. 234–238). San Francisco: Jossey-Bass.

Wachtel, P. L. (1991). From eclecticism to synthesis: Toward a more seamless psychotherapeutic integration. *Journal of Psychotherapy Integration, 1,* 43–54.

Wagner, L., Davis, S., & Handelsman, M. M. (1998). In search of the abominable consent form: The impact of readability and personalization. *Journal of Clinical Psychology, 54*(1), 115–120.

Warner, M. (1997). Does empathy cure? A theoretical consideraton of empathy, processing, and personal narrative. In A. Bohart & L. Greenberg (Eds.), *Empathy reconsidered* (pp. 125–140). Washington, DC: American Psychological Association.

Watkins, H. H., & Watkins, J. G. (1990). *Ego-states: Theory and therapy.* New York: W. W. Norton.

Watson, J. C., & Greenberg, L. S. (1994). The alliance in experiential therapy: Enacting the relationship conditions. In A. O. Horvath & L. S. Greenberg (Eds.), *The working alliance* (pp. 152–172). New York: John Wiley & Sons.

Watzlawick, P., Weakland, J., & Fisch, R. (1974). *Change.* New York: W. W. Norton.

Weinberger, J., & Eig, A. (1999). Expectancies: The ignored common factor in psychotherapy. In I. Kirsch (Ed.), *How expectancies shape experience* (pp. 357–382). Washington, DC: American Psychological Association.

Weinberger, J., & Weiss, J. (1997). Psychoanalytic and cognitive conceptions of the unconscious. In Stein, D. J. (Ed.), *Cognitive science and the unconscious* (pp. 23–54). Washington, DC: American Psychiatric Press.

Weiss, J. B., & Weiss, L. (1998). Perspectives on the current state of contractual regressive therapy. *Transactional Analysis Journal, 28,* 45–47.

Wile, D. B. (1984). Kohut, Kernberg, and accusatory interpretations. *Psychotherapy, 21,* 353–364.

Wolpe, J. (1969). *The practice of behavior therapy.* New York: Pergamon.

Yalom, I. (1985). *The theory and practice of group psychotherapy.* New York: Basic Books.

Yalom, I. (1999). Momma and the meaning of life. New York: Basic Books.

# Name Index

# Subject Index